3rd edition

the behavioral sciences in psychiatry

in psychiatry

National Medical Series

In the basic sciences

anatomy, 2nd edition
the behavioral sciences
    in psychiatry, 3rd edition
biochemistry, 3rd edition
clinical epidemiology and
    biostatistics
genetics
hematology
histology and cell biology,
    2nd edition

human developmental anatomy
immunology, 3rd edition
introduction to clinical medicine
microbiology, 2nd edition
neuroanatomy
pathology, 3rd edition
pharmacology, 3rd edition
physiology, 3rd edition
radiographic anatomy

In the clinical sciences

medicine, 2nd edition
obstetrics and gynecology,
    3rd edition
pediatrics, 2nd edition
preventive medicine and
    public health, 2nd edition
psychiatry, 2nd edition
surgery, 2nd edition

In the exam series

review for USMLE Step 1,
    3rd edition
review for USMLE Step 2
geriatrics

The National Medical Series for Independent Study

3rd edition

the behavioral sciences in psychiatry

EDITORS

Jerry M. Wiener, M.D.

*Leon Yochelson Professor
and Chairman*
*Department of Psychiatry and
Behavioral Sciences*
*George Washington University
School of Medicine*
Washington, District of Columbia
President, American Psychiatric Association
Washington, District of Columbia

Nancy A. Breslin, M.D.

Assistant Professor of Psychiatry and Behavioral Sciences
Director of Psychiatric Clerkship
Department of Psychiatry and Behavioral Sciences
George Washington University School of Medicine
Attending Psychiatrist
George Washington University Medical Center
Washington, District of Columbia

Williams & Wilkins

Philadelphia • Baltimore • Hong Kong • London • Munich • Sydney • Tokyo

A Waverly Company

Williams & Wilkins

Development Editor: Karla M. Schroeder
Project Editor: Amy G. Dinkel
Production Manager: Laurie Forsyth

Copyright © 1995
Williams & Wilkins
Suite 5025
Rose Tree Corporate Center
Building Two
1400 N. Providence Road
Media, PA 19063 USA

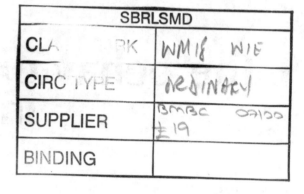

SBRLSMD	
CLA ... BK	WM18 WIE
CIRC TYPE	ordinary
SUPPLIER	BMBC 07100 £19
BINDING	

The chapters in this book were written in a private capacity by the authors. No official support by the NIH or FDA is intended nor should be inferred.

Printed in the United States of America

First Edition 1986
Library of Congress Cataloging-in-Publication Data
The Behavioral sciences in psychiatry / [edited by] Jerry M. Wiener,
  Nancy Breslin. — 3rd ed.
      p.   cm.—(National medical series for independent study)
  Rev. ed. of: Behavioral science. 2nd ed. c1990.
  Includes bibliographical references and index.
  ISBN 0-683-06203-4 (alk. paper)
  1. Medicine and psychology—Outlines, syllabi, etc.   2. Medicine
and psychology—Examinations, questions, etc.   3. National Board of
Medical Examiners—Examinations—Study guides.   I. Wiener, Jerry
M., 1933-   . II. Breslin, Nancy.   III. Behavioral science.   IV. Series.
  [DNLM: 1. Behavior—examination questions.   2. Behavior—outlines.
3. Behavioral Medicine—examination questions.   4. Behavioral
Medicine—outlines.   5. Psychiatry—examination questions.
  6. Psychiatry—outlines.   WM 18 B4193 1994]
R726.5.B4267   1994
616'.001'9—dc20
DNLM/DLC   93-23682
for Library of Congress   CIP

95 96 97 98
10 9 8 7 6 5 4 3 2

Dedication

To the medical students of the George Washington University School of Medicine.

Table 3-1 was adapted with permission from Dunner DL: *Current Psychiatric Therapy.* Philadelphia, WB Saunders, 1993.

Table 15-1 was adapted with permission from American Psychiatric Association: *Diagnostic and Statistical Manual of Mental Disorders,* 4th ed. Washington, DC, American Psychiatric Association, 1994.

Contents

Contributors   xi
Preface   xv
To the Reader   xvii

Part I   The Bio-behavioral Sciences

1   Behavioral Neurochemistry   3
     I.   Introduction   3
     II.   Neuronal transmission of information   3
     III.   Catecholamines   6
     IV.   Serotonin   11
     V.   Acetylcholine   13
     VI.   Amino acids   15
     VII.   Other nonpeptide neurotransmitter candidates   16
     VIII.   Neuropeptides   17

2   Neuroanatomy and Behavior   25
     I.   Introduction   25
     II.   Neuroanatomy   25
     III.   Special neuroanatomic functions   29
     IV.   Neuroimaging techniques   35
     V.   Neuroanatomy and behavioral functioning   42

3   Pharmacology and Behavior   47
     I.   Introduction   47
     II.   Antipsychotic agents   47
     III.   Antidepressant agents   51
     IV.   Antimanic agents   53
     V.   Antianxiety agents   56
     VI.   Hypnotic agents   58
     VII.   Eating Disorders   59
     VIII.   Psychopharmacology in children and adolescents   60
     IX.   Psychopharmacology in the elderly   61
     X.   Drugs of abuse   62
     XI.   Behavioral effects of nonpsychiatric drugs   65
     XII.   Principles of prescribing   66

4   Genetics of Behavioral Disorders   73

    I.   Basic principles of human genetics   73
    II. Methods of studying genetics   76
    III. Genetics of psychiatric disorders   78
    IV. Therapeutic implications   82

5   Animal Models and Human Behavior   87

    I.   Evolution   87
    II. Motivation and consummatory behaviors   88
    III. Learning   94
    IV. Conflict situations   97
    V. Animal models of psychiatric disorders   99

6   Statistics and Research Design   107

    I.   Introduction   107
    II. Measurement and statistics   107
    III. Research design   112
    IV. Examples of research design   116

7   Theories of the Mind   121

    I.   Introduction   121
    II. Psychoanalytic (psychodynamic) theory   121
    III. Learning theory (behaviorism)   124
    IV. Cognitive theory   126
    V. Psychosocial theory   128
    VI. Biomedical theory   130
    VII. Summary   131

8   The Life Cycle   135

    I.   Definition of terms   135
    II. Infancy to toddlerhood   135
    III. Childhood   138
    IV. Adolescence   140
    V. Adulthood   141
    VI. Later adulthood and old age   143
    VII. Death and dying   144

Part II   The Psychosocial Behavioral Sciences

9   Human Sexuality   151

    I.   Development of sexuality   151
    II. Sexual physiology   153
    III. Cultural and psychological influences on sexual expression   155
    IV. Homosexuality   155
    V. Sexual dysfunction   156
    VI. Paraphilias and gender identity disorders   161
    VII. Sexuality in medical practice   161

10   Social and Family Behavior   **171**
    I.   Introduction   171
   II.   Interpersonal behavior   172
  III.   Large group behavior   177
  IV.   Family behavior   178

11   The Physician–Patient Relationship   **189**
    I.   Definition and components of the physician–patient relationship   189
   II.   Models of the physician–patient relationship   191
  III.   Transference and countertransference   192
  IV.   Personality types found in medical practice   192
   V.   The physician–patient relationship under stress   195

12   Communication and Interviewing   **203**
    I.   Introduction   203
   II.   Rapport-building skills   203
  III.   Information-gathering skills   205
  IV.   Patient education and treatment planning skills   206
   V.   Components of the medical history   207
  VI.   Variations in technique   210

13   The Mental Status Examination   **219**
    I.   Introduction   219
   II.   Applications   219
  III.   Structure of the examination   222
  IV.   Components of the examination   222

14   Psychological Assessment and Psychometric
Evaluation   **237**
    I.   Introduction   237
   II.   Specific psychological tests   240
  III.   Analysis and reporting of test data   250

15   Clinical Syndromes   **259**
    I.   Introduction   259
   II.   Disorders usually first diagnosed in infancy, childhood, or adolescence   259
  III.   Cognitive disorders   260
  IV.   Mental disorders due to a general medical condition   262
   V.   Substance-related disorders   262
  VI.   Psychotic disorders   265
  VII.   Mood disorders   266
 VIII.   Anxiety disorders   268
  IX.   Somatoform disorders   270
   X.   Factitious disorder   271
  XI.   Dissociative disorders   271
  XII.   Sexual and gender identity disorders   272
 XIII.   Eating disorders   272

XIV.   Sleep disorders 272
XV.   Impulse control disorders 273
XVI.   Adjustment disorder 274
XVII.   Personality disorders 274
XVIII.   Conclusion 274

16   Ethics in Medicine   279
   I.   Introduction 279
   II.   The character of ethical conflict 280
   III.   General ethical theory 281
   IV.   Major ethical principles 283
   V.   Fundamental issues and controversies in medical ethics 284

17   The Health Care System   295
   I.   Health care delivery in the United States 295
   II.   Management, economics, and politics 304
   III.   Health care reform 309

Case Studies in Clinical Decision Making   317

Comprehensive Exam   343

Index   367

Contributors

Robert C. Alexander, M.D.
Associate Professor of Psychiatry and Human
   Behavior
Department of Psychiatry and Human Behavior
Jefferson Medical College of Thomas Jefferson
   University
Philadelphia, Pennsylvania

Joan K. Barber, M.D.
Associate Professor of Psychiatry and Behavioral
   Sciences
Department of Psychiatry and Behavioral Sciences
George Washington University School of Medicine
Washington, District of Columbia

Philip S. Birnbaum, M.S.
Former Dean of Administrative Affairs
Professor of Administrative Medicine
Department of Health Sciences
Department of Medicine
George Washington University School of Medicine
Washington, District of Columbia

Nancy A. Breslin, M.D.
Assistant Professor of Psychiatry and Behavioral
   Sciences
Director of Psychiatric Clerkship
Department of Psychiatry and Behavioral Sciences
George Washington University School of
   Medicine
Attending Psychiatrist
George Washington University Medical Center
Washington, District of Columbia

David DeGrazia, Ph.D.
Assistant Professor of Philosophy
Department of Philosophy
George Washington University
Assistant Professor of Health Care Sciences
Department of Health Care Sciences
George Washington University School of
   Medicine
Washington, District of Columbia

James H. Egan, M.D.
Clinical Professor of Psychiatry and Pediatrics
Departments of Psychiatry and Pediatrics
George Washington University School of
   Medicine
Washington, District of Columbia

Lois M. Freed, Ph.D.
Pharmacologist
Division of Neuropharmacological Drug Products
Food and Drug Administration
Rockville, Maryland

William J. Freed, Ph.D.
Chief, Section on Preclinical Neuroscience
Neuropsychiatry Branch
National Institute of Mental Health
Neuroscience Center at St. Elizabeths
Washington, District of Columbia

Magda Giordano, Ph.D.
Assistant Professor
Department of Physiology
National Autonomous University of Mexico
Mexico City, Mexico

Madeline M. Gladis, Ph.D.
Assistant Professor of Psychiatry
Department of Psychiatry
Medical College of Pennsylvania
Philadelphia, Pennsylvania

Warren Greenberg, Ph.D.
Professor of Health Economics and of Health
  Care Sciences
Department of Health Services Management
  and Policy
George Washington University
Washington, District of Columbia

Robert L. Hendren, D.O.
Professor of Psychiatry
Department of Psychiatry
Associate Professor of Pediatrics
Department of Pediatrics
University of New Mexico School
  of Medicine
Director of the Division of Child
  and Adolescent Psychiatry
University of New Mexico Medical Center
Albuquerque, New Mexico

Fuad Issa, M.D.
Senior Staff Fellow
Neuropsychiatry Branch
Division of Intramural Research Programs
National Institute of Mental Health
National Institutes of Health
Washington, District of Columbia

Dilip V. Jeste, M.D.
Professor of Psychiatry and Neurosciences
Department of Psychiatry
University of California, San Diego,
  School of Medicine
La Jolla, California
Director, Geriatric Psychiatry Clinical
  Research Center
San Diego Veteran's Affairs Medical Center
San Diego, California

Robert L. Jenkins, Ph.D.
Associate Professor and Chief Psychologist
Department of Psychiatry and Behavioral
  Sciences
George Washington University Medical
  Center
Washington, District of Columbia

Darrell G. Kirch, M.D.
Dean, School of Medicine
Professor of Psychiatry
Department of Psychiatry and Health Behavior
Professor of Pharmacology
Department of Pharmacology and Toxicology
Medical College of Georgia School
  of Medicine
Augusta, Georgia

Kala Ladenheim, M.S.P.H.
Ph.D. Candidate
Senior Research Associate
Intergovernmental Health Policy Project
George Washington University
Washington, District of Columbia

Bradley Lewis, M.D.
Associate Professor of Psychiatry
Department of Psychiatry and Behavioral
  Sciences
George Washington University School of
  Medicine
Medical Director of Psychiatric Day Treatment
  Program
George Washington University Medical Center
Washington, District of Columbia

James B. Lohr, M.D.
Associate Professor of Psychiatry
Department of Psychiatry
University of California, San Diego,
  School of Medicine
La Jolla, California
Chief, Psychiatry Service
San Diego Veteran's Affairs Medical Center
San Diego, California

Leslie D. Manley, Ph.D.
Instructor
Department of Pharmacology
University of California, San Diego,
    School of Medicine
La Jolla, California

Michael S. Manley, M.D.
Assistant Research Psychobiologist
Department of Psychiatry
University of California, San Diego,
    School of Medicine
La Jolla, California

James R. Phelps, M.D.
Assistant Professor of Psychiatry
Department of Psychiatry
Primary Care Psychiatry/Behavioral Consultant
University of New Mexico School of Medicine
Albuquerque, New Mexico

Alison Reeve, M.D.
Assistant Professor
Department of Psychiatry
Research Assistant Professor
Department of Neurology
University of New Mexico School of Medicine
Clinical Director
Neuropsychiatry Clinic, Outpatient Division
University of New Mexico Mental Health Center
Albuquerque, New Mexico

Barry Sarvet, M.D.
Assistant Professor of Psychiatry
Department of Psychiatry
Division of Child and Adolescent Psychiatry
University of New Mexico School of Medicine
Attending Child and Adolescent Psychiatrist
Medical Director
University of New Mexico Partial Hospital
    Program
University of New Mexico Psychiatric Hospital
Albuquerque, New Mexico

Janell Schweickert, Ph.D.
Psychology Associate
Department of Psychiatry and Behavioral
    Sciences
George Washington University Medical
    Center
Washington, District of Columbia

Richard F. Southby, Ph.D.
Chairman and Friesen Professor of International
    Health and Health Policy
Professor of Health Care Sciences
Department of Health Services Management
    and Policy
George Washington University
Washington, District of Columbia

Frederick S. Wamboldt, M.D.
Associate Professor of Psychiatry
Department of Psychiatry
University of Colorado Health Sciences
    Center
Associate Faculty Member
Division of Adult Psychosocial Medicine
Department of Medicine
National Jewish Center for Immunology and
    Respiratory Medicine
Denver, Colorado

Marianne Z. Wamboldt, M.D.
Assistant Professor of Psychiatry
Associate Director, Division of Child
    Psychiatry
Department of Psychiatry
University of Colorado Health Sciences
    Center
Assistant Faculty Member
Department of Pediatrics
Director, Division of Pediatric Psychiatry
National Jewish Center for Immunology and
    Respiratory Medicine
Denver, Colorado

Jerry M. Wiener, M.D.
Leon Yochelson Professor and Chairman
Department of Psychiatry and Behavioral
  Sciences
Professor of Pediatrics
Department of Pediatrics
George Washington University School of
  Medicine
President, American Psychiatric Association
  (1994-1995)
Washington, District of Columbia

Thomas N. Wise, M.D.
Professor and Vice Chairman
Department of Psychiatry
Georgetown University School of Medicine
Washington, District of Columbia
Chairman
Department of Psychiatry
Fairfax Hospital
Falls Church, Virginia

Preface

The third edition of *The Behavioral Sciences in Psychiatry* follows the second by 4 years. Major advances continue in the exploding fields of genetics, psychopharmacology, and biochemistry, and a new edition of the *Diagnostic and Statistical Manual of Mental Disorders* was released earlier this year. The last several years also have seen the initiation of major reforms in the health care system of this country.

This book has incorporated these expanded and new areas of information, with updated sections on neuroimaging, psychopathology, and health care reform, and a new chapter on biostatistics. Many chapters feature new tables and figures to improve the presentation of material.

In response to the move at many medical schools toward problem-based learning paradigms, a series of clinical cases have been added to this edition. Many of these demonstrate the ties between the basic and clinical sciences in approaching and understanding behavior.

Finally, we would like to thank the superb group of authors—previous contributors along with new writers—who have made this third edition an exciting sequel to the second.

Jerry M. Wiener, M.D.
Nancy A. Breslin, M.D.

To the Reader

Since 1984, the *National Medical Series for Independent Study (NMS)* has been helping medical students meet the challenge of education and clinical training. In this climate of burgeoning knowledge and complex clinical issues, a medical career is more demanding than ever. Increasingly, medical training must prepare physicians to seek and synthesize necessary information and to apply that information successfully.

The *National Medical Series* is designed to provide a logical framework for organizing, learning, reviewing, and applying the conceptual and factual information covered in basic and clinical studies. Each book includes a concise but comprehensive outline of the essential content of a discipline, with up to 500 study questions. The combination of an outlined text and tools for self-evaluation allows easy retrieval of salient information.

All study questions are accompanied by the correct answer, a paragraph-length explanation, and specific reference to the text where the topic is discussed. Study questions that follow each chapter use current USMLE format to reinforce the chapter content. Study questions appearing at the end of the text in the Comprehensive Exam vary in format depending on the book. Wherever possible, Comprehensive Exam questions are presented as a clinical case or scenario intended to simulate real-life application of medical knowledge. The goal of this exam is to challenge the student to draw from information presented throughout the book.

All of the books in the *National Medical Series* are constantly being updated and revised. The authors and editors devote considerable time and effort to ensure that the information required by all medical school curricula is included. Strict editorial attention is given to accuracy, organization, and consistency. Further shaping of the series occurs in response to biannual discussions held with a panel of medical student advisors drawn from schools throughout the United States. At these meetings, the editorial staff considers the complicated needs of medical students to learn how the *National Medical Series* can better serve them. In this regard, the staff at Williams & Wilkins welcomes all comments and suggestions.

Part I
The Bio-behavioral Sciences

Chapter 1

Behavioral Neurochemistry

Dilip V. Jeste
Michael S. Manley
Leslie D. Manley
James B. Lohr

I. **INTRODUCTION. Certain chemical substances influence mood, thought, and action.**
The mind-altering properties of amphetamines, cocaine, opiates, barbiturates, and lysergic acid diethylamide (LSD), as well as other drugs that have a profound effect on normal and abnormal behavior, have stimulated the field of psychopharmacology. Interest in the basic biochemistry of behavior has grown as well. The neurochemistry of the brain is only beginning to be understood, and additional neuroactive substances and transmitter candidates are continually being discovered.

A. **Neurotransmitter disturbances.** Many behavioral disorders, particularly psychiatric and movement disorders, are believed to be associated with disturbances of specific neurotransmitters.

B. **Response to drugs** is a complex issue because few psychopharmacologic agents affect only a single transmitter system.

II. **NEURONAL TRANSMISSION OF INFORMATION.** Nearly a century ago, Ramon y Cajal developed the **"neuron doctrine,"** which states that **the neuron is the basic unit of the nervous system**. Information basic to behavior is transferred in the form of specific chemicals and energy within and between neurons.

A. **The neuron** is the cell type that is responsible for unilateral **transfer of information**. The **dendrites** and the **cell body** integrate information from many neuronal sources. If the neuron is sufficiently depolarized (i.e., by an influx of positive ions), an **action potential** is initiated at the **axon hillock** (a region joining the cell body and axon) and travels down the **axon** to the **nerve terminal**. The nerve terminal contains neurotransmitters packaged in membrane-bound vesicles. Some neurons have axons that are periodically encircled by layers of a lipid known as **myelin**. The points of the axon between the myelin are called the **nodes of Ranvier**. Myelinated neurons convey information much faster than do unmyelinated neurons. Action potentials jump from node of Ranvier to node of Ranvier. This mode of information transfer is called **saltatory conduction**.

1. **The action potential** is the sweeping wave of depolarization that passes down the length of the neuron's membrane when it is stimulated above a threshold voltage.
   a. **Depolarization.** During the action potential, **voltage-dependent sodium ion (Na^+) channels** in the membrane open, and Na^+ rushes into the axon. This influx of positive charge causes depolarization, in which the electrical potential difference across the membrane increases from approximately -70 mV (the **resting potential**) to approximately -15 mV.
   b. **Repolarization.** This increase is followed by repolarization toward the resting potential as **positively charged potassium ions (K^+) leak out** of the cell. These changes are then propagated down the length of the axon until they reach the axon terminal.

2. **Neurotransmitter release.** When the wave of depolarization spreads into the nerve terminal, **voltage-dependent calcium ion (Ca^{2+}) channels** open. Extracellular Ca^{2+} flows into the terminal and causes the vesicles to fuse with the plasma membrane. Thus, the neurotransmitter is released into the synapse.

B. **The synapse.** Synapses are specialized contacts between neurons. Interneuronal communication of information occurs at these sites. Synapses that use chemical neurotransmission are called **chemical synapses**. Synapses in which cells are directly electrically connected are known as **electrotonic synapses**.

1. **Chemical synapses** are the best understood and most important type. They appear under the electron microscope as discrete areas of apposition of neuronal membranes. The **presynaptic bouton** ("button," or axon terminal) contains vesicles that are filled with stored neurotransmitter. On the arrival of an action potential, the neurotransmitter in the presynaptic bouton is released into the **synaptic cleft** between the two neurons. The neurotransmitter acts at **receptors** that are located on the **postsynaptic or presynaptic cell**.

2. **Electrotonic (electrical) synapses** are specialized junctions between neurons. These synapses permit charge to flow directly from cell to cell. The release of neurotransmitter is not required. Electronic synapses are poorly understood.

C. **Receptors** are protein structures that are located in the plasma membrane. They transduce information from the outside to the inside of the neuron. Different families of receptors exist. Two important receptor families found in the brain are ligand-gated ion channels and G-protein–coupled receptors.

1. **Ligand-gated ion channels** are receptors and are composed of several **peptide subunits** surrounding a central core through which ions flow. When certain neurotransmitters bind to a particular subunit of the receptor, a conformational change occurs that allows the ions to flow through the channel.
   a. Typically, channels that allow positive ions (Na^+ or Ca^{2+}) to flow inward yield **excitatory** responses. These receptors include the **nicotinic acetylcholine receptor; the amino-4-phosphonobutyric acid (AMPA), kainate,** and **N-methyl-D-aspartate (NMDA) glutamate receptors;** and the **5-hydroxytryptamine$_3$ (5-HT$_3$)** receptor.
   b. Channels that allow the flow of negative chloride ions (Cl^-) produce **inhibitory** effects. These receptors include **γ-aminobutyric acid (GABA)** and **glycine receptors**.

2. **G-protein–coupled receptors** consist of one long peptide that traverses the plasma membrane seven times. They interact with other proteins in the membrane. These proteins are called **G-proteins** because they hydrolyze guanosine triphosphate (GTP). G-proteins interact with a variety of cellular enzymes. These enzymes produce a product inside the cell known as a **second messenger**. The neurotransmitter is the first messenger. This receptor type includes **muscarinic acetylcholine** and **dopamine** and **adrenergic, opiate,** and **most serotonin receptors (5-HT$_1$** and **5-HT$_2$ types)**.
   a. **Cyclic nucleotides** include **cyclic adenosine 3',5'-monophosphate (cAMP)** and **cyclic guanosine 3',5'-monophosphate (cGMP)**. The enzymes that produce these substances are **adenylate cyclase** and **guanylate cyclase,** respectively.
      (1) Certain neurotransmitters **activate adenylate cyclase** by binding to specific receptors. This enzyme catalyzes the formation of cAMP from **adenosine triphosphate (ATP)**. The increase in cAMP concentration may activate **cAMP-dependent protein kinase,** which regulates intracellular components by phosphorylation. Receptors that increase cAMP formation include **β-adrenergic receptors** and **dopamine D$_1$ receptors**. cAMP is subsequently broken down by the enzyme **phosphodiesterase,** which terminates the effects of this second messenger.
      (2) Activation of other receptors inhibits the activity of adenylate cyclase. These receptors include **α_2-adrenergic receptors, dopamine D$_2$ receptors,** and certain **muscarinic** and **opiate receptors**.

   b. Phosphatidylinositol is a membrane phospholipid that is hydrolyzed by **phospholipase C** after receptor occupation. **Diacylglycerol** and **inositol triphosphate** are produced. These second messengers activate **protein kinase C** and increase intracellular **calcium** concentration, respectively.

   c. Calcium. When depolarization occurs, a significant amount of calcium enters the neuron. Phosphatidylinositol hydrolysis also increases the level of available intracellular calcium. Calcium, which is considered a second messenger, binds to intracellular calcium-binding proteins (e.g., calmodulin, calbindin). These proteins modulate a number of calcium-dependent enzymes, such as a calcium-calmodulin–dependent protein kinase, adenylate cyclase, phosphodiesterase, and adenosinetriphosphatase (ATPase).

3. Autoreceptors are located on the neuron. These receptors are sensitive to the neurotransmitter of the neuron. These receptors can detect the release of neurotransmitter and decrease the firing rate of the neuron or transmitter synthesis by a process called **self-inhibition**.

D. **Neurotransmitters**

1. Types. Five main types of neurotransmitters are present in the central nervous system (CNS). They fall into two classes: monoamines and amino acids.

   a. Monoamines include catecholamines, acetylcholine (ACh), and indolealkylamines (serotonin). Monoamines have complex and subtle actions that are dependent on the type of receptor with which they interact.

   b. Amino acids include the major excitatory and inhibitory neurotransmitters.

      (1) Excitatory amino acid neurotransmitters (glutamate, aspartate) increase the likelihood of the firing of the postsynaptic neuron.

      (2) Inhibitory amino acid neurotransmitters (GABA, glycine) decrease the likelihood of the firing of the postsynaptic neuron.

2. Classification. To be considered a neurotransmitter, a neurochemical must meet specific criteria.

   a. Criteria

      (1) The neurotransmitter must be present in nerve terminals.

      (2) Stimulation of the nerve must cause the transmitter to be released in sufficient amounts to exert its actions on the postsynaptic neuron.

      (3) The effects of the exogenously applied transmitter on the postsynaptic membrane must be similar to those produced by stimulation of the presynaptic nerve.

      (4) Pharmacologic agents should alter the dose–response curve of the neurotransmitter in the same magnitude and direction that they alter the naturally occurring synaptic potential.

      (5) A mechanism for inactivation or metabolism of the transmitter must exist in the vicinity of the synapse.

   b. Classification system

      (1) Neurotransmitters that meet all of the criteria are considered **proven, or definite, neurotransmitters**. This category includes **ACh, dopamine, norepinephrine, epinephrine, GABA, serotonin, and glycine**.

      (2) Those that meet some, but not all, of the criteria are considered **putative neurotransmitters**. This category includes **glutamate, aspartate, and substance P**.

      (3) Those that meet only one or two criteria are considered **neurotransmitter candidates**. This category includes **adenosine, cAMP, prostaglandins, and most peptides**.

3. Steps in neurochemical transmission and targets for pharmacological intervention

   a. Synthesis of a neurotransmitter occurs either near the presynaptic membrane where the neurotransmitter is to be released or in the cell body of the neuron.

      (1) For many **classic neurotransmitters** (e.g., catecholamines, ACh, 5-HT, GABA), the **synthesizing enzymes** are manufactured in the cell body. They are transported down the axon to the **nerve terminal,** where neurotransmitter synthesis occurs. Peptide neurotransmitters, however, are synthesized in the soma of the neuron then transported along the axon to the nerve terminals.

    (2) The synthesis of some neurotransmitters can be interrupted by specific **enzyme inhibitors**. This process leads to neurotransmitter depletion. These inhibitors include **α-methyltyrosine (AMPT)** for catecholamines and **p-chlorophenylalanine (PCPA)** for serotonin.

b. Storage of a neurotransmitter usually occurs in membrane-bound **vesicles** that are located near sites of neurotransmitter release. Neurotransmitters are usually taken up into the vesicles by uptake carriers. Storage can be disrupted by the administration of **reserpine,** which prevents neurotransmitter uptake into the vesicles. High doses of reserpine can cause destruction of the vesicles.

c. Release into the **synaptic cleft** occurs next. The mechanism of release is controversial, but it depends on calcium and may involve exocytosis of the contents of the synaptic vesicles.

d. Binding of the neurotransmitter to specific receptors occurs next. Specific **antagonists** can prevent the action of a neurotransmitter at a receptor. Agents that act as receptor **agonists** mimic the actions of the neurotransmitter at the binding site. Table 1-1 lists the agonists and antagonists for many neurotransmitters.

e. Transduction is the process by which the binding of a transmitter with a receptor causes a biologic response of the neuron. Transduction occurs through the **opening of ion channels** or the **production of second messengers** (see II C 2). Transduction amplifies the signal of the neurotransmitter. The transduction process **can be modulated**.

    (1) Phosphodiesterase inhibitors (e.g., caffeine) can produce an accumulation of cAMP.

    (2) Pertussis toxin interferes with G-protein action.

f. Termination. The action of a specific neurotransmitter may be terminated by re-uptake (usually into the presynaptic neuron), **metabolism,** or **diffusion**. Reuptake is probably the most important termination process for catecholamines and indolealkylamines. Metabolism is more important for ACh and peptides.

    (1) The metabolism of ACh can be prevented by **acetylcholinesterase inhibitors (e.g., physostigmine)**.

    (2) The uptake of catecholamines and serotonin can be prevented by **uptake blockers (e.g., cocaine, trycyclic antidepressants)**.

    (3) Monoamine oxidase (MAO) inhibitors prevent the metabolism of catecholamines by MAO.

III.   **CATECHOLAMINES.** These compounds are related to 1,2-dihydroxybenzene (catechol). They include **dopamine, norepinephrine, and epinephrine (adrenaline)**.

A.   **Synthesis and metabolism of catecholamines**

    1. Synthesis (Figure 1-1). The ability of a neuron to synthesize dopamine versus norepinephrine versus epinephrine depends on the synthesizing enzymes that the neuron contains. For instance, a norepinephrine neuron contains all of the enzymes except phenylethanolamine N-methyltransferase (PNMT).

    a. Hydroxylation of the amino acid tyrosine by **tyrosine hydroxylase** to produce **L-dihydroxyphenylalanine (L-dopa)** is the **rate-limiting step** in the synthesis of all major catecholamines. This enzyme can be inhibited by AMPT.

    b. The L-dopa is converted to **dopamine** by **aromatic L-amino acid decarboxylase**. L-dopa crosses the blood–brain barrier, but dopamine cannot.

    c. Dopamine is converted to **norepinephrine** by **dopamine β-hydroxylase,** which is the only catecholamine-synthesizing enzyme that is located inside the neurotransmitter vesicles. The rest of the enzymes are located in the cytoplasm.

    d. Norepinephrine is converted to epinephrine by **PNMT**.

TABLE 1-1. Neuroregulator Agonists and Antagonists

Regulator	Receptor	Agonist	Antagonist
Dopamine	D-nonspecific	Dopamine Bromocriptine Apomorphine	Neuroleptics[†]
	D_2	Quinpirole*	L-sulpiride Raclopride*
Norepinephrine	Nonspecific	Norepinephrine	Labetalol
	α-Nonspecific	Ephedrine . . .	Phenoxybenzamine Phentolamine
	$α_1$	Phenylephrine	Prazosin
	$α_2$	Clonidine	Yohimbine
Serotonin	5-HT-nonspecific	Serotonin* LSD* . . .	Methysergide Cyproheptadine
	5-HT_{1A}	Buspirone	. . .
	5-HT_{1D}	Sumatriptan	. . .
	5-HT_2	. . .	Ketanserin
	5-HT_3	. . .	Odansetron
ACh	ACh-nonspecific	ACh*	. . .
	Nicotinic	Nicotine*	D-tubocurarine
	Muscarinic-nonspecific	Muscarine* Pilocarpine	Atropine Scopolamine
	M_1	. . .	Pirenzepine
GABA	GABA-nonspecific	GABA*	. . .
	GABA-A	Muscimol*	Bicuculline* Picrotoxin*
	GABA-B	Baclofen	. . .
Glycine	Glycine	Glycine*	Strychnine*
Glutamate	Glutamate-nonspecific	Glutamate*	. . .
	Kainate	Kainate*	. . .
	AMPA	AMPA*	. . .
	NMDA	NMDA*	MK-801* Phencyclidine*
Adenosine	A-nonspecific	Adenosine*	Methylxanthines
Opioid peptides	μ	Morphine Met-enkephalin*	Naloxone
	κ	Dynorphin*	Naloxone
	ε	B-Endorphin*	Naloxone
	δ	Leu-enkephalin*	Naloxone
	σ	Phencyclidine*	. . .
	κ and σ	Pentazocine	. . .
Other peptides	CCK	CCK*	Lorglumide
	Somatostatin	Somatostatin*	. . .
	Vasopressin	AVP	. . .

*Not used clinically.
[†]Including haloperidol, fluphenazine, trifluoperazine, thiothixene, thioridazine, mesoridazine.
ACh = acetylcholine; *AMPA* = amino-4-phosphonobutyric acid; *AVP* = arginine vasopressin; *CCK* = cholecystokinin; *GABA* = γ-aminobutyric acid; *5-HT* = 5-hydroxytryptamine; *LSD* = lysergic acid diethylamide; *NMDA* = N-methyl-D-aspartic acid.

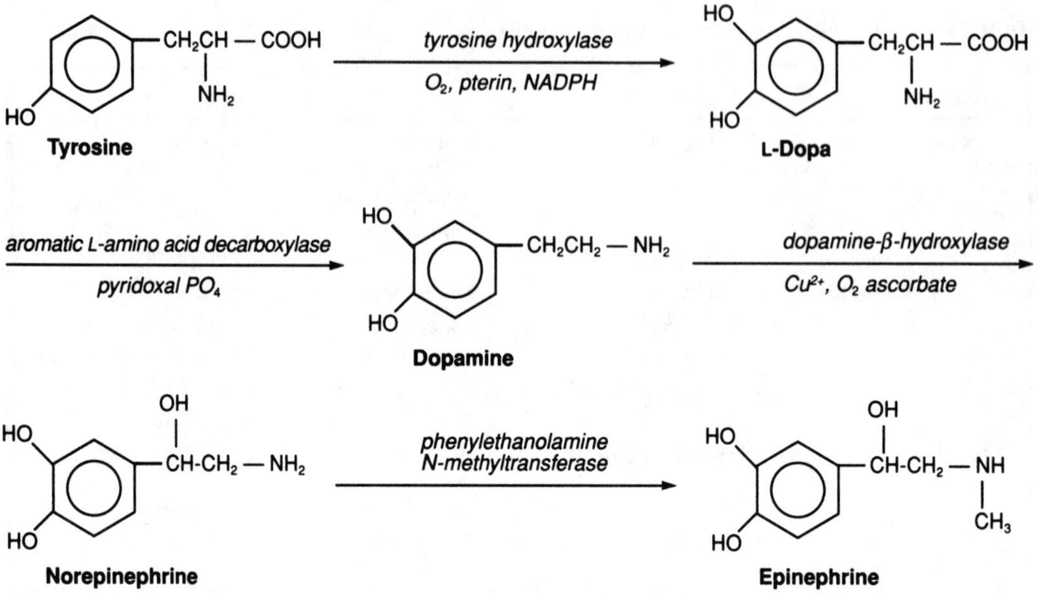

FIGURE 1-1. Catecholamine synthesis.

2. **Metabolism.** Two enzymes are important for the inactivation of catecholamines.
    a. **MAO** is located on the outer membrane of the mitochondria. MAO is important for the oxidative deamination of intracellular cytoplasmic catecholamines. There are two forms of MAO: MAO-A and MAO-B.
    b. **Catechol-O-methyltransferase (COMT)** is located on the outer plasma membranes of most cells. It methylates most extracellular catecholamines.

B. **Dopamine**

1. **Termination and metabolism.** After dopamine is released, it is cleared from the synapse by a specific reuptake process. Dopamine is metabolized by deamination by either MAO-A or MAO-B, or by methylation by COMT. A major metabolite of dopamine in urine and plasma is **homovanillic acid (HVA),** which is formed through the actions of MAO and COMT.

2. **Receptors.** Five types of dopamine receptors are known.
    a. **D_1 receptors** are believed to be **postsynaptic**. They activate adenylate cyclase.
    b. **D_2 receptors** are probably **both presynaptic and postsynaptic**. They are believed to inhibit adenylate cyclase.
    c. **D_3, D_4, and D_5 receptors** were recently identified. Little is currently known about the pharmacology of these receptors, however.

3. **Important brain tracts**
    a. **Nigrostriatal pathway.** This tract originates in the dopaminergic cells of the **substantia nigra** ("black substance") pars compacta. It travels to the **striatum** in the median forebrain bundle. The nigrostriatal pathway is important in the initiation of movement in animals and humans. Its destruction causes a reduction or loss of movement. This pathway degenerates in **Parkinson's disease**.
    b. **Mesolimbic and mesocortical tracts.** The dopaminergic neurons that form these tracts are located in the **ventral tegmental area (VTA),** which lies superior and medial to the substantia nigra. VTA neurons project to the limbic system, which includes the amygdala, nucleus accumbens, septum, and cingulate gyrus. These neurons also project to the **cerebral cortex,** predominantly to the frontal lobes. In humans, these tracts are important in affect, cognition, and motivation. Hyperactivity of this pathway is important in **schizophrenia**.

    c. Tuberoinfundibular (tuberohypophyseal) tract. The dopaminergic neurons of this tract are located in the **arcuate and periventricular nuclei of the hypothalamus**. The neurons project to the median eminence of the hypothalamus and to the intermediate lobe of the pituitary gland. In this area, dopamine inhibits the release of prolactin.

4. Effects on behavior
  a. Parkinsonism
    (1) Pathogenesis
      (a) Nigrostriatal dopaminergic tract degeneration in Parkinson's disease causes akinesia, tremor, rigidity, and loss of postural reflexes.
      (b) A similar syndrome was observed when drug addicts injected **methylphenyltetrahydropyridine (MPTP),** which destroys dopamine cells in the substantia nigra.
      (c) Parkinsonism is also caused by **antipsychotic drugs,** which block postsynaptic dopamine receptors, and by **reserpine,** which depletes dopamine.
    (2) Therapy
      (a) Exogenous **L-dopa** is given to patients with Parkinson's disease. Subsequently, L-dopa is converted to dopamine, probably by the remaining dopamine cells in the patient's brain. Dopamine cannot be given because it does not cross the blood–brain barrier. L-Dopa is given in combination with **carbidopa,** an inhibitor of dopa decarboxylase that does not cross the blood–brain barrier. Therefore, when these drugs are used together, L-dopa is converted to dopamine only in the brain and not in the periphery. Thus, many unwanted peripheral side effects are eliminated.
      (b) Normal control of voluntary movement requires a balance between dopamine and ACh in the neostriatum. A deficiency of dopamine leads to an overabundance of ACh. Thus, restoration of the balance of dopamine and ACh in the striatum requires an increase in the level of dopamine and a decrease in ACh tone by ACh receptor antagonists. The antagonists most frequently used in the treatment of Parkinson's disease are **benztropine** and **trihexyphenidyl**.
      (c) Another drug that is useful in the treatment of Parkinson's disease is **deprenyl (selegiline).** This drug, which is an **MAO-B inhibitor,** helps to prevent the onset of symptoms.
    (3) Side effects of therapy. The underlying problem in Parkinson's disease is the degeneration of the nigrostriatal tract. Ideally, treatment would increase the dopamine level only in this tract. Unfortunately, when the dopamine levels are raised pharmacologically in the nigrostriatal tract, they are increased also in the mesolimbic, mesocortical, and tuberoinfundibular tracts as well. Therefore, the side effects of L-dopa therapy include hallucinations (mesolimbic and mesocortical tracts) and hypoprolactinemia (tuberoinfundibular tract).
  b. Other movement disorders. Certain hyperkinetic disorders (e.g., Huntington's disease, tardive dyskinesia) are believed to be related to excessive dopamine transmission. **Tardive dyskinesia** occurs after long-term treatment with antipsychotic drugs. It usually causes choreoathetoid movements of the mouth and hands. One hypothesis about tardive dyskinesia is that long-term treatment with antipsychotic drugs causes supersensitivity of the postsynaptic D_2 receptors. This hypothesis has been questioned, because D_2 receptor sensitivity appears to be a universal consequence of the use of antipsychotic drugs. Therefore, the hypothesis may not explain the development of tardive dyskinesia in some patients and not others.
  c. Schizophrenia. Dopamine is also believed to be important for the organization of thought and feeling and has been implicated in the psychotic disorder schizophrenia.
    (1) Pathogenesis. Schizophrenia is believed to be related to abnormalities in transmission in the mesolimbic and possibly mesocortical dopamine systems (**the dopamine hypothesis of schizophrenia**).
    (2) The **psychotic symptoms** of schizophrenia are believed to result from a **hyperdopaminergic state.**

    (a) The ability of antipsychotic drugs to block D_2 receptors correlates significantly with their antipsychotic potency.

    (b) Drugs that enhance dopaminergic transmission (e.g., amphetamine, L-dopa) tend to intensify the symptoms of schizophrenia. They also cause hallucinations and delusions in normal individuals.

    (c) Increases in dopamine concentration and dopamine receptor binding are found in patients with schizophrenia. However, in some cases, these increases are caused by treatment with neuroleptic drugs.

  (3) Certain negative symptoms of schizophrenia (e.g., affective blunting, poverty of thought) may be related to reduced dopamine activity in some areas of the brain.

  (4) Antipsychotic drug therapy

    (a) Antipsychotic drugs, also called **neuroleptics,** are primarily dopamine antagonists. Because they interfere with the extrapyramidal systems (e.g., nigrostriatal tract), these drugs cause motor side effects, such as **parkinsonism, akathesia, dystonia, and tardive dyskinesia**.

    (b) Some antipsychotic drugs, called **atypical antipsychotics,** cause fewer extrapyramidal side effects than the typical neuroleptics. The best example of this type of drug is **clozapine**. It is not known why these drugs cause fewer motor side effects, but atypical drugs are more effective at blocking $5\text{-}HT_2$ receptors than that of D_2 receptors. However, clozapine causes agranulocytosis, a potentially fatal reaction, in some patients.

C. **Norepinephrine**

  1. Metabolism

    a. Two metabolites of norepinephrine are commonly measured in plasma or urine: **3-methoxy-4-hydroxyphenylglycol (MHPG)** and **3-methoxy-4-hydroxymandelic acid (vanillylmandelic acid, or VMA)**. Thirty to fifty percent of urinary MHPG is formed in the brain. Both MHPG and VMA are formed through the **oxidative deamination** of norepinephrine by MAO-A.

    b. After norepinephrine is released into the synaptic cleft from storage vesicles, an **active reuptake** process occurs. This process removes norepinephrine from the synaptic cleft.

  2. Receptors

    a. α-Receptors

      (1) α_1-Receptors are postsynaptic. They act by raising the intracellular calcium level. In the periphery, α_1-receptors are located in the smooth muscle of blood vessels, where they mediate vasoconstriction. **Prazosin** exerts a relatively selective α_1-receptor blockade.

      (2) α_2-Receptors are both presynaptic and postsynaptic, are negatively linked to adenylate cyclase, and decrease the synthesis of norepinephrine in the presynaptic neuron when stimulated. Clonidine is an α_2-agonist. Piperoxan and yohimbine are selective α_2-antagonists.

    b. β-Receptors

      (1) β_1-Receptors

        (a) β_1-Receptors are mainly, but not exclusively, **postsynaptic**. They are positively linked to **adenylate cyclase**.

        (b) In the **periphery** (i.e., tissues outside the brain and spinal cord), β_1-receptors are found predominantly in the heart.

      (2) β_2-Receptors

        (a) β_2-Receptors are also **postsynaptic** and are positively linked to **adenylate cyclase**.

        (b) In the **periphery,** β_2-receptors are found mainly in the lungs, blood vessels, and vascular beds in skeletal muscle.

      (3) Nonselective β-agonists and -antagonists

        (a) Nonselective β-agonists include **epinephrine and norepinephrine**. These agents are equally potent on β_1-receptors, but epinephrine is much more potent than norepinephrine on β_2-receptors.

(b) **Nonselective β-antagonists** include **propranolol, alprenolol, nadolol, and timolol**.

3. **Important brain tracts**
   a. Much of the norepinephrine in the brain originates from the **locus coeruleus ("blue spot"),** which is a cluster of pigmented neurons located within the pontine central gray area along the lateral aspect of the fourth ventricle. Additionally, some norepinephrine-producing cells are scattered throughout the ventral brain stem.
   b. Noradrenergic neurons project widely to the brain. Fibers innervate the cerebellum and spinal cord. Through the median forebrain bundle, they project to the hippocampus, ventral striatum, septum and amygdala, and cerebral cortex.

4. **Effects on behavior**
   a. **Neuromodulatory functions**
      (1) Norepinephrine is believed to play a role in various **physiologic functions,** including arousal and attention, olfaction, the sleep–wake cycle, response to pain, and anxiety.
      (2) The norepinephrine system may mediate the **orientation of an organism to the environment**. When unexpected external sensory stimuli occur, noradrenergic neuronal firing increases. It decreases during tonic vegetative activities.
   b. **Mood.** Norepinephrine is important in mood, and it may be related to **mood and anxiety disorders**.
      (1) **The catecholamine theory of mood disorders** states that reduced activity of catecholaminergic systems (usually the noradrenergic system) in certain areas of the brain is associated with depression and that increased activity is associated with mania. This theory is based on indirect pharmacologic evidence.
         (a) **Reserpine,** which depletes catecholamine and indolealkylamine levels, causes a state similar to depression.
         (b) **MAO inhibitors** (e.g., iproniazid, phenelzine), which increase catecholamine availability, have antidepressant properties.
         (c) **Amphetamines,** which cause the release of norepinephrine, dopamine, and serotonin, also cause an elevation of mood.
         (d) **Tricyclic antidepressants,** at least transiently, increase the availability of norepinephrine in the cleft by blocking its active reuptake.
         (e) **Propranolol,** a nonselective β-blocker, causes improvement of symptoms in some patients with mania, but also worsens depression.
      (2) **Inconsistencies in the catecholamine hypothesis** include the existence of agents that improve depression, but do not block monoamine reuptake or inhibit MAO activity, and the ineffectiveness of cocaine as an antidepressant, even though it blocks the reuptake of catecholamines.

IV. SEROTONIN

A. **Synthesis.** Figure 1-2 shows the synthesis of serotonin (5-HT).

B. **Metabolism**

1. **Serotonin catabolism** involves oxidation of the amino group. This step is catalyzed by MAO (primarily MAO-A) yielding to 5-hydroxyindoleacetic acid (**5-HIAA**).
   a. **Melatonin** is an N-acetylated derivative of serotonin. It is produced in the pineal gland.
   b. **N-Methylated** and **N-formylated derivatives** are formed in the brain. They also may be related to psychosis.

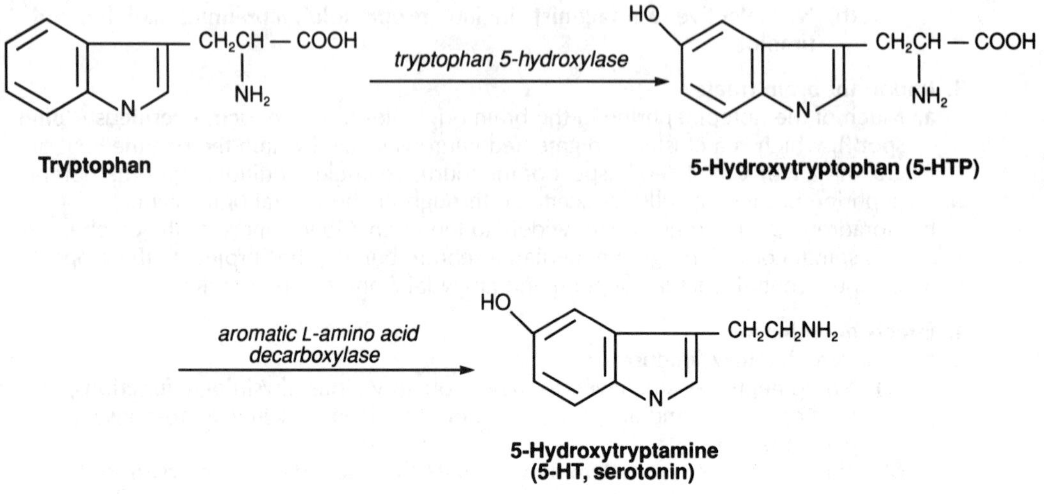

FIGURE 1-2. Serotonin synthesis.

2. **Serotonin inactivation** occurs by reuptake into the presynaptic neuron. This process is inhibited by tricyclic antidepressants and cocaine. Drugs such as reserpine and tetrabenazine deplete serotonin from the vesicles. After serotonin is internalized, it can be metabolized by MAO.

C. **Receptors**

1. **Types**
    a. **5-HT$_1$ receptors** preferentially bind serotonin. They are categorized into several subclasses.
        (1) **5-HT$_{1A}$ receptors** are located in the **raphe nuclei**. They are believed to function there as **somatodendritic autoreceptors**. They are also found in the **hippocampus,** and they **inhibit the production of cAMP**. 5-HT$_{1A}$ agonists, such as **buspirone** and **gepirone,** are used clinically as antidepressants and antianxiety agents.
        (2) **5-HT$_{1B}$ receptors** occur in high density in the **striatum**. They function as **terminal autoreceptors** (i.e., autoreceptors located on the axon terminals). They are negatively linked to the production of cAMP.
        (3) **5-HT$_{1C}$ receptors** are found in the **choroid plexus**. They are linked to phosphatidylinositol turnover.
        (4) In humans, the 5-HT$_{1D}$ receptor is similar to the 5-HT$_{1B}$ receptor. The 5-HT$_{1D}$ agonist, **sumatriptan,** is used clinically as an antimigraine agent.
    b. **5-HT$_2$ receptors** preferentially bind spiperone, which is a drug that is also a D$_2$-antagonist. They are believed to be important in mediating the behavioral effects of serotonin. They are found in the neocortex and hippocampus and also on platelets. 5-HT$_2$ receptors are linked to phosphatidylinositol turnover, and they share much sequence homology with 5-HT$_{1C}$ receptors. 5-HT$_2$ receptors are believed to play an important role in the mechanism of action of hallucinogenic drugs, such as **lysergic acid diethylamide (LSD)**.
    c. **Other serotonin receptors** (e.g., 5-HT$_3$, 5-HT$_4$) exist, but little is known about their function. **Odansetron,** a 5-HT$_3$ antagonist, is an effective antiemetic.

2. **Action.** The primary action of serotonin on receptors is **inhibition,** although excitation occurs in some cases.

D. **Important brain tracts.** The most important serotonergic neurons in the brain originate in clusters in or around the midline (raphe) of the pons and the mesencephalon, especially the **median and dorsal raphe nuclei**. The raphe nuclei send fibers to most areas of the brain.

1. The **median raphe neurons** innervate the cerebral cortex, hippocampus, thalamus, and amygdala.

2. The **dorsal raphe neurons** innervate the striatum, cerebral cortex, thalamus, amygdala, and cerebellum.

E. **Effects on behavior.** Serotonin is believed to be important for many central processes, including pain perception, aggression, appetite, thermoregulation, blood pressure control, heart rate, and respiration. It is probably important for induction of sleep and wakefulness.

1. **Mood disorders**
   a. **Pathogenesis**
      (1) Low activity of serotonin in the brain may be associated with depression. High activity is associated with mania.
      (2) Another theory, known as **the permissive serotonin hypothesis,** states that reduced serotonin activity permits low levels of catecholamines to cause depression and high levels to cause mania.
   b. **Therapy. Specific serotonin reuptake inhibitors (SSRIs)** (e.g., fluoxetine, sertraline, paroxetine) are powerful new agents that show clinical efficacy as antidepressants. **Fluoxetine (Prozac)** is one of the most widely prescribed drugs today.

2. **Schizophrenia.** The **transmethylation hypothesis of schizophrenia** states that certain methylated derivatives of serotonin may cause psychosis. These derivatives are formed as a result of errors in metabolism.
   a. This theory is supported by the finding that LSD and serotonin derivatives (e.g., dimethyltryptamine, harmaline, psilocybin) cause hallucinations and behavioral abnormalities.
   b. There is no direct proof of this hypothesis, however. Overall, evidence of serotonin involvement in schizophrenia is much weaker than that of catecholamine involvement.

3. **Obsessive-compulsive disorder.** Serotonin is probably involved in the pathogenesis of obsessive-compulsive disorder. SSRIs show considerable efficacy in the treatment of this debilitating syndrome.

V. ACETYLCHOLINE

A. **Synthesis.** Choline is not synthesized in neurons; it is transported into the brain by high-affinity and low-affinity transport processes. The high-affinity process, which is inhibited by hemicholinium-3, appears to be the primary factor that regulates the amount of ACh in neurons. ACh is formed by the condensation of choline with acetylcoenzyme A (acetyl-CoA), which is catalyzed by the enzyme **choline acetyltransferase (ChAT)**. Figure 1-3 shows the synthesis of ACh.

B. **Metabolism**

1. ACh is inactivated by **cholinesterases,** such as acetylcholinesterase, and by butyrylcholinesterase (pseudocholinesterase). Cholinesterases are reversibly inhibited by physostigmine and irreversibly inhibited by organophosphorus compounds, such as those used in insecticides.

2. The choline produced by ACh hydrolysis is reabsorbed and reused in the cell.

C. **Receptors.** There are two main types of ACh receptors: **nicotinic and muscarinic receptors**. Both occur in the brain.

1. **Nicotinic receptors** are channels that allow sodium ions to enter the neuron, thus bringing the membrane closer to the threshold. Therefore, these receptors are **excitatory.**

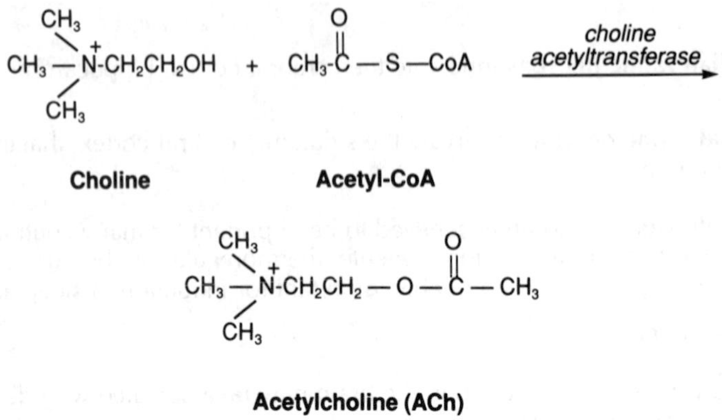

FIGURE 1-3. Acetylcholine synthesis. *Acetyl-CoA* = acetyl coenzyme A.

   a. Sites
   (1) Nicotinic receptors in the peripheral nervous system are located on the cell bodies of postganglionic neurons of both the sympathetic and parasympathetic divisions of the **autonomic nervous system**.
   (2) Nicotinic receptors are also located at the junctions of motor nerves and **skeletal muscle**.
   (3) Nicotinic receptors are found in the brain, but less is known about them than about muscarinic receptors.
   b. Agonists include nicotine, and **antagonists** include D-tubocurarine, which is derived from curare.

   2. Muscarinic receptors. Presynaptic ACh receptors are primarily muscarinic.
   a. Sites. Muscarinic receptors are located in the peripheral ganglia of the sympathetic and parasympathetic nervous systems. They modulate the predominantly nicotinic transmission. They are also located on the end organs of the parasympathetic nervous system (i.e., smooth muscle, glands).
   b. Muscarinic receptor agonists include muscarine (a mushroom alkaloid), pilocarpine, and oxotremorine. Antagonists include atropine and scopolamine.
   c. Types. Muscarinic receptors are divided into five types: M1 through M5. All appear to operate through G-proteins (see II C 2).
   (1) **M1 receptors** are postsynaptic and excitatory. They appear to be widespread throughout the neocortex.
   (2) **M2 receptors** are concentrated in cortical laminae that show significant choline acetyltransferase activity. They may be presynaptic and modulate the release of ACh, probably through the inhibition of adenylate cyclase.
   (3) **M3 through M5 receptors** are found in the CNS as well.

D. **Important brain tracts.** An important cholinergic pathway extends from the basal forebrain (the nucleus basalis) to the hippocampus and probably to the cerebral cortex. The striatum is rich in ACh, which is located mainly in large interneurons. Few cholinergic neurons appear to be located in the cortex.

E. **Effects on behavior.** In animals, ACh is believed to be important in movement, sleep, aggression, exploratory behavior, sexual behavior, and memory. For humans, the most significant effects involve movement and memory.

   1. Movement. ACh is important in movement, both peripherally and centrally.
   a. Peripherally, ACh is the main neurotransmitter for skeletal muscles; many powerful neurotoxins (e.g., curare, α-bungarotoxin) paralyze by blocking ACh receptors.
   b. Centrally, ACh and dopamine exist in a reciprocal balance in the extrapyramidal motor system. Cholinergic hypoactivity may be associated with tardive dyskinesia, although the evidence is weak.

   2. Memory and cognition. Dementing illnesses such as **Alzheimer's disease** appear to be associated with a loss of cholinergic transmission in the brain, both to the hippocampus and to the cerebral cortex. A decreased number of cholinergic neurons in the nucleus basalis of Meynert (located in the basal forebrain) is found in patients with Alzheimer's disease and certain other dementing disorders. **Tetrahydroaminoacridine (tacrine),** a moderately long-acting cholinesterase inhibitor, improves cognitive functioning in some demented patients. Tacrine was recently approved by the Food and Drug Administration for use in the United States.

VI. AMINO ACIDS

A. Inhibitory neurotransmitters

1. **GABA,** the first amino acid identified as a neurotransmitter, has proved to be **purely inhibitory** in all studies. Unlike most other neurotransmitters, GABA is limited to the CNS. GABA is present in as many as 60% of synapses, and is 200 to 1000 times more abundant than dopamine, ACh, or norepinephrine.

   a. **Synthesis.** Figure 1-4 shows the synthesis of GABA.

   b. **Metabolism.** GABA is catabolized through transamination (catalyzed by GABA transaminase) to succinic semialdehyde. Succinic semialdehyde is oxidized to succinic acid, which enters the citric acid cycle.

   c. **Receptors.** At least two types of GABAergic receptors are found in the CNS.

      (1) **GABA-A receptors** are the classic postsynaptic GABA receptors. They are ligand-gated **chloride channels.** Muscimol is a selective agonist, and bicuculline (a convulsant) and picrotoxin are selective antagonists. Some GABA-A receptors are coupled to a recognition site for **benzodiazepines** and **barbiturates.** These drugs potentiate the inhibitory action of GABA at the GABA-A receptor. This action makes these drugs effective anxiolytics, hypnotics, and anticonvulsants.

      (2) **GABA-B receptors.** Baclofen, a drug used to treat spasticity, is a selective agonist.

   d. **Important brain tracts.** Many brain pathways contain GABA.

      (1) GABA is the primary neurotransmitter for **Purkinje cells,** which are the only efferent neurons for the entire cerebellar cortex.

      (2) **Inhibitory interneurons** in almost all areas of the brain (brain stem, striatum, amygdala, cerebral cortex, spinal cord) contain GABA.

      (3) GABAergic pathways extend from the **striatum** to the **substantia nigra** and to the **globus pallidus.** These pathways may be important in movement disorders, such as Parkinson's and Huntington's diseases. These tracts may be regulated by endogenous opiates because morphine and β-endorphin cause a decrease in GABA turnover.

2. **Glycine** has the simplest structure of all of the amino acids.

   a. Like GABA, glycine is an **inhibitory neurotransmitter.** It is the major inhibitory neurotransmitter of the spinal cord.

   b. The alkaloid strychnine is a glycine antagonist that causes convulsions.

$$HOOC — CH_2CH_2CH — COOH \xrightarrow{\textit{glutamic acid decarboxylase}} HOOC — CH_2CH_2CH\ NH_2$$
$$\underset{NH_2}{|}$$

Glutamic acid **γ-Aminobutyric acid (GABA)**

FIGURE 1-4. γ-Aminobutyric acid (GABA) synthesis.

B. **Excitatory neurotransmitters.** The only amino acids that are believed to act as excitatory neurotransmitters are **glutamate** and **aspartate**. These neurotransmitters and some of their analogues (e.g., kainate) are neurotoxic under certain conditions.

1. **Synthesis.** Both glutamate and aspartate are synthesized from glucose, but the source of these compounds as neurotransmitters is unclear.

2. **Inactivation** occurs by rapid uptake.

3. **Receptors.** Four receptor subtypes for glutamate are known.
   a. **Kainate** and **AMPA receptors** are ligand-gated channels and allow the influx of Na^+.
   b. The **NMDA receptor** is a ligand-gated channel and allows the influx of Ca^{2+} and Na^+. This receptor is normally blocked by a magnesium ion (Mg^{2+}). After depolarization, the Mg^{2+} leaves the receptor, allowing the influx of Ca^{2+} and Na^+.
   c. The **metabotropic receptor** is a G-protein–coupled receptor that is linked to phosphatidylinositol hydrolysis.
   d. **Phencyclidine (PCP, angel dust),** a common drug of abuse, is an antagonist at the NMDA receptor. It affects the σ-opioid receptor.

4. **Important brain tracts.** It is believed that glutamate is present in the corticostriatal pathway and in cerebellar granule cells. Aspartate is believed to exist in the hippocampal commissural pathway. Both transmitters probably exist in many other pathways as well. Glutamate and aspartate seem to be the primary excitatory transmitters of the brain.

5. **Effects on behavior.** The NMDA receptor is involved in at least three processes: **long-term potentiation** of neurons in the hippocampus, a process important for memory storage; **kindling,** a phenomenon related to epilepsy, in which repeated subthreshold electrical stimulation causes a **seizure;** and **neurotoxicity and cell death** caused by ischemia.

VII. OTHER NONPEPTIDE NEUROTRANSMITTER CANDIDATES

A. **Prostaglandins and thromboxanes**

1. **Synthesis and biochemistry.** Prostaglandins and thromboxanes belong to a family of substances known as **eicosanoids,** which are products of arachidonic acid metabolism.
   a. These hormone-like substances are among the most abundant of **autacoids** (i.e., compounds synthesized at or close to their site of action, in contrast to circulating hormones, which act on tissues distant from their site of synthesis).
   b. Prostaglandins and thromboxanes are found in virtually every tissue and body fluid. Their synthesis is increased in response to widely varied stimuli, and they have diverse and complex biologic actions.

2. **Nervous system effects**
   a. **Prostaglandins** do not appear to function as neurotransmitters, but they may play a neuromodulatory role. **Prostaglandin E_2 (PGE_2)** may inhibit the stimulated release of dopamine and norepinephrine in rodents. PGD_2 seems to modulate the serotonin system.
   b. **Eicosanoids** are released from brain tissue after ischemia or trauma. They may contribute to the development of edema and the deterioration of the blood–brain barrier.

B. **Purines. Adenosine** may be an **inhibitory neuromodulator** of excitatory cells in the cerebellum, hippocampus, medial geniculate body, and septum. Adenosine receptors are also concentrated in the striatum, where adenosine may help to modulate dopaminergic transmission.

VIII. **NEUROPEPTIDES.** These peptides function principally as **neurohormones** and are important in psychoneuroendocrinology. Neuropeptides may also serve as **neuromodulators**. In some cases, they act as **neurotransmitters**.

A. Endogenous opioid peptides

1. **Overview and terminology. Opium** has been used as a pain reliever and psychotomimetic drug for millennia. In the nineteenth century, it was determined that most of this action is caused by the alkaloid morphine. In the 1970s, stereospecific binding of opiates to animal brain homogenates was discovered, and a class of **endogenous neuropeptides** that bind to these receptors was identified. These substances were called **enkephalins** ("in the head"). Other substances that bind to the receptors were discovered later. They were called **endorphins** (a contraction of "endogenous" and "morphine").

2. **Endogenous opioid families**
   a. Endogenous opioids fall into one of three families: **enkephalins** [e.g., methionine and leucine enkephalin (met- and leu-enkephalin)], **endorphins** (e.g., α-, β-, and γ-endorphins), and **dynorphins** (e.g., dynorphin A, dynorphin B).
   b. These substances are synthesized as parts of larger, **precursor polypeptides**. They are derived from proopiomelanocortin (POMC), proenkephalin, or prodynorphin. For example, β-endorphin is derived from POMC, which also produces adrenocorticotropic hormone (ACTH), melanocyte-stimulating hormone (MSH), and β-lipotropin.

3. **Opioid receptors.** Several opioid receptors are found in the CNS.
   a. **Mu (μ) receptors** mediate supraspinal **analgesia,** respiratory depression, and **euphoria**. Morphine and met-enkephalin are agonists at these receptors.
   b. **Kappa (κ) receptors** mediate spinal analgesia and pupillary miosis. Dynorphins are agonists at these receptors.
   c. **Delta (δ) receptors** in the CNS appear to be associated with mood components of opioid action. Leu-enkephalin is an agonist at these receptors.
   d. **Epsilon (ε) receptors** may produce catatonia, especially in rodents. β-Endorphin is an agonist at these receptors.
   e. **Sigma (σ) receptors** are associated with the psychotomimetic effects of certain opiates. However, these receptors probably are not opiate receptors because traditional opiate antagonists do not block σ-receptors. Pentazocine binds to both κ-receptors and σ-receptors.

4. **Effects on behavior**
   a. Many behavioral states, some movement disorders, analgesia, thermoregulation, and certain neuropsychiatric disorders (alcoholism, schizophrenia, seizures) may be associated with alterations in endogenous opioids, particularly β-endorphin.
   b. Naloxone and naltrexone are opiate antagonists that are useful in the management of narcotic overdose. These agents may also be helpful in cases of self-mutilatory behavior.

B. **Gut peptides** are found in both the brain and the digestive tract.

1. **Substance P** is an 11-amino acid peptide that was discovered in 1931 in extracts of brain and intestine. It is also found in the spinal cord, substantia nigra, striatum, amygdala, hypothalamus, and cerebral cortex. Substance P may be the principal neurotransmitter for the primary afferent sensory fibers that travel through the dorsal roots to the substantia gelatinosa of the spinal cord and carry information about **pain**. It is also involved in a major inhibitory outflow tract from the striatum to the substantia nigra and globus pallidus. Thus, it may be important for **movement**.

2. **Cholecystokinin (CCK)** is a polypeptide that is released from the gut. It stimulates gallbladder motility and the secretion of pancreatic enzymes. CCK is found in the hippocampus and neocortex as well as in the brain stem, basal ganglia, hypothalamus, and amygdala.

     a. Behaviorally, CCK is associated with **satiety**. The polypeptide may be useful in appetite reduction.

     b. CCK coexists with dopamine in the neurons in the VTA of the brain stem and in the nucleus accumbens. These brain regions are believed to be important in the pathophysiology of **schizophrenia**.

  3. Vasoactive intestinal polypeptide (VIP) is a 29-amino acid peptide that was discovered in the intestine. It is named for its ability to alter blood flow in the gut.

     a. VIP is common in the neocortex, where its distribution shows that VIP neurons may be localized to single cortical columns.

     b. VIP appears to be excitatory and positively coupled with adenylate cyclase.

  4. Somatostatin, a 14-amino acid peptide, was isolated and characterized in the early 1970s.

     a. Somatostatin is found in the gastrointestinal tract, in the islets of Langerhans, and in several areas in the nervous system (e.g., dorsal root ganglia, amygdala, striatum, cerebral cortex).

     b. Somatostatin suppresses the release of **growth hormone (GH)** and **thyroid-stimulating hormone (TSH)** in the brain and glucagon and insulin in the pancreas.

     c. Somatostatin is thought to be important in the production of slow-wave and rapid eye movement (REM) sleep and also in appetite and motor control.

     d. Injection of somatostatin in animals is associated with decreased spontaneous motor activity.

     e. Increased somatostatin levels are found in the corpus striatum of patients with Huntington's disease. Decreased levels are found in the cortex of patients with Alzheimer's disease.

  5. Neurotensin is a 13-amino acid peptide found in the substantia gelatinosa of the spinal cord. It is also found in the brain stem (especially in the motor nucleus of the trigeminal nerve and substantia nigra), hypothalamus, amygdala, nucleus accumbens, septum, and anterior pituitary gland. Neurotensin appears to be **excitatory,** and may play a role in arousal, thermoregulation, and pain perception.

C. | **Pituitary, hypothalamic, and pineal peptides**

  1. Pituitary hormones. The pituitary gland has two main lobes.

     a. The **anterior lobe of the pituitary gland** secretes six hormones, most of which have tropic properties (i.e., affinity for a specific gland). Anterior pituitary hormones include: ACTH, GH, TSH, **luteinizing hormone (LH), follicle-stimulating hormone (FSH),** and **prolactin**.

     (1) ACTH (corticotropin) is found in several areas of the brain (e.g., limbic system, brain stem, thalamus). It may be important in learning, memory, and attention. ACTH regulates the release of the adrenal steroid, cortisol. ACTH is regulated by the hypothalamic **corticotropin-releasing factor (CRF)**. The levels of ACTH and cortisol show a diurnal variation. Cortisol levels peak at approximately 7 A.M.

       (a) Excess amounts of cortisol are seen in **Cushing's syndrome,** which may be associated with depression, mania, hallucinations, delusions, and delirium.

       (b) A deficit of cortisol is seen in **Addison's disease,** which may be accompanied by depression, lethargy, and fatigue.

       (c) Some patients with **major depression** have high cortisol levels, loss of the normal diurnal variation in cortisol levels, and "early escape" from the suppression of cortisol secretion by administration of dexamethasone (a synthetic glucocorticoid) in the dexamethasone suppression test. However, other patients may also exhibit these effects. These patients often respond well to antidepressants.

       (d) CRF is found in the paraventricular nucleus of the hypothalamus, the median eminence, and other areas of the brain. In addition to its role in ACTH secretion, CRF appears to be involved in the **response to stress**. It may interact with norepinephrine in this role.

(2) GH (somatotropin) is a protein with 190 amino acids. GH secretion and synthesis are controlled by GH-releasing factor and **GH-release-inhibiting factor (somatostatin)**. GH has a diurnal pattern of release, with higher levels secreted during sleep. **Depressed patients** show a reduced GH response to clonidine (an α_2-agonist) stimulation.

(3) TSH (thyrotropin) causes the release of the thyroid hormones **triiodothyronine (T_3)** and **thyroxine (T_4)**. The release of TSH is controlled by **thyrotropin-releasing hormone (TRH)**.

   (a) TRH is believed to be localized in the dorsomedial and periventricular nuclei of the hypothalamus. These nuclei send processes to other hypothalamic nuclei as well as to the anterior pituitary, median eminence, medial forebrain bundle, septum, nucleus accumbens, and motor cranial nerve nuclei (i.e., III, V, VII, XII).

   (b) TRH is largely inhibitory to postsynaptic neurons. In addition to its role in thyroid function, it is believed to affect **mood and behavior**. Some patients with **major depression** show a decreased TSH response to intravenous infusion of TRH. This finding suggests hypothalamic–pituitary dysfunction in major depression.

(4) LH and **FSH** regulate ovarian follicle growth, spermatogenesis, and testosterone secretion. Release of LH and FSH from the anterior pituitary is regulated by **gonadotropin-releasing hormone (GnRH)**.

   (a) GnRH injection in men causes an increase in sexual arousal. Injections are used with some success to treat delayed puberty.

   (b) GnRH may function as a neurotransmitter or neuromodulator as well as a hormone. It may be excitatory or inhibitory.

(5) Prolactin, a 198-amino acid protein released from the anterior pituitary, is controlled by prolactin-inhibiting factor (PIF) and prolactin-releasing factor (PRF).

   (a) Prolactin regulates the activity of the mammary glands during lactation. Sleep, exercise, pregnancy, and breast-feeding increase the circulating levels of prolactin.

   (b) Dopamine functions physiologically as PIF. Most antipsychotic medications block dopamine receptors in the tuberoinfundibular dopamine tract. The result is an increase in the circulating prolactin level, which causes breast enlargement and lactation. This side effect of antipsychotic drugs is common in women. It can also occur in men.

b. The **posterior pituitary secretes vasopressin** and **oxytocin**. They are 9–amino acid peptides that are formed from larger precursor hormones known as neurophysins. Vasopressin and oxytocin are synthesized in large neurons in the supraoptic and paraventricular hypothalamic nuclei as well as in the suprachiasmatic, arcuate, dorsomedial, and ventromedial nuclei of the hypothalamus. The neurons from the supraoptic and paraventricular nuclei project to the posterior pituitary, where the hormones are released into the circulation. Neurons containing vasopressin and oxytocin also project to the medial amygdaloid nucleus, lateral septum, hippocampus, thalamus, nucleus of the solitary tract, VTA, area postrema, and locus coeruleus.

(1) Vasopressin is also known as **antidiuretic hormone (ADH)** because it facilitates water absorption in the distal tubule of the nephron. Its release is increased by stress, pain, exercise, and a variety of drugs (e.g., morphine, nicotine, barbiturates). Alcohol decreases its release and causes diuresis. Vasopressin is believed to be mainly inhibitory, and it may be important in learning, memory, and attention. Treatment with vasopressin has been reported to improve memory in patients with dementia and brain damage, although results are inconsistent. Vasopressin may also be important in depression and psychosis.

(2) Oxytocin release is stimulated by estrogens, vaginal and breast stimulation, and psychic stress. Oxytocin release is inhibited by severe pain, increased temperature, and loud noise.

   (a) The main peripheral effects of oxytocin include the expression of milk and induction of uterine smooth muscle contraction during parturition.

       (b) Centrally, oxytocin may be an inhibitory neurotransmitter or neuromodulator. In contrast to vasopressin, it causes amnesia.

    c. Melanocyte-stimulating hormone (MSH). The intermediate lobe is vestigial in adult humans. MSH is believed to be secreted from this part of the pituitary gland in animals, but it may be secreted from the anterior pituitary in humans. MSH is **structurally similar to ACTH**. Its release is regulated by dopamine and possibly by MSH-inhibiting factor and MSH-releasing factor.

       (1) MSH is found in the pituitary gland and a number of other brain areas, including the hypothalamus and cerebral cortex.

       (2) MSH is important in the **control of pigmentation** in animals. Its behavioral function is unclear, although it may have a role in **learning** and **memory**. Paradoxically, MSH and MSH-inhibiting factor have antidepressant effects.

  2. Hypothalamic hormones, or releasing factors, control the release of anterior pituitary hormones. The anterior pituitary hormones control the release of hormones from target endocrine glands.

  3. Pineal hormones. Melatonin is synthesized from serotonin in the pineal gland.

    a. Although it is not a peptide, melatonin has important endocrinologic effects. It is thought to be involved in the regulation of circadian rhythms. Melatonin synthesis is regulated by the day–night or light–dark cycle, and levels are increased during darkness.

    b. Because the pineal gland transforms information contained in light into chemical information contained in melatonin, the pineal gland has been called a neuroendocrine transducer.

    c. Some **depressed patients** have low nocturnal levels of melatonin.

    d. Individuals with **seasonal affective disorder** have regularly occurring seasonal depressions, usually in the fall and winter. Early morning therapy with bright light (phototherapy) can help these patients. This therapy may be associated with normalization of the dim-light onset of melatonin secretion. The role of melatonin in seasonal mood disorder, however, is not known.

STUDY QUESTIONS

DIRECTIONS: Each of the numbered items or incomplete statements in this section is followed by answers or by completions of the statement. Select the ONE lettered answer or completion that is BEST in each case.

1. The ion that is most important for the release of a neurotransmitter is

(A) sodium
(B) potassium
(C) calcium
(D) iron
(E) manganese

Questions 2–5

A 27-year-old man is brought to the emergency room by a friend. Physical examination findings are inconclusive; the only significant findings are sinus tachycardia (105 beats/min), rapid respiration, and diaphoresis. The patient appears disoriented and reports hearing voices. Treatment with haloperidol is begun. After 48 hours, the patient's symptoms are improved, but he walks slowly and rigidly and has a slow resting tremor. These symptoms gradually subside. His condition progressively improves, and he eventually leaves the hospital. He receives injections of neuroleptics in depot form to ensure compliance. He is re-evaluated after several years. Physical examination findings show choreoathetoid movements of his hands, and repetitive grimacing.

2. This patient's disorientation and auditory hallucinations are believed to be caused by

(A) a hypercholinergic state
(B) a hyperdopaminergic state
(C) a hypocholinergic state
(D) a hypodopaminergic state
(E) none of the above

3. The tremor, rigidity, and akinesia observed after 48 hours are probably caused by

(A) schizophrenia
(B) Parkinson's disease
(C) exhaustion secondary to cardiac arrhythmia
(D) dopamine receptor blockade
(E) dopamine receptor supersensitivity

4. Which of the following neuroanatomical pathways is believed to be important in this patient's thought disorder?

(A) Nigrostriatal pathway
(B) Mesolimbic and mesocortical pathway
(C) Incertohypothalamic pathway
(D) Tuberoinfundibular pathway
(E) None of the above

5. The abnormal movements exhibited by the patient during his last visit suggest that he has

(A) Huntington's disease
(B) Parkinson's disease
(C) akinesia
(D) tardive dyskinesia
(E) neuroleptic overdose

DIRECTIONS: Each of the numbered items or incomplete statements in this section is negatively phrased, as indicated by a capitalized word such as NOT, LEAST, or EXCEPT. Select the ONE lettered answer or completion that is BEST in each case.

6. The following associations exist between neuropsychiatric disorders and disturbances in specific neurotransmitter systems EXCEPT

(A) Parkinson's disease and dopaminergic dysfunction
(B) sleep disturbances and glutamatergic dysfunction
(C) Alzheimer's disease and cholinergic dysfunction
(D) depression and noradrenergic dysfunction
(E) schizophrenia and dopaminergic dysfunction

7. All of the following statements about glutamate neurotransmission are true EXCEPT

(A) glutamate is involved in the neurotoxic effects of ischemia
(B) glutamate is a major central nervous system (CNS) excitatory neurotransmitter
(C) glutamate is involved in learning and memory
(D) glutamate is involved in seizure activity
(E) glutamate causes long-term potentiation by binding to the kainate receptor

DIRECTIONS: Each set of matching questions in this section consists of a list of four to twenty-six lettered options (some of which may be in figures) followed by several numbered items. For each numbered item, select the ONE lettered option that is most closely associated with it. To avoid spending too much time on matching sets with large numbers of options, it is generally advisable to begin each set by reading the list of options. Then, for each item in the set, try to generate the correct answer and locate it in the option list, rather than evaluating each option individually. Each lettered option may be selected once, more than once, or not at all.

Questions 8–12

Match each receptor with the type of signal transduction.

(A) Ligand-gated ion channel permitting the influx of sodium
(B) Ligand-gated ion channel permitting the influx of chloride
(C) G-protein-coupled receptor positively linked to adenylate cyclase
(D) G-protein-coupled receptor negatively linked to adenylate cyclase
(E) G-protein-coupled receptor linked to the breakdown of phosphatidyl inositol

8. β-Adrenergic receptors

9. 5-Hydroxytryptamine-2 (5-HT$_2$) receptor

10. Glycine receptor

11. Nicotinic acetylcholine receptor

12. D$_2$ receptor

ANSWERS AND EXPLANATIONS

1. The answer is C [II A 1–2]. Sodium and potassium are important for the depolarization and repolarization, respectively, that occur during an action potential. The release of neurotransmitters from synaptic vesicles requires calcium. Iron and manganese are found in moderate concentrations in some brain areas. Their functions are not well understood, but may involve oxidation and reduction reactions.

2. The answer is B [III B 4 c (1)]. The original symptoms are caused by a hyperdopaminergic state.

3. The answer is D [III B 4 c (4) (a)]. The acute extrapyramidal symptoms of tremor, rigidity, and akinesia are caused by dopamine receptor blockade in the neostriatum.

4. The answer is B [III B 3 a–b]. The neuronal pathway involved in these symptoms is the nigrostriatal pathway. The symptoms of acute schizophrenia are believed to result from overactivity in the mesolimbic and mesocortical dopamine pathways.

5. The answer is D [III B 4 b]. Long-term administration of neuroleptics can cause tardive dyskinesia, a disorder characterized by choreoathetoid movements and oral–buccal–lingual dyskinesias (manifested as repetitive grimacing in this patient).

6. The answer is B [III B 3 a–b, C 4 b; V E 2]. Specific associations are known for Parkinson's disease and severe deficiency of dopamine, for Alzheimer's disease and hypofunction of the cholinergic system, for depression and decreased levels of monoamines such as norepinephrine, and for schizophrenia and hyperactivity of the mesolimbic and mesocortical dopamine systems. No known association exists between glutamate abnormalities and sleep disorders.

7. The answer is E [VI B 5]. Glutamate is the major excitatory neurotransmitter in the brain. There are several types of glutamate receptors. The N-methyl-D-aspartate (NMDA) subtype is believed to mediate the action of glutamate in the processes of long-term potentiation (involved in learning and memory), kindling (involved in epilepsy), and neurotoxicity and cell death secondary to ischemia and other pathologic processes.

8–12. The answers are: 8-C, 9-E, 10-B, 11-A, 12-D. [II C 1, 2 a (1); III B 2 b, C 2 b (2); IV C 1 b; V C 1]. β-Adrenergic receptors are positively linked to cyclic adenosine 3',5'-monophosphate (cAMP) production through a specific G-protein.

5-Hydroxytryptamine-2 (5-HT$_2$) receptors elicit the breakdown of phosphatidylinositol.

Glycine receptors allow the passage of chloride ions, and hence are inhibitory.

Nicotinic acetylcholine receptors are ligand-gated ion channels that allow the passage of sodium ions, and hence are excitatory.

Dopamine D$_2$ receptors are negatively linked to cAMP production.

Chapter 2

Neuroanatomy and Behavior

Alison Reeve
Nancy A. Breslin

I. INTRODUCTION. The anatomy of the normal and abnormal brain has been of interest to neuroscientists for at least a century. The last 10 to 15 years have seen the introduction of new tools that have greatly expanded our knowledge of the function of the anatomic structures of the brain. Direct links between anatomic structure and function and behavior are becoming increasingly clear. Research is currently active in this area.

II. NEUROANATOMY. The order in which brain structures are presented in this chapter stems from embryology, with the most anterior parts of the central nervous system (CNS) (telencephalic structures) listed first, and proceeding posteriorly. Because of the confined space of the cranium, this order becomes distorted in the fully formed human brain. This section is not a review of all neuroanatomy, but a discussion of the structures and systems that significantly affect behavior and behavioral disorders.

A. Telencephalon. The telencephalon develops into the **cerebral cortices, basal ganglia, and basal forebrain. The components of these structures are paired, with more or less mirror images found in the right and left hemispheres.**

1. **Cortex**
    a. **Structure.** The cortex has four lobes, the **frontal, parietal, temporal, and occipital lobes**. The cingulate and parahippocampal gyri are sometimes referred to as the **limbic lobe** (see II B 3). Prominent afferents include the sensory fibers from the thalamus and striatum. Many intracortical connections occur within lobes, between lobes, and between hemispheres through the corpus callosum.
    b. **Function.** The various cortical lobes have some common functions. Sensory information is received by the thalamus and processed, integrated, and interpreted in the cortex. **Association areas** of the cortex allow multimodal sensory input to trigger memories (e.g., a certain pattern of shape and color is recognized as a friend's face). Table 2-1 lists the functions of individual lobes.

2. **Basal ganglia**
    a. **Structure.** The basal ganglia are paired structures of gray matter that consist of the **caudate nucleus, putamen, globus pallidus,** and depending on the reference, often the substantia nigra, subthalamic nuclei, amygdala, and nucleus accumbens.
        (1) The caudate, putamen, and globus pallidus are often referred to as the **corpus striatum**.
        (2) The putamen and globus pallidus form a pair of oval structures known as the **lentiform nuclei** because they resemble lentils. These structures sit lateral and somewhat rostral to the thalamus on each side.
        (3) The **caudate** has a head structure that is located anterobasally in the brain. It also has a tail, or cauda, which loops around, following the course of the lateral ventricles, to end in the amygdala, which is embedded in the medial temporal lobe.
    b. **Functional role in movement.** The basal ganglia are the center of the **extrapyramidal motor system**. This term is used to differentiate the system from the corticospinal motor pathways that pass through the pyramids of the medulla.

TABLE 2-1. Function and Dysfunction of the Cortical Lobes

Cortical Lobe	Function	Dysfunction
Frontal	Voluntary movement (posterior frontal cortex)	Contralateral hemiplegia (motor strip lesions)
	Problem solving, planning, immediate memory (prefrontal cortex)	Motor (Broca's) aphasia (lesion of dominant hemisphere)
		Disinhibition, mood lability (orbital prefrontal lesions)
		Flat affect, apathy (dorsolateral prefrontal lesions)
Temporal	Hearing and auditory language comprehension	Sensory (Wernicke's) aphasia (lesion of dominant hemisphere)
	Learning and memory (hippocampus)	Korsakoff's amnesia (bilateral hippocampal lesions)
	Motivation and emotion (limbic system)	Klüver-Bucy syndrome (placidity, fearlessness, hypersexuality, and orality in animals after bilateral amygdala lesions)
		Auditory hallucinations
		Complex partial seizures
Parietal	Somatosensation, both superficial (touch, temperature) and deep (proprioception, pain)	Contralateral sensory impairment
		Apraxia, neglect of left half of body (nondominant hemisphere lesions)
	Sensory discrimination	Gerstmann's syndrome (inability to write, calculate, identify fingers, and tell left from right, from dominant hemisphere lesions)
	Sensory–motor and multisensory integration	
Occipital	Sight and interpretation of visual information	Contralateral homonymous hemianopia (unilateral lesion)
		Inability to recognize objects (left-sided lesion)
		Illusions, hallucinations, loss of visual orientation (right-sided lesions)
		Cortical blindness, agnosia (bilateral lesions)

    (1) Acting in conjunction with the cerebellum, frontal cortex, and thalamus, the basal ganglia are involved with **muscle tone** and the initiation and smooth **coordination of movement**.

    (2) Lesions and neurochemical alterations of this system, such as the dopaminergic blockade caused by antipsychotic drugs, can result in symptoms such as **tremor, rigidity,** and choreoathetotic **dyskinesia**.

  c. Functional role in memory. The basal ganglia are important for a type of memory known as **procedural memory,** which is used when learning motor skills, such as dancing or tying shoes (see III E 2).

 3. Basal forebrain. These structures are located ventromedially in each hemisphere. They include the **olfactory tubercle, septal nuclei, and substantia innominata,** also known as the **nucleus basalis of Meynert.** The substantia innominata is important because it contains the cholinergic neurons that project widely to the cortex. These neurons degenerate in patient's with **Alzheimer's disease.**

B. **Diencephalon.** The diencephalon develops into two structures with key **integrating roles**: the thalamus and the hypothalamus. Each has widespread connections in the brain.

 1. Thalamus

  a. Structure. The thalamus is an oval mass of nuclei located at the anterior end of the brain stem. It is subdivided into nuclei on the basis of differing cytologic characteristics, connections, and functional roles.

  b. Function. The thalamus relays all **sensory information,** except smell, from the periphery to the cortex, and plays an important **gating** role (i.e., filtering what would otherwise be an overload of information before it reaches the cortex). Messages from the basal ganglia and cerebellum pass through the thalamus before entering the motor cortex. Because it is part of the limbic system, the anterior nucleus has a role in **emotions and memory.** The mediodorsal nucleus is involved with **affective behavior.**

2. Hypothalamus
  a. Structure. The hypothalamus is a smaller, central structure located beneath the thalamus. Its **mammillary bodies** can be seen on the ventral surface of the brain, just posterior to the pituitary gland.
  b. Function. The hypothalamus has several important functions, including maintenance of the **sleep–wake cycle,** control of **autonomic functions** (i.e., sympathetic and parasympathetic), and **regulation of pituitary** gland activity, food intake, and **aggression.**

3. Limbic system. The limbic system is not all diencephalic in origin. However, because of the central role of the hypothalamus in the system, it is described here.
  a. Structure. Papez described a **circuit** that contains elements that are important to the integration of the subjective and physiologic components of emotion, now considered part of the limbic system. This circuit is: hippocampus through the fornix to the mammillary bodies through the mammillothalamic tracts to the anterior nucleus of the thalamus through the internal capsule to the cingulate gyrus, and back to the hippocampus. Table 2-2 describes the elements of the limbic system in more detail.
  b. Function. The interconnections of the limbic system "provide part of the mechanism by which sensory stimuli and psychic phenomena influence emotional aspects of behavior."[1] Lesions of parts of the limbic system can produce a number of emotional difficulties, including rage attacks, anxiety, placidity, and hyper- and hyposexuality.

C. **Mesencephalon (midbrain).** This small area contains cell bodies of neurons that supply **dopamine and serotonin** to synapses located elsewhere in the brain. Dopamine has an important role in the symptoms of schizophrenia, and serotonin is implicated in mood disorders. The midbrain, pons, and medulla are also the locations of the **reticular formation.** Other mesencephalic structures that are not discussed here are the tectum (colliculi), the tegmentum, and the crura cerebri.

  1. Substantia nigra and ventral tegmental area (VTA). These structures contain the cell bodies of most **dopamine-producing neurons** in the brain. Dopaminergic cells are also seen in the eye and in the hypothalamus. In the hypothalamus, they inhibit prolactin secretion from the pituitary.
    a. Structure. The paired dark bands of the substantia nigra and the more central VTA are located in the dorsal half of the midbrain.
    b. Function. The cell bodies of the substantia nigra send their axons to synapse in the caudate and putamen (**nigrostriatal tract**). These connections are important in controlling movement (see II A 2 b). The cell bodies of the VTA send axons to the frontal cortex, amygdala, and other limbic structures (**mesocortical and mesolimbic tracts**). Excessive dopaminergic function in some limbic structures is hypothesized to cause the hallucinations seen in **schizophrenia.** The drugs most commonly used to treat schizophrenia block dopamine at the postsynaptic receptor.

  2. Raphe nuclei. These largely serotonergic neurons are also found in the metencephalon and myelencephalon.
    a. Structure. The raphe nuclei consist of a number of midline cell groups in the midbrain, pons, and medulla. These cell groups **project widely** within the CNS, particularly to the substantia nigra, thalamus, limbic system, frontal cortex, and spinal cord.
    b. Function. Serotonin is the predominant neurotransmitter produced by this group of cells, but dopaminergic and cholecystokinin (CCK)-producing cells are also seen. Enkephalin is coproduced by some serotonergic cells. The functions of this system include **sleep regulation** and the control of **mood and aggressive behavior.** Some serotonin agonists are effective antidepressants (see Chapter 3 III B 2, C 1).

TABLE 2-2. The Limbic System

Limbic Structure	Location	Function
Hippocampus	Medial temporal lobe	Learning and memory
Subiculum	Superior parahippocampal gyrus	Sends hippocampal input on to the cortex
Fornix	Pair of white fiber bands; each exits the posterior hippocampus and arches over the thalamus and under the corpus callosum to terminate in the mammillary body of the hypothalamus	Tract from the hippocampus to the hypothalamus (some fibers to the thalamus), tying cortical input to the autonomic and endocrine systems
Hypothalamus (mammillary bodies)	Lies below and anterior to the thalamus, just behind the optic chiasm	Receives input from the hippocampus, amygdala, and brain stem; projects reciprocally and also to the spinal cord and pituitary; regulates the physiologic (autonomic and endocrine) correlates of emotion; also important for water and weight balance, reproduction, and growth
Anterior nuclei of the thalamus	Rostral thalamus	Receives input from the mammillothalamic tract and fornix and projects to the cingulate cortex, providing a key connection between hypothalamus and cortex
Cingulate gyrus	Medial aspect of each hemisphere between the corpus callosum and the cingulate sulcus.	Projects to the hippocampus through the entorhinal cortex, completing the circuit that starts at the hippocampus
Septum	Just rostral to the anterior commissure	Connects to the hippocampus, amygdala, and hypothalamus
Amygdala	Medial temporal lobe, rostral to the hippocampus	Receives input from the hypothalamus, locus ceruleus, and substantia nigra and projects to the cortex, striatum, and many limbic structures; modulates hypothalamic function and has a role in the integration of emotional, behavioral, and autonomic responses

3. **Reticular formation**
   a. **Structure.** This system consists of several nuclei in the midbrain, pons, and medulla that receive input from the cortex and raphe nuclei. It projects to the cerebellum, spinal cord (through the reticulospinal tracts), diencephalon (thalamus and the hypothalamus), and cortex.
   b. **Function.** This system influences a number of body functions, including voluntary and reflex **movement and muscle tone, respiration, blood pressure, and sensory input. The ascending reticular activating system (RAS) is critical to consciousness.** Decerebration (lesions at the midbrain level) leads to coma because of the loss of these ascending reticular fibers to the thalamus. This condition is functionally observed by changes in the electroencephalogram (EEG) reading from awake to sleeping patterns [see III A 1, IV B 1 a (1)].

D. **Metencephalon.** The **pons and cerebellum** are the major metencephalic structures. This area also includes the **locus ceruleus,** which contains the cell bodies of the **noradrenergic** neurons in the brain, as well as a continuation of the **raphe nuclei,** which contain **serotonergic** cell bodies. The **locus ceruleus** projects widely to the cortex, limbic system, thalamus, cerebellum, and spinal cord. It affects **rapid eye movement (REM) sleep, physical and emotional responses to stress, the sensory system, and cortical activation**.

E. **Myelencephalon.** The myelencephalon develops into the medulla oblongata. Recent work suggests that pH-sensitive neurons in the medulla may play a role in the onset of panic attacks (see Chapter 15 VIII A 1).

III. SPECIAL NEUROANATOMIC FUNCTIONS

A. **Sleep. Sleep is a normal and restorative function of the human organism.** It is a time during which memory traces are consolidated, experiences are reviewed (such as in dreams), general energy and vitality are renewed, and cellular changes, such as neuronal selection and elimination (pruning) occur. Normal sleep consists of cycles of REM and non-REM stages that last approximately 70 to 120 minutes.

1. **Normal sleep architecture** is characterized by EEG findings and behavior. Sleep occurs as a consequence of decreased activity in the RAS and increased activity in areas of sleep generation. EEG characteristics of non-REM sleep stages are listed in Table 2-3.

2. **Non-REM sleep** is believed to be controlled by neurons in the raphe nuclei and median forebrain bundle. Serotonergic neurons of the raphe nuclei are thought to inhibit neurons in the pons that are responsible for REM sleep.

3. **REM sleep** occurs approximately every 90 to 100 minutes. It increases in duration as the sleep time progresses. As the duration of REM sleep increases, the interval between episodes of REM sleep decreases.
   a. During REM sleep, the brain is physiologically and metabolically active (62% to 173% increase in blood flow), with accompanying generalized muscle atonia.
   b. Phasic bursts of rapid eye movement are accompanied by fluctuations in respiration and heart rate, increased gastric secretion, penile and clitoral enlargement, lowered body temperature, and vivid dreaming.
   c. The pons contains cholinergic gigantocellular tegmental neurons that are thought to generate REM sleep.

TABLE 2-3. Non–Rapid Eye Movement (REM) Sleep Stages

Stage	Description	Electroencephalogram Pattern
0	Awake	Low-voltage fast activity, with a mix of alpha and beta waves
1, non-REM	Transition between wakefulness and sleep	Alpha waves disappear; theta waves appear
2, non-REM		Background of theta waves; sleep spindles appear briefly; K complexes are seen
3, non-REM		20% or greater high-amplitude delta waves
4, non-REM	Deepest sleep	50% or greater high-amplitude delta waves

4. **Sleep stage sequence.** In the ideal state, a person progresses through stages 1, 2, 3, 4, 3, 2, REM, then repeats the cycle. Later in the sleep period, stages 3 and 4 are short-ened and eventually may be omitted completely, and both the duration and frequency of REM sleep increase (Figure 2-1). Several measurements are used to analyze sleep patterns (Figure 2-2).
   a. **Mean latency sleep-onset time.** The interval between the time at which an individual attempts to fall asleep and the onset of sleep (i.e., stage 0 to stage 1) is known as mean latency sleep-onset time.
   b. **REM latency.** The interval between sleep onset and the first period of REM sleep is known as REM latency.
   c. **Polysomnography.** Nocturnal EEG recording is usually performed in a sleep laboratory. Between 2 and 28 electrodes are placed, always including the top of the head and sites C_3 and C_4 [see IV B 1 a (1)]. Also measured are electrocardiogram (EKG) reading, respiratory effort (chest wall electrode), oxygenation (oximeter on earlobe or finger), peripheral muscle activity (electrode on leg muscle), and body temperature. The study may also include a measure of penile tumescence. Polysomnography is used most often in the evaluation of insomnia, nocturnal myoclonus, sleep apnea, functional enuresis, impotence, and somnambulism.

5. **Sleep cycles vary with age.**
   a. **Infancy.** Newborns spend as many as 20 hours per day asleep. Non-REM and REM sleep are not fully differentiated until 3 to 6 months of age. A circadian rhythm is developed over the first 3 years of life (as opposed to an established sleep–wake cycle at 3 months).
   b. **Childhood.** From infancy into childhood, a progressive decrease in total sleep time occurs, primarily because of a **reduction in REM sleep time**. Prepubertal children have large percentages of REM and high-amplitude slow-wave sleep. The decrease in slow-wave sleep that occurs in adolescence is hypothesized to correspond to the neuronal pruning that occurs during this period.
   c. **Adulthood.** Adults typically sleep approximately 7 hours per day, although reported norms range from 4 to 10 hours. A **decrease in slow-wave sleep** accounts for the decrease in total sleep time in the third through sixth decades of life.
   d. **Senescence.** Increased age corresponds to increased stages 1 and 2 non-REM sleep and **decreased stages 3 and 4 and REM sleep**. Older individuals have more transient arousals and a redistribution of sleep (loss of diurnal sleep–wake pattern) in the form of frequent naps.

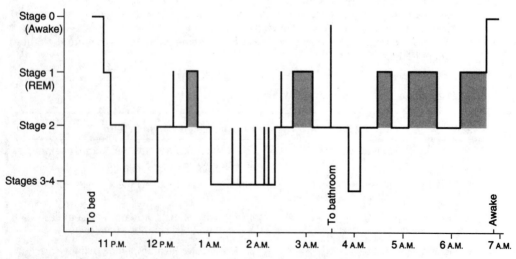

FIGURE 2-1. Relative distribution of sleep stages. *Shaded areas* represent REM sleep. *REM* = rapid eye movement.

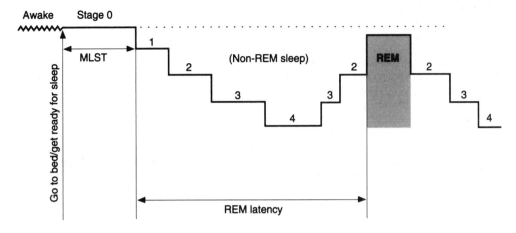

FIGURE 2-2. Sleep stages. *MLST* = mean latency sleep-onset time; *REM* = rapid eye movement; *non-REM* = non–rapid eye movement.

6. **Sleep history.** During the evaluation of a patient with sleep problems, a comprehensive history requires persistence on the part of both examiner and patient.
   a. The examiner should obtain a detailed record of exact times, duration, and types of behavior.
   b. The examiner should ask the patient about specific medical conditions, medications, sexual habits (function and dysfunction), psychological stressors, environmental stressors, and family patterns of sleep.

7. **Disorders of sleep**
   a. Sleep disorders can be grossly divided into difficulties in falling asleep and maintaining an effective sleep state and problems with excessive sleepiness or sleep time. This classification allows treatment to be directed toward the appropriate problem. Sleep disorders, as defined in the ***Diagnostic and Statistical Manual of Mental Disorders,*** 4th edition (***DSM-IV***) of the American Psychiatric Association, are discussed elsewhere (see Chapter 15 XIV).
   b. Many **psychiatric disorders** have a sleep disturbance as the first identifiable or most significant symptom.
      (1) Patients with **major depressive** episodes typically have decreased REM latency. They frequently report awakening during the night and early morning. First-degree relatives of patients with endogenous depression also appear to have shorter REM latency. REM latency is used experimentally as a marker to predict treatment response to antidepressants.
      (2) **Atypical depression** includes hypersomnolence, with both increased duration of the major sleep period and more frequent naps or desire to sleep throughout the day.
      (3) **Schizophrenia** causes prolonged sleep latency, with sleep fragmentation (many awakenings), decreased stages 3 and 4 sleep, and variable REM latency.
      (4) **Anxiety disorders** and depression may produce similar symptoms, but REM latency is usually normal in patients with anxiety disorders. However, these patients often have increased sleep latency and frequent interruption of sleep. **Panic attacks** may occur during non-REM sleep, especially during the transition from stage 2 to stage 3 sleep. It is not clear whether the traumatic and vivid dreams that occur with **post-traumatic stress disorder (PTSD)** are caused by dysfunctional REM sleep or whether they occur during a specific phase of sleep (e.g., only after one complete cycle).
      (5) **Dementia** accelerates the changes in sleep pattern that are seen with normal aging. REM and slow-wave (delta) sleep, spindles, and K complexes are significantly reduced. There is a commensurate increase in indeterminate sleep,

which is stage 2 sleep with few or no sleep spindles. Unlike patients with depression, patients with true dementia experience no improvement in mood after sleep deprivation.

(6) Many patients with **epilepsy** experience seizures during sleep or at arousal. Non-REM sleep has an activating effect on seizures. This effect may be caused in part by increased synchronization of brain activity. Hypersomnolence occurs after seizures and may be caused by disruption of a sufficient sleep period.

c. Medication. Many medications affect sleep efficiency and efficacy.

(1) The **tricyclic antidepressants** have direct sedative properties and suppress REM sleep. When tricyclics are abruptly discontinued, patients experience increased amounts and duration of REM sleep. This condition is known as **REM rebound**.

(2) **Benzodiazepines** bind to a benzodiazepine receptor of the γ-aminobutyric acid (GABA) receptor complex, leading to inhibition of monoamine systems in the locus ceruleus. These agents increase stage 2 sleep and sometimes decrease the amount of REM sleep. Efficacy at the initial dosage usually decreases after approximately 2 weeks because tolerance to the drug develops.

(3) **Antipsychotic medications** induce sleep because of their antihistaminergic and antiserotonergic properties. Because the activity of the RAS is decreased, activity of other sleep generators is permitted.

(4) **Antihistamine medications** also produce sedation and can effectively reduce sleep-onset latency.

B. **Pain.** Pain is a complicated sensation. It is "felt" by the thalamus, but the cortex has an important role in its localization and interpretation.

1. Anatomy. Peripheral pain receptors relay messages to the brain through either **C (thin, unmyelinated)** or **A-delta (thinly myelinated) fibers,** which synapse in the dorsal horn of the spinal cord.

a. Most messages proceed rapidly up the **lateral spinothalamic tract** to the thalamus and then to the cortex, providing identification and localization of the pain.

b. A slower route follows the more central **reticulothalamic tract,** which travels to the hypothalamus and thalamus and then to the frontal and limbic lobes, producing the subjective sensation of pain.

c. Descending raphe neurons release serotonin and enkephalin in the spinal cord and modulate pain.

2. Role of opiates. Opiates are effective pain relievers. Their effectiveness is the result of opiate receptors in the dorsal horn of the spinal cord that respond to **enkephalin,** an endogenous opiate. Enkephalin is also present in other brain areas, including the basal ganglia, the spinal trigeminal nucleus, the midbrain periaqueductal gray, and the raphe nuclei.

3. Types of pain

a. Surface pain can be pricking (A-delta) or burning (C) and is well localized.

b. Visceral or musculoskeletal pain is usually felt as aching and diffuse. It can be felt on the skin surface that is innervated by the same level of the spinal cord (**referred pain**).

c. Neuropathic pain is a burning or stabbing sensation that is caused by pathology of the sensory system itself. Neuropathic pain may be caused by peripheral nerves (e.g., trigeminal neuralgia, face pain caused by fifth cranial nerve compression), the spinal cord, or the thalamus.

d. Much **chronic pain** is of undetermined cause. Environmental factors (e.g., leave from work, attention from spouse, euphoria produced by prescribed narcotic analgesics) tend to reinforce both the pain and pain-related behavior. This phenomenon is known as **secondary gain**.

4. Pain in association with mental disorders

a. Major depressive disorder is often accompanied by pain (e.g., chronic headache). Conversely, chronic pain can lead to depression. Some tricyclic antidepressants help

to relieve pain, regardless of whether depression is present, possibly through serotonergic effects.

b. Pain can also be a feature of several **somatoform disorders** (see Chapter 15 IX).
Generally, these disorders feature chronic pain.

c. Pain in patients with **delusional disorder or psychosis** is often best treated by antipsychotic agents. When evaluating pain of suspected psychiatric origin, a thorough
evaluation for an organic cause must often be completed. Doing so in stages may
avoid overemphasizing pain as an effective means of communicating distress.

C. **Stress responses.** Exposure to **emotional or physical stress** leads to a variety of responses.
These responses are adaptive in the short run, but can lead to pathology if stress is prolonged or dysregulation of the system occurs. The two major components of the stress system are the autonomic nervous system and the hypothalamic–pituitary–adrenal (HPA)
axis.

1. **Autonomic nervous system.** One response to stress is the activation of the locus ceruleus and the diffuse release of **norepinephrine** in the brain. The result is **arousal, vigilance,** and **anxiety.** Norepinephrine also stimulates the **dopaminergic system (enhancing cognitive function** through its effects on the frontal cortex) and the amygdala and
hippocampus (enhancing memory retrieval). The sympathetic nervous system stimulates adaptive peripheral responses to stress, such as tachycardia and slowing of gastrointestinal function.

2. **HPA axis.** Secretion of corticotropin-releasing hormone (CRH), which is stimulated by
stress, **heightens arousal** and inhibits feeding and sexual function. Prolonged stress inhibits growth hormone (GH) secretion and **immune function,** probably through the
HPA axis.

3. **Abnormality of the stress system.** The adaptive value of the stress response is obvious,
but this system can lead to abnormality when stress is unremitting or when the system
malfunctions.

a. **Chronic emotional or physical stress** can lead to weight loss, depression, loss of
sexual function (e.g., loss of libido), amenorrhea, and immune suppression.

b. Some **mental disorders,** such as melancholic depression and anorexia nervosa, may
be caused in part by abnormal response to stress.

D. **Neuroendocrinology.** The endocrine system directly and indirectly affects the functioning
of the nervous system, and vice versa. An important aspect of this relation is the **maintenance of homeostasis in response to environmental change.** Examples include temperature regulation, appetite regulation, stress responses, and thyroid function.

1. **Thyroid.** Minute changes in brain thyroid hormone levels may produce marked mood
changes. Thyroid hormone is postulated to help maintain neuronal structure and central adrenergic transmission.

a. **Hyperthyroidism.** Psychiatric symptoms associated with hyperthyroidism may include sudden tearfulness, insomnia, persistent anxiety, depressed mood (often more
prominent in the elderly), difficulty in concentration and memory, and, in extreme
cases, delirium accompanied by psychosis. Treatment to reduce thyroid hormone
levels will eventually reverse symptoms.

b. **Hypothyroidism** is most often caused by damage to the thyroid gland as a result of
ablation, autoimmune disease, or the use of drugs, such as lithium. Pituitary or
hypothalamic disease can cause decreased production of thyroid hormone. Hypothyroidism will develop in approximately 10% of patients who take lithium.
Women and rapid cycling bipolar patients are at increased risk. Mild hypothyroidism (Table 2-4) frequently presents as a psychiatric disorder only, with patients
experiencing anxiety and depression. Cognitive impairment is often more severe
than with depressive disorder. In elderly patients, this condition must be differentiated from primary dementia. Irritability, emotional lability, and difficulty with sleep
also occur. In severe cases, psychosis occurs as part of delirium.

TABLE 2-4. Diagnostic Profile of Hypothyroidism

Grade	Severity	T_4 and Free T_3	Thyroid-Stimulating Hormone	Thyrotropin-Releasing Hormone	Psychiatric Symptom Severity
I	Mild	Normal	Normal	↑	+
II	Moderate	Normal	↑	↑	+ +
III	Severe	↓	↑	↑	+ + +

↑ = increased; ↓ = decreased; + = mild; + + = moderate; + + + = severe.

2. **Cortisol.** Patients with a variety of psychiatric disorders, but particularly depression, demonstrate **nonsuppression** with the **dexamethasone suppression test** (i.e., the adrenal continues to release cortisol after administration of an exogenous steroid). This offers a further **link between endocrine and monoamine systems**.
   a. **Hypercortisolism** may cause mood changes, anxiety, personality change, or delirium. Cushing's disease and Cushing's syndrome can cause psychiatric change that occurs before physical symptoms are seen. Physical symptoms include moon facies, muscle weakness, buffalo hump, hypertension, and hyperglycemia. Corticotropin-releasing factor (CRF) receptor downregulation is thought to be related to the depressive symptoms.
   b. **Hypocortisolism** is associated with psychiatric symptoms of fluctuating severe anxiety or depression and paranoia. The diagnosis of hypocortisolism should be considered in patients with major medical illness, such as tuberculosis, carcinoma, or autoimmune disease.

3. **Glucose and insulin**
   a. **Hypoglycemia** is a common complaint, but the diagnosis should be made by biologic markers. The blood glucose level after a 24-hour fast or during an attack must be 50 mg/dl to meet the criteria for hypoglycemia. This condition is often misdiagnosed as hysteria, epilepsy, or intoxication.
   b. **Hyperglycemia** occurs in patients who take insulin for type II diabetes mellitus when injections do not correspond to the blood glucose load. Polydipsia and polyuria occur acutely. The lasting effects of poorly controlled diabetes, such as microvascular and macrovascular changes, may produce decrements in cognition, memory, and modulation of affect.

E. **Memory.** Memory is not a single function involving a single brain region or circuit. Rather, different memory systems exist to handle various memory functions. Two recently defined systems are declarative memory and procedural memory.

1. **Declarative memory.** This type of memory involves conscious recall of events and facts.
   a. Information must first be learned and consolidated. These functions appear to require an intact medial **hippocampus** and intact midline diencephalic structures. These structures include the mediodorsal nucleus of the thalamus and the mammillary bodies of the hypothalamus, areas that are damaged in **Korsakoff's syndrome** (see Chapter 15 V F). However, this area does not appear to be the actual site of storage because hippocampal lesions do not erase all old memories.
   b. Recall of stored memories appears to involve frontal–subcortical circuits. These circuits also appear to be responsible for **immediate memory** (e.g., ability to recall a new telephone number long enough to dial it).

2. **Procedural memory.** This memory is unconscious and includes learning motor skills (e.g., juggling, touch typing), classic conditioning, and habits. People cannot recall these memories except by performing them. This memory is mediated by the **basal ganglia**. Damage to this area (e.g., in patients with Huntington's chorea or Parkinson's disease) causes difficulty in learning new motor skills.

IV. NEUROIMAGING TECHNIQUES

A. **Structural neuroimaging.** Several techniques provide information about the anatomic structure of the brain.

1. **Computed tomography (CT)** (Table 2-5)
   a. **Technique.** CT is a graphic display of a pattern in a plane. Many thousands of x-ray readings of the head are processed by computer to make a CT image.
      (1) A collimated x-ray source rotates around and passes thin beams of radiation through the head while detectors collect the nonabsorbed x-rays on the opposite side. These emitters and detectors are oriented in a plane perpendicular to the longitudinal axis (i.e., **transaxial**). The computer applies an algorithm to recreate slices from the multiple linear x-ray projections.
      (2) Images can be enhanced with electron-dense **iodinated contrast materials** in the bloodstream to show lesions that involve abnormal vascular structures or breakdown of the blood–brain barrier.
      (3) Tissues with differing electron density differentially absorb x-rays. **Bone, air, and fluid are particularly well visualized** with this technique because of the relatively high contrast between them.
   b. **Findings.** Enlarged ventricular systems, as measured by either the ventricular–brain area on a single slice or by the ventricular–brain volume, are reported in many chronic mental illnesses. Pathognomonic anatomic changes are found only for disorders such as neoplasms, vascular diseases, and specific neurologic illnesses, some of which also produce behavioral changes.
      (1) **Schizophrenia. Lateral and third ventriculomegaly** is consistently found in studies of schizophrenia. However, it does not appear to be progressive or affected by medication status, movement disorder, or clinical symptoms. The significance of the reported loss of normal cerebral asymmetry in patients with schizophrenia is unclear, but it may be linked to structural and functional imaging findings.
      (2) **Dementia. Normal pressure hydrocephalus,** a reversible cause of dementia, has characteristic changes on CT of anterior ventriculomegaly and periventricular lucencies. **Multi-infarct dementia** is usually better visualized with magnetic resonance imaging (MRI).
      (3) A decreased area of caudate nuclei is seen in men with **obsessive-compulsive disorder**.

TABLE 2-5. Comparison of Computed Tomography and Magnetic Resonance Imaging Scans of the Brain

Characteristic	Computed Tomography	Magnetic Resonance Imaging
Visualizes	Bone, air, blood	Brain/soft tissue, water
Exposure	X-ray	Magnetic field
Contrast	Yes	Yes
Indication	Extent of bleed	Enhance tumor
Resolution	Fair	High
Best use	Hemorrhage, vascular anomaly, ring-enhancing tumor, abscess	Dementia, white matter, volumetric analysis of cortex, old hemorrhage, plaques, arteriovenous malformation
Cost	$300	$450–$1300
Contraindications	Allergy to iodine in contrast material	Metal in head, welding history, pacemaker
Risk	3–5 rad ionizing radiation, iodinated contrast agents	Magnetic field exposure, unknown metal being moved, claustrophobia

(4) CT detects brain tumors that cause behavioral disturbances. Edema, shift of midline structures, and other changes in the ventricular system are well visualized.

2. MRI

a. Technique. The electromagnetic properties of biologic tissue are used to generate images. Dipoles result when atoms with unpaired electrons exhibit net magnetization.

   (1) When exposed to a strong **magnetic field** (0.15–2.0 tesla), as in an MRI scanner, the **dipoles become aligned** in one net direction.

   (2) While in the aligned field, dipoles are exposed to a pulse of short-wave radiofrequencies. For each atom at a given magnetic field strength, there is a unique radiofrequency, known as the Larmor frequency, at which nuclei absorb energy.

   (3) From this excited state, the **nuclei are allowed to relax back** to the original aligned state in the magnetic field.

   (4) The radio wave **signals emitted** during the relaxation phase **are measured and processed** by computer to create an image. The **resonance** of magnetic nuclei passing from relaxed to excited to relaxed state gives the technique its descriptive name.

   (5) **Contrast agents** can enhance visualization of the circulatory system. **Gadolinium** does not normally cross the blood–brain barrier. Pathologic tissue processes that disrupt the blood–brain barrier are easily identified by the increased intensity of the contrast agent.

b. Three methods of analysis

   (1) **T1 relaxation time** is the constant describing the interval between excitation and the return of 63% of magnetization to the original axis of the externally applied field (the longitudinal axis). This process involves energy loss because of local spin–lattice interaction between nuclei. Such scans are most useful for identifying **contrast between brain densities** (e.g., borders of tumors) and detecting paramagnetic substances, such as methemoglobin or melanin.

   (2) **T2 relaxation time** is the constant describing the interval between excitation and the loss of 63% of net magnetization in the tranverse plane (i.e., perpendicular to the applied magnetic field). T2 is the result of energy produced by spin–spin interactions between nuclei. T2 scans are most useful for detecting **edema, ischemia, and plaques,** which show as hyperintensities. The relative weighting of T1 and T2 can be altered to maximize the image.

   (3) A **proton-weighted** scan is based on the number of protons in the tissue. Proton-weighted scans are useful for visualizing anatomy and **differentiating between white and gray matter**.

c. Findings in neurologic diseases that may have behavioral symptoms

   (1) **Arteriovenous vascular malformation** can be well visualized and may cause behavioral disruption, particularly in the setting of chronic seizure disorder.

   (2) **Huntington's disease** is associated with bilateral atrophy of the head of the caudate nucleus, with concomitant widening of the frontal horn of the lateral ventricles.

   (3) **Multiple sclerosis** is caused by demyelination that may evolve into plaques, or focal lesions that appear as white areas on T2-weighted images.

   (4) Some patients with **Parkinson's disease** show narrowing of the pars compacta of the substantia nigra.

   (5) MRI is used to monitor for **iron deposits** in patients with **hemachromatosis** and for **copper deposits** in patients with **Wilson's disease**.

d. Psychiatric disorders. MRI is not useful in the diagnosis of most psychiatric illness. However, certain findings are replicable and are easily related to the clinical condition.

   (1) **Schizophrenia** is the mental disorder that has been studied the most extensively with MRI. Findings include increased ventricular system size (lateral ventricles and third ventricle), decreased temporal lobe gray matter (left hemisphere tissue loss is greater than right hemisphere loss), and dilation of the cortical sulci. Other changes are also reported.

(2) Lesions that are characteristic of **multi-infarct dementia** are best shown with T2-weighted images.

(3) **Neurodegenerative dementias,** such as Alzheimer's disease, cause diffuse frontal atrophy and ventricular enlargement. Clinical findings and MRI changes are usually used to make a presumptive diagnosis because a tissue sample (brain biopsy) is required for a definitive diagnosis. Because of overlap in the degree of atrophy with the normative aging population, repeat scans may be necessary.

(4) An increased number of high-intensity areas is reported in patients with **bipolar (manic-depressive) disorder,** at least at the time of acute exacerbation.

(5) Patients with **anorexia nervosa** have apparent atrophy during the acute stages of illness. This problem may resolve with the return to a reasonable body weight. **Bulimia nervosa** may cause ventriculomegaly, but the variation in findings may reflect vascular and fluid–osmotic changes secondary to endocrine changes caused by the illness.

B. **Functional neuroimaging.** In addition to studies that provide anatomic information, techniques are available to measure properties that are directly or indirectly related to brain function.

1. EEG and evoked potentials

a. Technique

(1) EEG is one of the least expensive, most portable tools that measures brain activity. Whether provided as paper tracings or computer-generated color images, the data are a measure of the difference in electric potential between two recording, or active, electrodes. In a standard array, **scalp electrodes** (Figure 2-3) are paired in different combinations, known as montages, that allow patterns of activity to be identified over different parts of the head (e.g., frontal, temporal, occipital). By convention, the frequency of electric activity is categorized into four bands: alpha, beta, theta, and delta (Table 2-6).

(2) **Evoked potentials.** The **signal-to-noise** ratio can be increased by compiling the responses over time to a predictable event, such as a click or a flash of light. By averaging traces, the response to the stimulus can be seen more clearly as different from the varying background activity (Figure 2-4).

b. Findings

(1) Generalized **low-grade dysrhythmia** is frequently found in patients with epilepsy or chronic brain illness and in those taking various medications. It does not predict behavioral disturbance, but it is a common finding in persons with persistent behavioral problems.

(2) Patients with **schizophrenia** have no pathognomonic EEG findings. However, as a group, these patients show decreased amplitude and increased latency of auditory evoked responses, especially for P300 and attentional tasks. **Sensory gating is impaired** in patients with schizophrenia and in their first-degree relatives, regardless of whether they exhibit symptoms. Sensory gating is measured by a lack of reduction of response (P50) to paired click stimuli. Antipsychotic medication produces large, often frontal, generalized sharp waves.

(3) Evoked responses in patients with **mania** show disruption of sensory processing that requires focused attention. During periods of remission, patients with bipolar illness have responses that fall within the normal distribution in the population.

(4) Patients with **borderline personality disorder** are differentiated from those with other personality disorders, but not from a comparison group of patients with schizophrenia, by decreased amplitude and latency as shown on P300 testing.

2. Magnetoencephalography (MEG) and evoked fields

a. Technique. Magnetic fields are produced by any electric current, and the current produced by neurons is no exception. MEG translates **absolute magnetic field strength** measured at the surface of the head (not a relative strength, as in EEG) into signals that can be amplified and digitally processed. Therefore, MEG and EEG reflect information from the same source, but detect different activity. The greater the

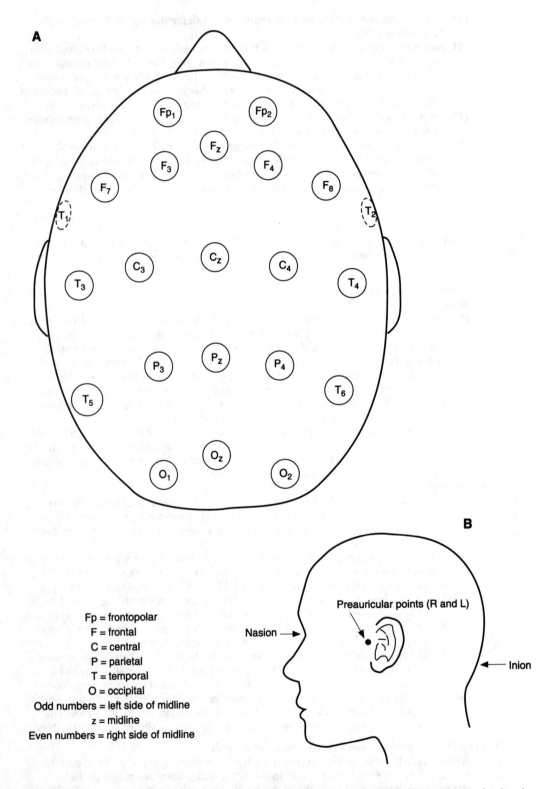

A

Fp₁ Fp₂
Fz
F₃ F₄
F₇ F₈
T₁ T₂
C₃ Cz C₄
T₃ T₄
Pz
P₃ P₄
T₅ T₆
Oz
O₁ O₂

B

Fp = frontopolar
F = frontal
C = central
P = parietal
T = temporal
O = occipital
Odd numbers = left side of midline
z = midline
Even numbers = right side of midline

Preauricular points (R and L)

Nasion →

Inion →

FIGURE 2-3. (*A*) International 10–20 system for electrode placement. The *circled* sites represent landmarks for electrode placement. This system is a proportionate placement of electrodes at 10% and 20% increments between anterior–posterior and right–left landmarks. (*B*) Bone landmarks.

TABLE 2-6. Electroencephalogram Frequency Band and Characteristics

Frequency	Name	Location	Characteristics
1–4 Hz	Delta	Frontal, central	Generalized in sleep; seen in encephalopathy, coma, toxic states
4–8 Hz	Theta	Central	Awake, task oriented
8–12 Hz	Alpha	Occipital	Awake, resting state with eyes closed (meditative); does not slow appreciably with increased age
12 + Hz	Beta	Frontal	Increased in drugged states

distance from the source, the weaker the magnetic field is likely to be. MEG instruments are housed in shielded rooms that screen out ambient magnetic fields, which are much stronger than brain signals.

b. Findings

   (1) Localization of functional tissue, such as the sensory or motor cortex, is an important application of MEG in preparation for neurosurgical excision of a mass.

   (2) MEG and EEG provide important and complementary information in the evaluation of the **epileptogenic source** in patients who have severe epilepsy and are candidates for neurosurgery.

   (3) The processing of auditory, visual, and sensory stimuli is being studied with greater resolution with MEG, increasing the utility of these studies in the evaluation of patients with neuropsychiatric disorders.

   (4) Slow-wave activity is seen at the margins of the affected cortex in patients with tumor and stroke. This information is useful in the evaluation of the extent of diseased tissue as well as in follow-up studies of blood clots.

3. Magnetic resonance spectroscopy (MRS)

   a. Technique. Nuclei in different molecules exhibit different magnetic field strengths. Disturbing these nuclei with a broadband pulse or continuous radiofrequency wave will cause them to **resonate**. A number of nuclei exhibit magnetic resonance (Table 2-7), which can then be measured. Phosphorus 31 is particularly useful to measure because phosphocreatine, adenosine triphosphate (ATP), and inorganic phosphorus are present in millimolar concentrations in cell nuclei, where they can easily be detected by MRS. Phosphorus measurements can also provide estimates of pH because many resonances of phosphorus are pH dependent.

   b. Findings

   (1) Examination of patients with both **stable and acute stroke** shows peaks of phosphorus that are consistent with dead tissue. Nearby signs of repair and regeneration are shown by increased energy metabolism.

   (2) Children with **autism** show characteristic patterns on phosphorus or hydrogen measurements. These patterns are thought to support the hypothesis that the loss of neuronal sprouting may contribute to the severity of symptoms.

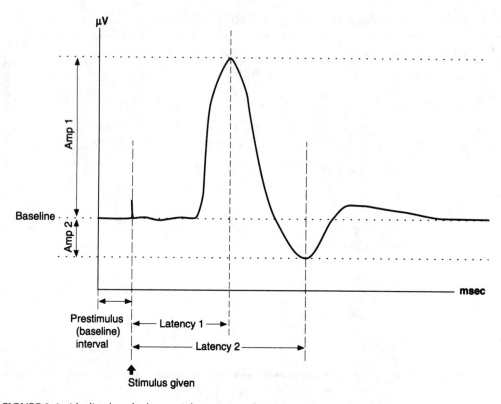

FIGURE 2-4. Idealized evoked potential, an averaged response. The stimulus is often auditory (e.g., a click) or visual (e.g., a flash) and is given repeatedly. Delays in latency 1 or latency 2 may help pinpoint problems in the auditory or visual pathway. *Amp* = amplitude.

     (3) Tumor growth and diminution in response to treatment can be followed with this technique.

     (4) Areas of active research include multiple sclerosis, developmental disorders, schizophrenia, panic disorder, and obsessive-compulsive disorder. Brain levels of some psychiatric drugs, including medications such as fluoxetine and lithium, may be measurable by MRS.

  4. Regional cerebral blood flow (rCBF). This technique is being largely supplanted by positron emission tomography (PET) and single-photon emission computer tomography (SPECT) because its advantage of low cost is outweighed by its poor spatial resolution and inability to measure subcortical functioning.

  a. Technique. After the patient inhales a **radioactive tracer,** such as xenon 133, and brain tissues become saturated, the rate of radioactive emission is used to calculate regional blood flow (assumed to correspond to regional cortical metabolism).

  b. Findings

     (1) Decreased activity over the frontal areas is seen in **frontal dementias,** such as Pick's disease.

TABLE 2-7. Nuclei with Potential for Clinical Studies

Hydrogen*	Fluorine
Carbon	Sodium
Nitrogen	Phosphorus*
Oxygen	

*Human studies.

    (2) Decreased parietal lobe activity is recorded in patients with **Alzheimer's dementia**. This decrease correlates with impairments in cognitive functioning.

    (3) Compared with normal matched controls, patients with **schizophrenia** show **decreased dorsolateral prefrontal cortical rCBF** during the Wisconsin card-sorting test, which requires trial-and-error learning over time.

5. SPECT

a. Technique. This tomographic technique measures either blood flow through the brain or receptor distribution.

    (1) SPECT captures images with the use of columnators that are arrayed perpendicularly around the head. Information about the radioactivity that is present and its decay is processed for different distances (depth toward the center of the head) from the probes. The tracers used are **single-photon–emitting radionuclides,** which have long half-lives, permitting their manufacture at one site and use at another.

    (2) The xenon 133 inhalation technique shows the blood flow distribution through the brain, especially at cortical levels.

    (3) Dopamine, serotonin, opiate, benzodiazepine, and muscarinic compounds, or receptor agonists, are labeled with iodine 123 to show **receptor binding and distribution patterns**. During the study time (30–60 minutes), regional brain function is stimulated by specific behavioral, sensory, or cognitive tasks.

b. Findings

    (1) Dementia. Patients with Alzheimer's disease show symmetric parietal cortex deficits with SPECT. In patients with Pick's disease, SPECT shows decreased blood flow and labeling in the frontal lobe.

    (2) Depression. Patients with pseudodementia, or depression presenting with the symptoms of dementia, show cortical activity comparable to that of normal control subjects. The findings are different in patients with true dementia.

    (3) Schizophrenia. In patients with schizophrenia, the resting blood flow rate is normal. However, when these patients attempt to perform tasks that require attention and cognitive manipulation, they do not show the normal increase in rCBF.

    (4) SPECT has the potential to become a useful and cost-effective clinical tool, but there are no established clinical indications for obtaining SPECT scans of psychiatric patients.

6. PET

a. Technique

    (1) The patient is injected with a **positron-emitting compound,** such as fluorine 18, that is **incorporated into an organic compound,** such as deoxyglucose. After it is injected into the bloodstream, the labeled compound is taken up by neurons in active brain areas. Thus, PET provides a pictogram of regional metabolic brain activity.

    (2) Repeated gamma ray emission sequences are collected by detectors that are arranged in a curve around the patient's head. The images are compiled, and the distribution of the radionuclide is reconstructed by computer as a dynamic picture of the brain.

    (3) A patient performs specific tasks during the study to demonstrate activity of different brain systems, such as those for auditory, attention, or memory functions.

    (4) Difficulties with the technique:

        (a) The discomfort of having both arterial and venous access established to estimate the relative rate of blood flow throughout the body

        (b) The need for a cyclotron located near the scanner so that the produced labeled compounds do not lose their potency

b. Findings

    (1) Anterior:posterior ratios of brain slices in the resting state show decreases in patients with **schizophrenia and bipolar disorder**. These decreases suggest that severe chronic mental illness affects resting brain function.

     (2) In **Alzheimer's dementia,** diffuse reduced metabolic activity is seen. Dementias caused by subcortical disease (e.g., Parkinson's disease) or focal lesions (e.g., brain tumor) may show areas of relatively intact metabolic activity and areas of inactivity.

     (3) Injection of lactate rapidly produces panic attacks in vulnerable individuals. PET scans demonstrate decreased right parietal metabolic activity during the attacks.

     (4) PET scans reveal increased brain activity in the basal ganglia and frontal lobes of patients with **obsessive-compulsive disorder**.

     (5) **Specific neurotransmitter labels** are used to show receptor patterns, such as the dopamine (D_2) binding of certain antipsychotic medications. This technique is becoming an important tool for evaluating the mechanisms responsible for differences in the clinical efficacy of different drugs.

 NEUROANATOMY AND BEHAVIORAL FUNCTIONING. Understanding the normally developed and functioning brain is as important as identifying changes that cause abnormal function. It is often difficult to determine whether neurochemical and other changes are responsible for the pathologic changes in behavior observed in patients with illnesses such as schizophrenia or whether these neurochemical changes result from an alteration in the state of the brain that is caused by a disease process. The use of a range of approaches to study the biologic function of the brain is essential to address these complex clinicopathologic problems.

REFERENCE

1. Carpenter MB: *Core Text of Neuroanatomy.* Baltimore, Williams & Wilkins, 1991.

BIBLIOGRAPHY

Adams RD, Victor M: *Principles of Neurology,* 5th ed. Companion Handbook. New York, McGraw-Hill, 1994.

Andreasen NC: *Brain Imaging: Applications in Psychiatry.* Washington, DC, APA Press, 1989.

Bloom FE, Lazerson A: *Brain, Mind and Behavior.* New York, WH Freeman, 1988.

Carpenter MB: *Core Text of Neuroanatomy.* Baltimore, Williams & Wilkins, 1991.

Chrousos GP, Gold PW: The concepts of stress and stress system disorders. *JAMA* 267:1244–1252, 1992.

Meltzer HY (ed): *Psychopharmacology: The Third Generation of Progress.* New York, Raven Press, 1987.

Yudofsky SC, Hales RE (eds): *APA Textbook of Neuropsychiatry,* 2nd ed. Washington, DC, APA Press, 1991.

▌STUDY QUESTIONS

DIRECTIONS: Each of the numbered items or incomplete statements in this section is followed by answers or by completions of the statement. Select the ONE lettered answer or completion that is BEST in each case.

1. Stimulation of corticotropin-releasing hormone (CRH) by physical or emotional stress causes which adaptive response?

(A) Tachycardia and slowing of gastrointestinal function
(B) Chronic immune suppression
(C) Enhanced memory retrieval
(D) Heightened arousal and inhibition of feeding and sexual function
(E) Anorexia nervosa

2. Which is the best description of Korsakoff's syndrome?

(A) Apathy and distractibility seen after frontal lobotomy
(B) Amnesia seen in alcoholic patients who have had thiamine deficiency
(C) Ataxia due to lithium toxicity
(D) Symptoms that accompany withdrawal from opiates
(E) Amenorrhea seen in women with anorexia nervosa

3. Sleep is best characterized by

(A) reticular activating system (RAS) activity; restorative trophic and psychological properties
(B) RAS increased activity; decreased muscle tone
(C) REM and non-REM stages that are stable over the life cycle
(D) changing patterns of arousal, characteristic for disorders

DIRECTIONS: Each set of matching questions in this section consists of a list of four to twenty-six lettered options (some of which may be in figures) followed by several numbered items. For each numbered item, select the ONE lettered option that is most closely associated with it. To avoid spending too much time on matching sets with large numbers of options, it is generally advisable to begin each set by reading the list of options. Then, for each item in the set, try to generate the correct answer and locate it in the option list, rather than evaluating each option individually. Each lettered option may be selected once, more than once, or not at all.

Questions 4–6

Match each neurotransmitter with its brain area origin.

(A) Substantia innominata
(B) Substantia nigra
(C) Raphe nuclei
(D) Globus pallidus
(E) Locus ceruleus

4. Serotonin

5. Dopamine

6. Norepinephrine

Questions 7–13

Match each descriptor with the associated technique.

(A) Magnetic resonance spectroscopy (MRS)
(B) Magnetoencephalography (MEG)
(C) Magnetic resonance imaging (MRI)
(D) Single-photon emission computed tomography (SPECT)
(E) Computed tomography (CT)
(F) Positron emission tomography (PET)
(G) Regional cerebral blood flow (rCBF)
(H) Electroencephalography (EEG)
(I) Pneumoencephalography (PEG)

7. Measure of real-time electric activity

8. Tomographic x-ray

9. Dynamic measure of hydrogen or phosphorus resonance

10. Static image of nuclear resonance

11. Dynamic measure of blood flow with tomography

12. Measure of absolute magnetic activity

13. Dynamic measure of brain metabolism

ANSWERS AND EXPLANATIONS

1. The answer is D [III C 2]. Stress causes the release of corticotropin-releasing hormone (CRH), which leads to heightened arousal and the inhibition of eating and sexual behavior, which is adaptive in dealing with acute stress. Tachycardia, slowing of gastrointestinal function, and enhanced memory retrieval are also adaptive responses to stress, but are caused by the release of norepinephrine. Chronic immune suppression can be caused by chronic stress, but it is not adaptive. Some mental disorders, such as anorexia nervosa, may be caused partly by malfunction, not adaptive function, of the stress response system.

2. The answer is B [III E 1 a]. Chronic alcohol abuse commonly leads to thiamine deficiency, which can lead to Wernicke's encephalopathy, a syndrome of ophthalmoplegia, ataxia, and confusion. Untreated, this can advance to an amnestic disorder known as Korsakoff's amnesia, Korsakoff's psychosis, or Korsakoff's syndrome.

3. The answer is A [III A]. Reticular activating system (RAS) activity decreases in order for the human brain to fall asleep. Over the life cycle, there are varying amounts and patterns of REM and non-REM sleep in each individual. Muscle tone is decreased during REM sleep, which is characteristic. Although there are no characteristic **arousal** patterns typical for different psychiatric disorders, specific **electroencephalography (EEG)** patterns are associated with the different stages of sleep. In addition, many consistent patterns of sleep disruption are associated with different psychiatric disorders (e.g., early morning awakening is associated with depression, although it is not pathognomonic for, or specific to, depression).

4–6. The answers are: 4-C, 5-B, 6-E [II A 3, C 1, 2, D]. The raphe nuclei of the midbrain, pons, and medulla contain serotonergic cell bodies. The substantia nigra and ventral tegmental area contain the cell bodies of dopaminergic neurons. The locus ceruleus contains noradrenergic neurons. The substantia innominata, also known as the nucleus basalis of Meynert, contains the cell bodies of cholinergic neurons. The globus pallidus is part of the corpus striatum, which **receives** dopaminergic input.

7–13. The answers are: 7-H, 8-E, 9-A, 10-C, 11-D, 12-B, 13-F [IV A 1 a, 2 a, 3 a (1)–(4), B 1 a (1), 2 a, 3 a, 4, 5 a, 6 a (1); Figure 2-3; Table 2-6; Table 2-7]. Real-time electric activity is measured by electroencephalography (EEG), which is a recording of the electric activity of cortical neurons by means of electrodes that are applied to the scalp.

Computed tomography (CT) is the computerized processing of information gathered by x-rays passed through an area of anatomy. A tomograph is a cross-sectional image, representing a particular plane in the body.

Magnetic resonance refers to the degree of disturbance of particular nuclei when a continuous radiofrequency wave causes them to vibrate. Magnetic resonance imaging (MRI) produces a static image of the brain, based on the nuclear resonance of various brain structures. A single wave of radiofrequency excites hydrogen nuclei, which are then allowed to relax. The signals emitted during the relaxation phase are processed by computer to create an image. In contrast, magnetic resonance spectroscopy (MRS) can measure the resonance of a variety of physiologically important nuclei, such as phosphorus, to yield regional information about metabolism, pH, and other indicators of brain function.

Single-photon emission computed tomography (SPECT) is a technique by which regional brain blood flow (a correlate of brain activity) is determined by use of single-photon emitting radionuclides, which have long half-lives, permitting relatively long (30–60 minutes) study of regional brain function. It can also be used to study receptor binding and distribution.

Magnetoencephalography (MEG) translates absolute magnetic activity at the surface of the head into signals that can be amplified and digitally processed.

Positron emission tomography (PET) is a dynamic measure of brain metabolism. It detects gamma rays from tissue after a patient has been injected with a positron-emitting compound (produced by a cyclotron). The paths of the gamma rays are detected by computer, and a tomographic image is created. Depending on the compound used, PET can be used to study blood flow (representing metabolic activity) or receptor occupancy and distribution.

Chapter 3

Pharmacology and Behavior

Darrell G. Kirch
Fuad Issa

I. INTRODUCTION

A. **Pharmacokinetic principles**

1. **Absorption** of a drug is a function of the **dose given** and the **route of administration** (i.e., alimentary, parenteral, topical, or via inhalation).

2. **Distribution** of a drug throughout the body occurs as a result of passage across membranes via diffusion, transport (active or passive), or endocytosis. Drugs that have a wide deposition throughout body fluids and tissues have a greater **volume of distribution,** which affects their relative availability to brain tissue. Lipid solubility of a drug enhances its ability to cross the **blood–brain barrier**.

3. **Elimination** of a drug is a function of **metabolism** within and **excretion** from the body. Metabolites of a drug may have pharmacologic activity. The half-life of a drug is the time required for its plasma concentration to decrease by 50%.

4. The **therapeutic index** of a drug is the ratio between a lethal dose and a clinically effective dose. Thus, the higher the therapeutic index, the safer a drug is in clinical use.

B. **Central nervous system (CNS) neurotransmitters and receptors**

1. **Behavior is the result of the transmission of messages through complex neuronal networks in the CNS.** The passage of a signal across the synaptic cleft depends on the release of a neurotransmitter from the presynaptic axonal terminal. This neurotransmitter then binds to a specific receptor on another neuron, causing a response in the postsynaptic cell.

2. **Primary neurotransmitters in the CNS are described in Chapter 1 and include:**
   a. **Monoamines**
      (1) **The catecholamines dopamine and norepinephrine**
      (2) **The indolamine 5-hydroxytryptamine (5-HT, or serotonin)**
   b. **Acetylcholine (ACh)**
   c. **γ-Aminobutyric acid (GABA)**
   d. **Glutamate and aspartate**
   e. **Various peptides,** such as the enkephalins, somatostatin, vasoactive intestinal polypeptide (VIP), and cholecystokinin (CCK)

3. **Drugs may act on one or more of the steps related to neurotransmission** (i.e., synthesis, release, degradation, reuptake, or postsynaptic receptor augmentation or blockade). This activity accounts for most of the therapeutic effects and side effects of a specific drug (Table 3-1).

II. ANTIPSYCHOTIC AGENTS

A. **General considerations**

1. **Psychosis** is a state of grossly impaired cognitive or perceptual ability that affects reality testing and is not accounted for by cultural factors. It involves deficits in the ability to think, remember, communicate, respond emotionally, behave appropriately, perceive sensory stimuli correctly, and interpret reality.

TABLE 3-1. Side Effects and Pharmacologic Properties of Psychotropic Medications

Pharmacologic Property	Side Effects
Dopamine D_2 receptor blockade	Extrapyramidal movement disorders
Serotonin 5-HT_2 receptor blockade	Orgasmic and ejaculatory disturbances, hypotension
Histamine H_1 receptor blockade	Sedation, drowsiness, weight gain
Muscarinic receptor blockade	Dry mouth, blurred vision, constipation, urinary retention, sinus tachycardia, memory disturbances
Adrenergic α_1 receptor blockade	Postural hypotension, dizziness, reflex tachycardia, ejaculatory disturbances
Adrenergic α_2 receptor blockade	Priapism
Dopamine reuptake inhibition	Psychomotor activation, aggravation of psychosis
Serotonin reuptake inhibition	Gastrointestinal disturbances, insomnia, restlessness, orgasmic disturbances
Norepinephrine reuptake inhibition	Tremor, tachycardia

   a. **Primary symptoms** of psychosis include disordered thought processes, hallucinations, and delusions.
   b. **Psychotic illnesses.** Psychosis is commonly seen in **schizophrenic disorders** and may also be present in **major affective disorders** (i.e., **depression, bipolar disorder**), **delirium,** and **substance-related disorders**.

2. **Antipsychotic agents** improve cognition, mood, and behavior in psychotic individuals without producing physical dependence. This antipsychotic effect is independent of any more general sedating effects. The **typical antipsychotics** tend to cause neurologic side effects; they are known as **neuroleptics**. Not all neuroleptics are antipsychotics (e.g., prochlorperazine and metoclopramide are antiemetics). The newer agents (**atypical antipsychotics**) are relatively free of potentially disabling neurologic side effects.

B. **Classes of drugs** (Table 3-2)

1. **Phenothiazines** are divided into three subgroups as determined by the side chain attached to the phenothiazine nucleus.

2. **Thioxanthene compounds** (e.g., thiothixene, chlorprothixene) chemically resemble the phenothiazines, with substitution of a carbon atom for a nitrogen atom in the central ring of the phenothiazine nucleus.

3. **Butyrophenone compounds** include haloperidol and pimozide.

4. **Other typical antipsychotics** include dibenzoxazepines (e.g., loxapine) and dihydroindolones (e.g., molindone).

5. **Atypical antipsychotics** include dibenzodiazepines (e.g., clozapine) and benzisoxizoles (e.g., risperidone).

C. **Pharmacology and pharmacokinetics**

1. **Mechanism of action.** All antipsychotic agents block dopamine receptors in the CNS. Some investigators believe that certain symptoms of schizophrenia (e.g., hallucinations, delusions, hyperactivity) may be the result of a hyperdopaminergic state.

2. **Pharmacologic properties,** in addition to the antipsychotic effects, are related to receptor blockade or reuptake inhibition (see Table 3-1).

3. **Absorption.** Antipsychotic agents are generally well absorbed after oral or parenteral administration, with rapid distribution throughout the body.

TABLE 3-2. Major Antipsychotic Medications and Their Pharmacologic Properties

	Chlorpromazine Equivalent* (mg)	Receptor Affinity				
		Dopamine D_2	Serotonin $5\text{-}HT_2$	Histamine H_1	Muscarinic M	Adrenergic α_1
Phenothiazines						
Alkylamino						
Chlorpromazine	100	+++	+++	+++	+++	+++
Piperidine						
Thioridazine	100	+	+++	+++	+++	+++
Piperazine						
Perphenazine	10	++	+++	++	++	++
Trifluoperazine	5	++	++	++	++	++
Fluphenazine	2	+++	+	+	+	+
Thioxanthenes						
Thiothixene	3	+++	+	+	+	+
Butyrophenones						
Haloperidol	2	+++	+	+	+	+
Dibenzoxazepines						
Loxapine	12.5	++	+++	++	++	++
Dihydroindolones						
Molindone	10	++	+	+	++	++
Dibenzodiazepines						
Clozapine	60	+	+++	+++	+++	+++
Benzisoxizoles						
Risperidone	1	+++	+++	+++	-	+++

+ = mild; ++ = moderate; +++ = strong; - = none.
*For example, a given patient is likely to respond similarly to 100 mg of chlorpromazine or 2 mg of haloperidol.

4. Metabolism may result in multiple active and inactive metabolites. Several metabolites are postulated for chlorpromazine, perhaps the agent that is best studied in this regard. Hydroxylation and formation of sulfoxides are common. For some antipsychotic agents, few metabolites are known.

5. Slow excretion occurs in urine and feces. For most compounds, a **relatively long half-life** allows once-daily dosing.

D. **Clinical use**

1. **Therapeutic uses.** Antipsychotic agents are used to treat several disorders, with specific target symptoms likely to be improved (e.g., hallucinations, delusions, flight of ideas, hyperactivity, combativeness, disorientation, insomnia). Improvement in insight, judgment, and logic is slower and more variable.
   a. Antipsychotics are used to control psychotic symptoms in **acute and chronic schizophrenia** and **schizoaffective disorder**. Clozapine is especially useful in treatment-resistant cases of schizophrenia.
   b. Antipsychotic agents are used to treat the **manic phase of bipolar illness**. However, lithium is the preferred maintenance agent for this disorder.
   c. Antipsychotics are used to treat **psychotic manifestations** of some severe major depressions, personality disorders, and dementia.
   d. **Haloperidol** is the current treatment of choice for the tics and involuntary vocalizations that occur with **Tourette's syndrome**.
   e. Antipsychotic agents can also be used to treat nausea, vomiting, and intractable hiccups.

2. **Dosage**
   a. The antipsychotic **potencies** of antipsychotic drugs and, therefore, their therapeutic doses **vary widely** (see Table 3-2). Dosage equivalent to 300 to 1000 mg/day chlorpromazine is usually sufficient. In general, antipsychotics have a **high therapeutic index,** which makes them relatively safe in case of an overdose.
   b. Assays to measure antipsychotic drug concentrations in the blood are available. Firm therapeutic ranges are not established for all drugs, but blood levels may help to identify patients who, because of noncompliance or pharmacokinetics, have subtherapeutic concentrations.
   c. Although divided doses may help to minimize sedation in the early phases of treatment, a **single daily dose** at bedtime is usually adequate in the maintenance phase of treatment.

E. **Side effects and toxicity** are related to the receptor blockade or reuptake inhibition involved (see Tables 3-1 and 3-2).

1. **Extrapyramidal side effects** (e.g., dystonia, akathisia, parkinsonism) may be treated with anticholinergic agents (e.g., trihexyphenidyl, benztropine) or the antiparkinsonian drug amantadine, or by reducing the dosage of the antipsychotic agent. Antipsychotic medications with high affinity for muscarinic receptors (e.g., chlorpromazine, thioridazine) usually have fewer extrapyramidal side effects. Compared with typical antipsychotics (neuroleptics), clozapine has few extrapyramidal side effects.

2. **Allergic reactions,** including agranulocytosis and cholestatic jaundice, occasionally occur with the use of conventional antipsychotic drugs. However, agranulocytosis occurs frequently enough with clozapine to require routine leukocyte count monitoring.

3. Antipsychotic drugs, especially low-potency phenothiazines and clozapine, may **lower the seizure threshold**.

4. **Impaired hypothalamic temperature regulation** may predispose patients to hypothermia or heat stroke.

5. **Pigmentary retinopathy** is associated with thioridazine in doses above 800 mg/day.

6. **Tardive dyskinesia** (i.e., late onset abnormal involuntary movements) is associated with the long-term use of antipsychotic agents. In many cases, it is irreversible. Vitamin E helps to reduce the symptoms in some cases. If the clinical status of the patient permits, gradual discontinuation of the drug should be considered. **Clozapine** and presumably risperidone, unlike other antipsychotics, do not appear to cause tardive dyskinesia.

7. **Neuroleptic malignant syndrome** has a significant mortality rate and requires immediate discontinuation of antipsychotic medication and intensive support measures. Signs include abnormalities in autonomic function, fever, rigidity, and deterioration in mental status, and laboratory studies usually reveal an elevated serum creatine phosphokinase.

8. An **overdose** of antipsychotic drugs may cause coma, anticholinergic delirium, hypotension, seizures, hypothermia, extrapyramidal reactions, and cardiac arrhythmia.

III. ANTIDEPRESSANT AGENTS

A. General considerations

1. **Depression** is an alteration of mood characterized by sadness or loss of interest or pleasure. It may be a normal reaction to a loss but may also occur spontaneously.
   a. As a psychiatric syndrome, major depression manifests itself in three spheres: **mood alterations** (e.g., dysphoric mood, loss of interest in usual activities, feelings of guilt or self-reproach), **cognitive disturbances** (e.g., impaired concentration, poor memory), and **neurovegetative signs** (e.g., appetite and sleep disturbances, psychomotor agitation or retardation, fatigue). DSM-IV criteria for major depression are found in Table 15-7.
   b. Depressive syndromes vary in severity, and may include psychotic symptoms (e.g., delusions, hallucinations).

2. **Antidepressants** improve mood and other manifestations of the major depressive syndromes. They have minimal value, however, in the short-term management of acute depression, or grief, as a normal emotional response to a loss.

3. **Other treatment modalities**
   a. **Psychotherapy** is also effective in the treatment of depression, especially when a significant loss, real or perceived, is identified. However, psychotherapy alone is less effective in major depressive syndromes in which disturbances of sleep, appetite, and libido are prominent. In these cases, **pharmacotherapy combined with psychotherapy** may be more effective than either modality alone.
   b. **Electroconvulsive therapy (ECT)** may be the most effective treatment approach for patients with severe depression who are unresponsive to antidepressant drugs or who exhibit active suicidal behavior.

B. Classes of drugs. Antidepressants are classified by their mode of action on neurotransmission.

1. **Nonselective monoamine reuptake inhibitors**
   a. **Tricyclic antidepressants** have two benzene rings linked through a central seven-member ring. They are structurally analogous to the tricyclic antipsychotic agents, including phenothiazines and thioxanthenes. Specific drugs include the tertiary amines, imipramine and amitriptyline, and demethylated secondary amines, desipramine and nortriptyline. Other tricyclic antidepressants include doxepin, clomipramine, trimipramine, and protriptyline.
   b. **Heterocyclic antidepressants** are variations on the basic tricyclic structure. These agents include the tetracyclic compound maprotiline, which contains an additional ethylene bridge across the central ring, and the dibenzoxazepine derivative amoxapine, which is structurally similar to loxapine, an antipsychotic drug.
   c. **Triazolopyridines** include trazodone and the newly developed drug nefazodone.

    d. The propiophenone bupropion is not structurally similar to the tricyclic antidepressants. It is a weak inhibitor of serotonin, norepinephrine, and dopamine reuptake.

  2. Selective serotonin reuptake inhibitors (SSRIs) include fluoxetine, sertraline, paroxetine, and fluvoxamine.

  3. Serotonin–norepinephrine reuptake inhibitors include venlafaxine.

  4. Monoamine oxidase inhibitors (MAOIs)
    a. Hydrazide derivatives, which include isocarboxazid and phenelzine
    b. Tranylcypromine, a nonhydrazide that structurally resembles dextroamphetamine

C. **Pharmacology and pharmacokinetics**

  1. Mechanism of therapeutic action. Antidepressants increase the concentration of different monoamines in the synaptic cleft by blocking reuptake mechanisms selectively (SSRIs) or nonselectively, or by inhibiting the degradation of these amines (MAOIs). Some antidepressants have other specific receptor blockade qualities. For example, tertiary amine tricyclics have potent muscarinic and histamine H_1 blockade qualities; nefazodone is a serotonin reuptake inhibitor and potently blocks postsynaptic $5\text{-}HT_2$ receptors; and tranylcypromine is an MAOI and a potent stimulant of norepinephrine release. Therefore, these drugs might reverse a deficiency in central amine neurotransmission. Although these drugs have immediate effects on amine concentrations, **antidepressant effects do not usually emerge until after 2 to 3 weeks of treatment**. Changes in adrenergic receptors appear to parallel the clinical actions of antidepressants.

  2. Special issues with MAOIs. MAOIs irreversibly inhibit the amine-degrading enzyme monoamine oxidase (MAO). An 85% or greater reduction in MAO activity in platelets is associated with therapeutic efficacy. MAOIs interact pharmacologically with many drugs, and can cause serious toxic reactions when combined with narcotic, sedative–hypnotic, anesthetic, stimulant, tricyclic antidepressant, and SSRI agents. They may block the degradation of tyramine from certain aged cheeses, wine, beer, and other foods, and may cause a massive release of stored catecholamines and **hypertensive crisis** after these foods are consumed.

  3. Absorption and elimination
    a. All antidepressants are **well absorbed** from the gastrointestinal tract.
    b. Generally, antidepressants have **long half-lives** and may be metabolized to active compounds by microsomal enzymes.
    c. There is wide individual variation in the efficacy with which MAOIs are inactivated by hepatic acetylation. Even after drug administration is discontinued, sufficient enzyme regeneration to restore normal levels of MAO activity may require 2 weeks or more.

D. **Clinical use**

  1. Therapeutic uses. Antidepressant drugs are clinically used to treat a number of disorders.
    a. All of these agents are effective in **major depression** and the **depressed phase of bipolar illness,** although in the latter case antidepressants may precipitate a switch from depression to mania if an antimanic agent is not being used.
    b. In **major depression with psychotic features,** combined treatment with a tricyclic antidepressant and an antipsychotic agent may be more effective than either agent alone.
    c. Antidepressants are used to treat **panic disorder**. Imipramine is the most studied, but newer antidepressants, such as the SSRIs, appear to be as effective.
    d. Antidepressants with strong affinity toward serotonin reuptake inhibition (e.g., clomipramine, fluoxetine) are particularly effective in the treatment of **obsessive-compulsive disorder**.
    e. The tricyclic antidepressants, particularly imipramine, are used to treat **enuresis**.
    f. MAOIs and imipramine are effective in the treatment of **narcolepsy**.

g. Antidepressants are also effective in some cases of **bulimia, chronic pain,** and **attention deficit disorder**. Protriptyline is useful in the treatment of sleep apnea.

2. Dosage. Antidepressant dosage is **limited by side effects and the clinical response** of the patient.

    a. The **typical daily dose** for most **tricyclic antidepressants** is 100 to 200 mg (less for nortriptyline and much less for protriptyline). Failure to respond to antidepressant therapy often results from inadequate dose or duration (at least 6 weeks) of treatment on a full dose. Divided doses may minimize the side effects early in treatment, but **once-daily dosing,** often at bedtime, is usually feasible because of the long half-life and sedating properties of many of these drugs. Therapeutic blood concentrations are known for the tricyclic antidepressants. This information may be useful for patients who are treated with nortriptyline, which appears to have a well-defined **therapeutic window** (i.e., a range of blood concentrations above and below which less than maximal clinical response occurs).

    b. The **SSRIs** have long half-lives and can be taken **once daily,** usually in the morning because of potential sleep disruption. They usually have a **high therapeutic index**. Fluoxetine may be taken less frequently, especially in the elderly and those who respond well to low doses. A range of therapeutic blood concentrations is not established for use in clinical practice.

    c. The usual **MAOI** dose ranges from 15 to 75 mg daily, depending on the drug. These agents are also usually taken in the morning to minimize sleep disruption.

E. Side effects and toxicity

1. Side effects are related to the receptor blockade and reuptake inhibition involved (Tables 3-1 and 3-3). Side effects are varied and may cause significant problems with patient compliance.

    a. Abrupt discontinuation of agents with significant anticholinergic effects (muscarinic affinity) may cause nausea, diarrhea, and lassitude.

    b. Tricyclic antidepressants have a quinidine-like effect on the heart that may cause conduction delay and arrhythmia, especially at higher doses. Less common side effects include cholestatic jaundice and agranulocytosis.

    c. Trazodone occasionally causes priapism.

    d. The **teratogenic effects** of tricyclic antidepressants are not well established. Most psychotropic drugs pass through the placenta and are secreted in breast milk. The effects of these drugs on CNS development, labor, delivery, and the postnatal period are not well known.

2. Acute poisoning. Tricyclic antidepressants have a **low therapeutic index** and may be toxic in cases of overdose. **Symptoms of overdose** include agitation, anticholinergic delirium, hyperpyrexia, seizures, and coma. Overdose often causes severe cardiac conduction abnormality and arrhythmia. Because of the **risk of suicide in depressed patients,** care must be exercised in prescribing antidepressants. In high-risk cases, a limited amount of medication should be prescribed at one time, a family member might be enlisted to monitor medication, or a drug with a higher therapeutic index (e.g., an SSRI) might be prescribed.

IV. ANTIMANIC AGENTS

A. General considerations

1. Mania is a condition characterized by elevated, expansive, or irritable mood in association with such symptoms as hyperactivity, pressured speech, grandiosity, decreased need for sleep, distractibility, and involvement in potentially self-damaging activities.

2. Manic states. The full manic syndrome is characteristic of **bipolar disorder** (i.e., alternating cycles of elevated and depressed mood, formerly known as manic-depressive

TABLE 3-3. Pharmacologic Properties of Selected Antidepressant Medications

	Maintenance Dose (mg)	Reuptake Inhibition			Receptor Affinity					
		Norepinephrine	Serotonin	Dopamine	Serotonin 5-HT$_2$	Dopamine D$_2$	Histamine H$_1$	Muscarinic M	Adrenergic α_1	Adrenergic α_2
Tricyclic: tertiary amines										
Imipramine	100–200	++	++	–	++	–	++	++	+++	+
Amitriptyline	150–200	++	++	–	++	+	+++	+++	+++	++
Doxepine	75–150	++	+	–	++	–	+++	++	+++	++
Tricyclic: secondary amines										
Desipramine	100–200	+++	+	–	++	–	+	+	++	+
Nortriptyline	75–100	++	+	–	++	–	++	++	++	+
Protriptyline	15–40	+++	+	–	+	–	++	+	++	++
Tetracyclic										
Maprotiline	100–150	++	–	–	+	+	++	+	++	+
Dibenzoxazepine										
Amoxapine	200–300	++	+	–	+++	+	++	+	++	+
Triazolopyridines										
Trazodone	150–400	–	+	–	++	–	+	–	+++	++
Propiophenones										
Bupropion	300	+	+	+	–	–	–	–	+	–
Selective serotonin reuptake inhibitors										
Fluoxetine	20–80	–	+++	–	+	NA	–	–	+	NA
Sertraline	50–200	–	+++	–	NA	NA	NA	NA	NA	NA
Paroxetine	20–50	–	+++	–	NA	NA	NA	NA	NA	NA
Serotonin–norepinephrine reuptake inhibitors										
Venlafaxine	75–375	+++	+++	+	NA	NA	–	–	–	NA

+ = mild; + + = moderate; + + + = strong; – = none; NA = data not available.

illness). Manic symptoms are also seen in other psychiatric illnesses, including **schizophrenia** and some **organic brain syndromes**.

B. **Classes of drugs**

1. **Lithium,** administered as lithium carbonate or lithium citrate, is effective in treating acute mania and controlling the mood swings of bipolar disorder.

2. **Carbamazepine,** an anticonvulsant that is structurally similar to imipramine, is effective as an adjunct or alone in the acute treatment and prophylaxis of manic episodes in patients in whom lithium is ineffective or poorly tolerated.

3. **Valproate** is an anticonvulsant that is used in the prophylaxis of manic episodes.

4. **Antipsychotic drugs** may be especially useful in treating acute mania (see II D 1 b).

5. Less established alternatives in patients with treatment-resistant bipolar disorder include the benzodiazepine anticonvulsant clonazepam and the calcium channel blocker verapamil.

C. **Pharmacology and pharmacokinetics**

1. **Lithium.** The mechanism of action by which lithium stabilizes mood is unknown, but the effect on the inositol phosphate second messenger system is apparently important in its therapeutic efficacy. Lithium is rapidly absorbed gastrointestinally and is primarily excreted by the kidney, where it is reabsorbed in the proximal tubule. The half-life of lithium is 20 to 24 hours.

2. **Carbamazepine.** The mechanism of action by which carbamazepine stabilizes mood is unknown, but it may involve suppression of subseizure threshold electrical kindling activity in the limbic system. Carbamazepine is metabolized by the liver and has a half-life of 12 to 17 hours.

3. **Valproate** appears to suppress the subseizure threshold electrical kindling activity in the limbic system. The presumed mechanism of action is the elevation of GABA levels throughout the brain. Valproate is rapidly absorbed after oral administration and is metabolized in the liver. It has a half-life of 6 to 16 hours.

D. **Clinical use**

1. **Lithium**
   a. **Screening** of leukocyte count, renal function, thyroid function, and cardiac conduction is required before lithium therapy is initiated, and periodically thereafter.
   b. The typical dose of lithium carbonate is 900 to 1500 mg/day, starting with a low dose and gradually increasing to a higher dose. Because the therapeutic index is low, serum lithium concentration must be monitored. A level of 0.9 to 1.5 mEq/L is usually required in the acute phase of bipolar disorder, although a lower serum concentration may be adequate for maintenance treatment.
   c. Although lithium has a **long half-life,** its **low therapeutic index** may necessitate administration in two or three divided doses, often with meals, to mitigate side effects.

2. **Carbamazepine**
   a. **Screening** of serum sodium concentration, blood and platelet counts, hepatic and renal function, and (in vulnerable patients) electrocardiogram (ECG) should be performed before the initiation of therapy and at regular intervals thereafter. The serum carbamazepine level should also be monitored.
   b. Maintenance doses are similar to those in seizure disorders, typically 600 to 1200 mg/day, with the aim of achieving serum levels of 6 to 12 mg/ml. However, the relations of dose to serum level and clinical effects are variable.

3. **Valproate**
   a. **Screening** of renal function, platelet count, and coagulation studies should be performed before the initiation of therapy and at regular intervals thereafter.

    b. Maintenance doses are similar to those used in seizure disorders, typically 750 to 3500 mg/day. A plasma concentration threshold of 50 μg/ml is necessary to obtain adequate response.

E. Side effects and toxicity

  1. Lithium

    a. Early side effects. Common early side effects, even at therapeutic serum concentrations, are nausea, diarrhea, polyuria, and tremor.

    b. Late side effects. Long-term administration of lithium causes several side effects, which may occur even if a therapeutic serum concentration is maintained. These side effects include edema and weight gain. Polydipsia and polyuria also are common. Chronic lithium treatment also may be associated with nephropathy. Renal function should be monitored during long-term treatment. Lithium may also interfere with thyroxine synthesis and lead to hypothyroidism.

    c. Contraindications. Lithium is contraindicated in the presence of significant cardiac conduction abnormalities. Lithium should not be given in the early months of pregnancy because of possible fetal cardiac abnormalities.

    d. Acute toxicity occurs at serum concentrations near 2 mEq/L. It includes slurred speech, drowsiness, coarse tremor, vertigo, and hyperreflexia. Severe toxicity may cause coma and convulsions.

  2. Carbamazepine. Gradual and reversible, but potentially fatal, suppression of bone marrow function rarely occurs. Patients may have easy bruising or fever. A transient mild decrease in neutrophil count is common and does not necessarily require discontinuation of the drug. Dermatologic reactions are also common; they may necessitate discontinuation of the drug. Antidiuretic effects may predispose patients to free-water retention and lead to hyponatremia.

  3. Valproate. Gastrointestinal symptoms (e.g., anorexia, nausea, vomiting) are the most common side effects. Clotting abnormalities and severe hepatic dysfunction rarely occur.

V. ANTIANXIETY AGENTS

A. General considerations

  1. Anxiety may be a normal response to a fear-inducing situation and therefore may require no pharmacologic intervention. Some anxiety is pathological **fear that is out of proportion to any external stimulus**. It is characterized by apprehension and may be accompanied by motor tension and autonomic responses (e.g., tachycardia, diaphoresis, dry mouth, urinary frequency, diarrhea). Endogenous anxiety, which is unprecipitated by external stimuli, usually occurs in anxiety disorders, mood disorders, and schizophrenia.

  2. Anxiety disorders. Symptoms of anxiety occur in several anxiety disorders, including panic disorder, generalized anxiety disorder, obsessive-compulsive disorder, posttraumatic stress disorder, and phobias.

B. Antianxiety agents

  1. Benzodiazepines are the most common drug treatment for anxiety disorders. These agents include alprazolam, chlordiazepoxide, clonazepam, clorazepate, diazepam, flurazepam, lorazepam, oxazepam, prazepam, temazepam, and triazolam. Alprazolam and clonazepam are widely used to treat panic disorder.

  2. Azaspirones. Buspirone, gepirone, and ipsapirone are structurally different from the benzodiazepines. They lack cross-tolerance with them, do not alter the seizure threshold, produce limited sedation, and have no known potential for abuse.

3. Other agents

a. Antihistamines (e.g., diphenhydramine, hydroxyzine) have some antianxiety properties.

b. β-Blockers have some antianxiety properties and are used to treat the autonomic manifestations of anxiety.

c. Of the **antidepressants,** tricyclics and MAOIs are useful in treating panic disorder, and the SSRIs and clomipramine are effective in treating obsessive-compulsive disorder.

d. Barbiturates, especially long-acting forms (e.g., phenobarbital), were used to treat anxiety. Problems of tolerance, dependence, and withdrawal led to diminished use of these drugs. Other barbiturates include amobarbital, mephobarbital, pentobarbital, and secobarbital.

e. Meprobamate, a glycerol derivative, was used widely until it was replaced by benzodiazepines.

C. Pharmacology and pharmacokinetics

1. Mechanism of action

a. The CNS activity of benzodiazepines and barbiturates involves the **facilitation of inhibitory GABA activity.** The two drug groups differ, however, in their ability to affect neuronal membrane ion channels in that barbiturates are more direct GABA agonists, whereas benzodiazepines only increase the affinity of GABA receptors for endogenous GABA.

b. Azaspirones are agonists of the serotonin receptor 5-HT$_{1A}$.

2. Pharmacologic properties

a. Benzodiazepines, meprobamate, and barbiturates share certain antianxiety and sedation properties. All act as hypnotic agents at higher doses. They also suppress rapid eye movement (REM) sleep. Long-term administration of these agents causes the induction of metabolic enzymes.

b. Azaspirones. Buspirone is well tolerated and does not cause drowsiness or impair psychomotor performance. Its anxiolytic effect occurs after approximately 1 week.

3. Absorption, metabolism, and excretion.
The absorption times and half-lives of antianxiety agents vary widely. In addition, some benzodiazepines are metabolized to a succession of active compounds. These drugs vary from short acting (e.g., pentobarbital, triazolam) to long acting (e.g., phenobarbital, diazepam).

D. Clinical use

1. Therapeutic uses

a. Anxiety

(1) **Benzodiazepines.** In the treatment of severe or prolonged anxiety, benzodiazepines are preferred over barbiturates and other agents. Alprazolam is widely used to treat **panic disorder.** Because of their potential for tolerance, habituation, and abuse, benzodiazepines are safest when used for limited periods. Benzodiazepines that act rapidly and produce euphoria (e.g., diazepam, alprazolam) are occasionally abused.

(2) **Buspirone** is safe and efficacious for the treatment of **generalized anxiety disorder**.

(3) Antidepressants and β-blockers are efficacious for the long-term treatment of certain anxiety disorders. They also produce fewer complications than benzodiazepines. Behavioral therapy is helpful in these cases.

b. Depression. Alprazolam and the 5-HT$_{1A}$ agonists, azaspirones, also have antidepressant properties.

c. Other uses. Benzodiazepines also are effective for the control of seizures, the treatment of alcohol withdrawal, and as preoperative medications and intravenous anesthetics. Diazepam is especially effective in the treatment of muscle spasm.

2. Dosage

a. Benzodiazepines vary in potency and typical therapeutic dose. Lower doses usually have antianxiety and sedative properties, and higher doses may be hypnotic. Dosing schedules depend on the half-life of the drug. Short-acting compounds may require several divided doses daily to avoid breakthrough anxiety or symptoms of withdrawal during long-term treatment. The benzodiazepines usually have a high therapeutic index.

   b. Buspirone does not seem to have hypnotic properties. It is given in a divided daily dose of 5 to 30 mg.

E. Side effects and toxicity

   1. **Sedation,** the primary side effect of benzodiazepines and barbiturates, may cause impaired judgment and slow the performance of motor tasks.

   2. **Tolerance,** which may lead to the use of increasing doses and the development of dependence, must be monitored with long-term use of barbiturates, meprobamate, and benzodiazepines. The time course of the development of withdrawal symptoms after a drug is discontinued depends on its half-life. Clonazepam is helpful in preventing the discomfort of benzodiazepine withdrawal because of its long half-life. Azaspirones do not appear to cause tolerance and dependence in humans.

   3. **Overdoses** of barbiturates and meprobamate may cause respiratory arrest, which may be fatal. An oral overdose of benzodiazepines may cause stupor or coma that must be managed medically, but ventilatory assistance is rarely needed. However, the sedative effects of **benzodiazepines in combination with other drugs,** particularly alcohol, may be lethal.

VI. HYPNOTIC AGENTS

A. General considerations

   1. **Insomnia** is the inability to initiate or maintain sleep.

   2. **Hypnotic agents** assist in inducing sleep. Benzodiazepines and barbiturates are sometimes used as hypnotics, although at a somewhat higher dose than that which is effective for treating anxiety. Sedating drugs with rapid absorption and relatively short half-lives are especially effective in this regard.

   3. **Differential diagnosis.** Before hypnotic drugs are used, other disorders associated with insomnia (e.g., nocturnal myoclonus, sleep apnea, chronic obstructive pulmonary disease, and psychiatric disorders) should be excluded.

B. Classes of drugs

   1. **Benzodiazepines.** As in the treatment of anxiety, the use of benzodiazepines (e.g., flurazepam, nitrazepam, temazepam, triazolam) as hypnotics has largely replaced the use of other sedating agents, such as barbiturates.

   2. **Zolpidem** is a newly approved drug that acts through the subunit modulation of the GABA$_a$ receptor.

   3. **Other agents.** Chloral hydrate, a halogenated hydrocarbon, was often used as a hypnotic agent, as were short-acting barbiturates, before the introduction of benzodiazepines. The antihistamine diphenhydramine is also used as a hypnotic agent.

C. Pharmacology and pharmacokinetics

   1. **Mechanism of action.** Hypnotic drugs cause CNS depression that involves not only the reticular activating system (RAS) but also multiple other levels from brain stem to cortex. One possible mode of action is their ability to **potentiate GABA-related inhibition.**

   2. **Pharmacologic properties.** Both barbiturates and benzodiazepines decrease REM and stage 4, or slow-wave, sleep. After long-term use, discontinuation of these agents may cause rebound insomnia. Zolpidem seems to preserve sleep architecture and does not appear to interfere with REM sleep.

3. **Absorption and excretion.** These drugs are well absorbed gastrointestinally and easily cross the blood–brain barrier. Zolpidem has a rapid onset of action. Some benzodiazepines, especially flurazepam and nitrazepam, may be metabolized to active compounds with relatively long half-lives. This activity allows accumulation of these agents and may cause chronic sedation if they are used nightly, particularly in elderly patients or those with hepatic insufficiency. Triazolam is short acting, temazepam is intermediate, and flurazepam is long acting.

D. Clinical use

1. **Therapeutic uses.** Zolpidem and short-acting benzodiazepines are the drugs of choice for the treatment of insomnia. Barbiturates and other hypnotic agents have significant toxicity, overdose lethality, and abuse potential.

2. **Dosage and administration.** The following guidelines should be followed in the clinical use of hypnotic drugs.
   a. The **lowest effective dose** should be used.
   b. **Long-term administration should be avoided.**
   c. **Nonpharmacologic approaches.** Sleep hygiene principles should be taught to patients. These include a regular awakening time, physical exercise early rather than late in the day, no food for 2 hours before going to bed, and using the bed for sleep and sex only.

E. Side effects and toxicity

1. **Oversedation** may occur with large doses of hypnotic drugs. Residual daytime sedation may occur after nighttime use and may cause impaired cognitive and motor performance. Memory loss sometimes occurs after ingestion of the drug. Zolpidem does not cause the memory disturbances that are associated with benzodiazepines.

2. **Dependence** may occur with habitual use, and subsequent discontinuation may cause a withdrawal syndrome.

3. **Rebound insomnia** may also occur after long-term use, particularly with shorter-acting benzodiazepines.

VII. EATING DISORDERS

A. Definition and classification.
Eating disorders involve gross disturbances in eating behavior that usually begin during adolescence. There are two types, **anorexia nervosa** and **bulimia nervosa**. Both types may occur in the same patient. These disorders are much more common in females than in males.

1. Patients with **anorexia nervosa** have an intense fear of being overweight and a distorted body image. They refuse to eat, even when they weigh less than the normal minimum.

2. **Bulimia** involves repeated eating binges, often accompanied by restrictive diets, self-induced vomiting, and the use of laxatives, emetics, or diuretics to maintain or lose weight.

B. Treatment
of eating disorders includes medical assessment, drug therapy, behavioral interventions, and psychotherapy.

1. **Anorexia nervosa.** The primary immediate treatment of anorexia nervosa involves medical management of fluids, electrolytes, and nutritional status combined with structured behavior modification programs. These programs often require inpatient treatment: Long-term treatment emphasizes the medical status of the patient, regular educational counseling by a dietician, and individual or group psychotherapy.

2. **Bulimia** treatment also involves medical management, cognitive therapy, and behavior modification. Drug therapy with SSRIs, tricyclic antidepressants, or MAOIs is effective in some patients.

VIII. PSYCHOPHARMACOLOGY IN CHILDREN AND ADOLESCENTS

A. General considerations

1. **Psychiatric symptoms in children** are often confused with behavior related to a developmental stage. The diagnoses of depression, anxiety, psychosis, and other general psychiatric problems are often difficult to establish because symptoms may appear indirectly as abnormal behavior (e.g., acting out behavior, substance abuse, poor school performance, impaired social interactions).

2. **Special considerations in children and adolescents**
   a. **Rates of absorption, metabolism, and excretion** may be significantly different in children compared with adults. Adult doses may not simply be converted by weight to determine appropriate doses for children. For example, renal clearance and hepatic metabolism are typically higher in children than in adults.
   b. **The ability of a child to accept and respond to a drug** is closely related to the child's level of psychosocial development and the family's attitude toward the use of the medication.
   c. **The long-term effects** of psychotropic drugs on psychological development as well as the development of the enzyme, neurotransmitter, and endocrine systems in children are unknown.

B. Mood disorders

1. **Depression**
   a. **Symptoms.** Prepubertal children who are depressed often exhibit somatic symptoms and agitated behavior. Older children usually exhibit social withdrawal, difficulty in school, sensitivity to rejection, anxiety, and aggressive or oppositional behavior.
   b. **Treatment.** SSRIs are used to treat depression in children. Tricyclic antidepressants, especially imipramine, are also used. Low starting doses are used, and serum concentrations are monitored in patients who do not respond to drug therapy. Side effects are described in III E.

2. **Mania**
   a. **Symptoms.** Adolescents and children with bipolar illness may exhibit cyclic expansiveness, impulsiveness, aggressiveness, or antisocial behavior, rather than the typical manic symptoms.
   b. **Treatment.** Lithium salts are used to treat mania in children and adolescents. Carbamazepine is used occasionally in adolescents. Side effects are described in IV E 1 a–d.

C. Psychosis

1. **Indications.** Antipsychotic drugs are used to treat schizophrenia, pervasive developmental disorders (such as autism), aggressive conduct disorders, and Tourette's syndrome.

2. **Side effects.** Children experience the full range of antipsychotic drug side effects. Sedation and weight gain are common. Children are also at risk for tardive dyskinesia.

D. Attention deficit hyperactivity disorder (ADHD)

1. **Clinical description.** ADHD was formerly referred to as hyperkinetic syndrome, hyperactivity, and minimal brain dysfunction. ADHD is characterized by an inability to focus attention that is manifested by distractibility, poor concentration, and impulsiveness. The disorder may be accompanied by motor hyperactivity.

2. Treatment

    a. Stimulants (e.g., methylphenidate, dextroamphetamine, pemoline) are used to treat ADHD. In most cases, these drugs decrease motor activity and increase attention span. In patients who are unresponsive to stimulants, tricyclic antidepressants may be effective. Side effects of stimulants include headache, nausea, anorexia, insomnia, and a decrease in the rate of growth. Because of the potential for abuse, adolescents who are given stimulants and sedatives should be monitored. Barbiturates and other sedatives may cause paradoxical excitement in patients with ADHD.

    b. Dietary manipulations do not appear effective in the control of ADHD.

    c. Additional nonpharmacologic treatment measures that may be effective in ADHD include psychotherapy, family therapy, behavior modification, and special educational approaches.

E. **Enuresis**

1. Definition. Enuresis is repeated involuntary urination, not caused by a physical disorder, after the age of 5 years.

2. Treatment involves medical and behavioral approaches. Before drug therapy is initiated, physical disorders (e.g., infection, urinary tract structural abnormalities, diabetes mellitus) must be excluded. The drug of choice is imipramine, although other tricyclic antidepressants are also effective in decreasing the frequency of enuresis. The most common side effects of imipramine in children are irritability, insomnia, and nightmares. Abrupt discontinuation of tricyclic antidepressants may cause excess cholinergic activity. Behavioral therapy is helpful in conjunction with drug treatment.

F. **Anxiety disorders**

1. School phobia and panic disorder in children may be a manifestation of separation anxiety. If psychotherapeutic and behavior modification techniques are unsuccessful, these disorders may respond to antidepressants.

2. Obsessive-compulsive disorder in children and adolescents often responds to treatment with SSRIs and clomipramine. Psychotherapy and behavior modification techniques are important adjuncts to drug therapy.

G. **Aggressiveness and impulsiveness**

1. The physician should consider psychosocial factors and the possibility that aggressiveness and impulsiveness are manifestations of another underlying disorder.

2. In severe cases, pharmacologic treatment includes β-blockers, lithium, carbamazepine, valproate, and antipsychotic medication.

IX. PSYCHOPHARMACOLOGY IN THE ELDERLY

A. **General considerations**

1. Pharmacokinetics. The elderly have slower metabolism and excretion rates as well as a different distribution volume than younger patients. These differences lead to **increased blood and tissue concentrations** after a given drug dose.

2. Toxicity. The elderly may also be more vulnerable to the side effects of psychopharmacologic agents (e.g., disorientation, urinary retention, cardiovascular effects), even at concentrations that are therapeutic in younger individuals (Table 3-1).

B. **Dementia**

1. Tacrine, a reversible cholinesterase inhibitor, improves cognitive functioning in some patients with Alzheimer's disease. Nimodipine, a calcium channel blocker, may be useful in the treatment of Alzheimer's dementia. Cerebrovasodilators and stimulants have a modest effect on emotional and social interactive variables. Agitation and confusion are common side effects of these stimulants.

2. **Psychotic symptoms** and behavioral agitation may improve with administration of a high-potency, less sedating antipsychotic drug, such as haloperidol. Lithium, β-blockers, and carbamazepine may help to prevent aggressive outbursts.

C. Other disorders

1. **Depression** in elderly patients may be accompanied by cognitive impairment known as pseudodementia. Treatment with an antidepressant agent may be indicated, although close monitoring for excessive sedation, hypotension, and anticholinergic side effects is necessary.

2. **Anxiety.** Benzodiazepines, specifically those with long half-lives, should be used with caution in the elderly because they impair cognitive and motor performance. In some cases, this effect leads to a toxic, confusional state. In this age group, buspirone is an alternative drug for the treatment of generalized anxiety disorders, and β-blockers can be used to treat episodic anxiety with peripheral manifestations or aggressive behavior.

X. DRUGS OF ABUSE

A. General considerations

1. **Drug abuse** involves a pattern of pathologic use of a substance, either prescription or nonprescription, that causes personal distress or social or occupational impairment. Drug abuse may cause or exacerbate other medical disorders. For example, sharing of needles by intravenous drug abusers is a significant mode of transmission of the human immunodeficiency virus (HIV).

2. **Drug dependence** involves the development of tolerance, the requirement for increasing amounts of a substance to achieve a given effect, and the presence of a specific syndrome, known as withdrawal, after discontinuation of the drug. This withdrawal syndrome may be accompanied by a continuing subjective desire for the drug. Animal models show that, even in the absence of physical dependence, drugs of abuse are strong reinforcers for continuing self-administration. Street drugs [e.g., phencyclidine (PCP)] are rarely pure.

B. Alcohol

1. Alcohol is used by approximately two-thirds of the adult population in the United States. The effects that are sought by users of alcohol include a sense of relaxation, euphoria, relief of anxiety or depression, and disinhibition of emotions.

2. Long-term alcohol abuse may lead to medical complications (e.g., hepatic dysfunction, malnutrition, myopathy, peripheral neuropathy, encephalopathic syndromes).

3. In individuals who are dependent on alcohol, withdrawal may cause a tremulous syndrome, seizures, hallucinosis, or delirium tremens. Benzodiazepines reduce the discomfort and diminish the medical complications of withdrawal because of their effects on the GABA receptors.

4. **Disulfiram** is given to patients with a history of alcohol abuse to help them to maintain sobriety. This agent alters the metabolism of alcohol, producing high concentrations of acetaldehyde. If an individual who is taking disulfiram ingests alcohol, a potentially dangerous reaction occurs because of the increased concentrations of acetaldehyde. The reaction is characterized by flushing, headache, nausea, and hypotension.

C. **Sedative hypnotic agents**

1. Abuse of barbiturates, benzodiazepines, and related drugs may vary from episodic intoxication to long-term use accompanied by dependence.

2. **Cross-dependence** occurs between these drugs and alcohol. Therefore, one drug may be substituted for another to ameliorate the effects of withdrawal. Abusers of alcohol or sedative–hypnotics may therefore misuse several drugs from this class.

3. **Withdrawal** from sedative–hypnotic drugs resembles withdrawal from alcohol.
   a. Symptoms range from tremor, mood lability, weakness, anxiety, irritability, and insomnia to delirium and seizures. In a drug with a long half-life (e.g., diazepam), withdrawal symptoms, including seizures, may not occur until several days after the drug is discontinued.
   b. Because of cross-dependence, symptoms of withdrawal from any sedative–hypnotic drug, including alcohol, may be alleviated by the administration of a gradual tapering equivalent dose of another long-acting sedative–hypnotic agent (e.g., chlordiazepoxide, clonazepam).

D. **Opioid drugs.** Patterns of use, degree of social and occupational impairment, and accompanying medical complications vary among opioid abusers.

1. **Agents and their effects**
   a. **Opioids** are ingested either orally or intravenously. Dependence involves naturally occurring compounds and synthetic drugs. Opioid drugs include heroin, morphine, methadone, codeine, and related compounds.
   b. These substances are analgesics, and they blunt sensory awareness. They also cause euphoria and sedation. High doses cause decreased respiratory drive.

2. **Withdrawal**
   a. Untreated **opioid withdrawal** causes a syndrome marked by yawning, piloerection, lacrimation, rhinorrhea, sweating, nausea, vomiting, diarrhea, abdominal cramps, and hypertension. Although unpleasant, this withdrawal syndrome is not as dangerous as that produced by barbiturates and benzodiazepines, and may be mitigated by clonidine administration or a tapering dose of methadone.
   b. **Cross-dependence** occurs among opioids. For example, a patient who is dependent on heroin may be given a maintenance dose of oral methadone or may be slowly withdrawn from heroin by the administration of a tapering dose of a long-acting opiate. Methadone and the related drug L-alpha-acetyl-methadol (LAAM) are used to treat opiate dependence. LAAM seems to have a longer half-life and will likely be easier to use in detoxification than methadone. Withdrawal symptoms may also be mitigated by the use of clonidine.
   c. In a dependent patient, the administration of an opioid antagonist, such as naloxone or naltrexone, which is available in an oral form, produces an immediate withdrawal syndrome that lasts approximately 2 hours.

3. **Overdose.** The characteristic symptoms of opioid overdose are pinpoint pupils, depressed respiration, and coma.

E. **Stimulant drugs**

1. **Agents and their effects**
   a. The most commonly abused stimulants are sympathomimetic drugs such as cocaine, amphetamine, and related compounds. Crack and freebase cocaine are potent, fast-acting cocaine derivatives that are ignited and inhaled.
   b. Although stimulants were once used medically to decrease appetite or combat drowsiness and fatigue, constraints have been placed on prescribing them. Abuse tends to occur in individuals seeking elevation of mood.
   c. The **CNS activity** of sympathomimetic drugs involves CNS amines, particularly dopamine and norepinephrine. For example, amphetamine appears to stimulate the release of dopamine and norepinephrine from presynaptic terminals, whereas cocaine blocks dopamine reuptake.

2. Tolerance to some effects of these drugs occurs. Withdrawal from stimulants may cause depressed mood, fatigue, sleep disturbance, and hyperphagia.

3. Medical complications include arrhythmia, hypertension, seizures, and pulmonary and nasal damage from insufflated drug.

4. Treatment of addiction and intoxication
   a. Bromocriptine (a dopamine agonist) and antidepressants (e.g., desipramine) may reduce the craving for cocaine in dependent individuals.
   b. High-potency antipsychotic drugs (e.g., haloperidol) are used to treat psychosis and agitation caused by amphetamine intoxication and the paranoid states that can follow intoxication.

F. **Hallucinogenic drugs**

1. Agents and their effects
   a. Hallucinogenic drugs cause dramatically altered perceptions, thought processes, and emotional states. Some individuals experience illusions (distortions of real stimuli) or hallucinations.
   b. Several groups of drugs have hallucinogenic properties:
      (1) Indolealkylamines, including lysergic acid diethylamide (LSD), dimethyltryptamine (DMT), and psilocybin
      (2) Phenylethylamines, including mescaline and 2,5-dimethoxy-4-ethylamphetamine (DOM, or STP).
      (3) Arylcyclohexylamines, primarily PCP

2. The **activity** of LSD-like compounds occurs at presynaptic serotonin receptors. PCP was initially developed as an anesthetic, but it has mixed analgesic, stimulant, depressant, and hallucinogenic properties. PCP may cause belligerence, assaultiveness, impulsiveness, and neurologic dysfunction characterized by nystagmus, dysarthria, and ataxia.

3. These drugs are used episodically. Therefore, although tolerance to their effects may develop, physical dependence and withdrawal syndromes are not common. They produce severe psychotic symptoms during intoxication and may also cause long-term cognitive impairment and psychiatric syndromes.

G. **MDMA, MDEA, and MDA.** 3,4-Methylenedioxymethamphetamine (MDMA, or ecstasy, or X), 3,4-methylenedioxyethamphetamine (MDEA, or Eve), and 3,4-methylenedioxyamphetamine (MDA) cause euphoria and enhanced sociability, but are apparently not hallucinogenic. The potential toxicity of these drugs is not known, but animal studies suggest that they may selectively damage serotonin nerve terminals.

H. **Cannabis (marijuana),** a drug derived from the hemp plant, contains a large number of cannabinoid compounds. Tetrahydrocannabinol (THC) is believed to be the primary active compound. The drug is usually self-administered by smoking.

1. Pharmacologic effects of THC
   a. Low doses induce a feeling of well-being, drowsiness, altered sensory and time perception, and impairment of short-term memory and complex motor function, such as that required for driving.
   b. Higher doses cause anxiety, hallucinations, delusions, paranoia, confusion, and depersonalization.
   c. Cardiovascular effects include tachycardia, increased supine blood pressure, and decreased standing blood pressure.

2. Tolerance develops with long-term use, and abstinence may cause withdrawal symptoms that include irritability, insomnia, anxiety, and anorexia.

3. Adverse effects of long-term use include an amotivational syndrome that is characterized by apathy and cognitive impairment. Smoking may also cause bronchitis and bronchospasm.

I. **Tobacco.** Although many gases and particles are contained in cigarette smoke, nicotine appears to be primarily responsible for the reinforcement of tobacco smoking. There is a higher than expected incidence of cigarette smoking among patients with chronic schizophrenia and major depression.

1. **Pharmacologic effects** of nicotine are paradoxical. They include an alerting response, with increased attention and memory, and skeletal muscle relaxation and decreased irritability.

2. Tobacco smoking increases the metabolism of antipsychotics and, conversely, quitting can lead to increased serum levels of these drugs if dosage is not adjusted.

3. **Long-term tobacco use** is linked to a number of diseases, including cardiac and peripheral vascular disease and cancer of the lung, oropharynx, and bladder.

4. **Tolerance** develops to nicotine, and tobacco withdrawal is associated with anxiety, irritability, impaired concentration, headache, and drowsiness. Nicotine, delivered by patch or gum, and clonidine may relieve withdrawal symptoms.

J. **Caffeine** is a methylxanthine compound that is found in several beverages, including coffee, tea, cocoa, and cola drinks. It is also included in many nonprescription drugs that are sold as stimulants.

1. **Pharmacologic effects** of caffeine include CNS stimulation, diuresis, cardiac stimulation, and smooth muscle relaxation.

2. **Caffeine intoxication** causes restlessness, agitation, insomnia, flushing, gastrointestinal disturbance, diuresis, muscle twitching, cardiac arrhythmia, and rambling speech.

3. **Physical dependence** is not well documented, but tolerance and psychological dependence occur with long-term use of caffeine-containing beverages.

XI. **BEHAVIORAL EFFECTS OF NONPSYCHIATRIC DRUGS.** Some nonpsychiatric medications have psychiatric side effects. Such drug effects should be considered in every patient who presents with behavioral changes.

A. **Cardiovascular drugs**

1. **Antihypertensive drugs,** especially reserpine, methyldopa, and propranolol, may cause depression.

2. Low doses of **digitalis** may cause weakness, apathy, and anorexia. Toxicity may occur at near-therapeutic blood levels, especially in the elderly. Patients exhibit delirium with hallucinations.

3. The **antiarrhythmic agents** quinidine, lidocaine, and procainamide may cause confusion and delirium.

4. **Calcium channel inhibitors,** including verapamil, nifedipine, and diltiazem, may cause depression.

B. **Anticholinergic drugs**

1. Many nonprescription drugs used to treat colds, motion sickness, and insomnia include anticholinergic agents that may cause drowsiness, impaired concentration, blurred vision, and dry mouth.

2. In higher doses, anticholinergic agents such as atropine and scopolamine may cause **toxic delirium** accompanied by fever and decreased sweating.

C. **Antimicrobial drugs**

1. The **antibacterial agents** nalidixic acid and nitrofurantoin may cause headache, drowsiness, and confusional states.

2. The **antitubercular drugs** isoniazid, iproniazid, and cycloserine may cause confusion, delusions, hallucinations, and delirium.

D. **Analgesic and anti-inflammatory drugs**

1. High doses of the analgesic agents propoxyphene and pentazocine may cause acute psychotic states. These drugs are also associated with the development of physical dependence.

2. The anti-inflammatory drug indomethacin may cause depression or, in rare cases, acute psychosis.

E. **Hormones**

1. Long-term treatment with **corticosteroids** and dose changes in either direction may cause depression. These agents also cause confusion, mania, delusions, and hallucinations in some patients.

2. **Oral contraceptives** often cause depression. Estrogen may augment the mood-elevating effects of tricyclic antidepressants. Occasionally, treatment with or withdrawal from oral contraceptives causes psychosis, especially in patients with a history of a psychotic disorder.

3. **Thyroid hormones** may cause anxiety, agitation, or symptoms of mania. In some patients with depression that does not respond to treatment, these agents are useful adjuncts to antidepressants.

F. **Dopaminergic drugs**

1. Drugs that increase CNS dopamine activity, including L-dopa, which is a precursor of dopamine, and bromocriptine, which is a dopamine receptor agonist, are used to treat Parkinson's disease.

2. Behavioral side effects are common with prolonged therapy. They include depression, euphoria, restlessness, hyperactivity, confusion, delirium, and dyskinesia.

G. **Antiemetic drugs.** Metoclopramide and phenothiazines may cause extrapyramidal symptoms (e.g., parkinsonism, akathisia, acute dystonia).

H. **Miscellaneous agents**

1. Theophylline, terbutaline, and albuterol may cause anxiety, agitation, and confusion.

2. Disulfiram inhibits dopamine β-hydroxylase activity and may cause depression, catatonia, psychosis, or delirium, even in the absence of interaction with alcohol.

3. Cimetidine and H_2 receptor antagonists used to treat peptic ulcer disease may cause depression, psychosis, and delirium.

4. Diphenhydramine and hydroxyzine frequently cause drowsiness.

5. Phenylephrine and phenylpropanolamine may cause agitation, anxiety, and psychosis.

XII. PRINCIPLES OF PRESCRIBING

A. **Informing the patient**

1. **Informed consent.** As with any medical procedure, when a drug is prescribed the physician should explain both the expected benefits and the potential side effects.

2. Patient noncompliance is a common cause of failure to respond to a prescribed drug regimen. Noncompliance may involve failure to take a drug or misuse of the drug. Several factors contribute to noncompliance.

    a. The physician may not explain both the nature of the disorder and the rationale for prescribing a specific drug.

    b. Outpatients, particularly if they are elderly or live alone, are much less likely to comply with a prescription than patients in a hospital setting.

    c. Side effects often lead to noncompliance, especially in patients who are not fully informed.

    d. Simple regimens, specifically once-daily dosing when pharmacokinetic factors allow it, facilitate compliance.

B. **Placebo effects**

  1. Nonspecific placebo effects (i.e., responses other than those caused by the pharmacologic properties of the drug) occur even when a patient is taking an active medication.

  2. These nonspecific effects may be positive or negative. They are affected by the quality of the physician–patient relationship and the expectations that the physician and patient have for the drug.

C. **Drug interactions.** Drugs can interact in beneficial or adverse ways. All drugs that the patient is taking, including nonprescription agents, must be considered before a new drug is prescribed. Drugs can have pharmacokinetic and pharmacodynamic interactions.

  1. An example of a **pharmacodynamic interaction** is the reduction of tremor and rigidity, which are common side effects of antipsychotic drugs, with the addition of an anticholinergic drug such as benztropine to the patient's regimen.

  2. A pharmokinetic interaction involves the effect of one drug on the plasma concentration of another drug. For example, it is necessary to lower a dose of haloperidol after the introduction of fluoxetine due to a **pharmacokinetic interaction**.

D. **Individualization of treatment**

  1. Basis of treatment. The decision to prescribe a specific dose of a specific drug depends on the physiologic and psychological characteristics of the patient.

    a. An **accurate diagnosis** is crucial. In psychiatry, a longitudinal, rather than a cross-sectional, view of the patient is often necessary. Medical disorders that cause psychiatric symptoms must also be excluded.

    b. Important **physiologic parameters** include patient age, weight, and cardiovascular, hepatic, and renal status. Other drugs that the patient is taking should be determined as well.

    c. A **patient's attitude** toward a drug may be influenced by past experience and by the patient's understanding of and reaction to illness.

  2. Frequent reevaluation of a prescribed regimen in terms of both therapeutic response and adverse reactions is crucial. Large prescriptions and frequent renewal without close monitoring should be avoided.

STUDY QUESTIONS

DIRECTIONS: Each of the numbered items or incomplete statements in this section is followed by answers or by completions of the statement. Select the ONE lettered answer or completion that is BEST in each case.

1. A 35-year-old cook with a 10-year-history of intravenous heroin abuse decides to stop using heroin by going "cold turkey." The most common withdrawal symptom is

(A) respiratory depression
(B) pinpoint pupils
(C) seizures
(D) piloerection and sweating
(E) hypotension

2. What is the initial management of insomnia that is not complicated by any other psychiatric or medical problem?

(A) Initiating treatment with zolpidem
(B) Advising the patient to exercise regularly at night
(C) Advising the patient to consume a small amount of alcohol before going to bed
(D) Teaching the patient basic principles of sleep hygiene
(E) Prescribing a low dose of a sedating antidepressant

DIRECTIONS: Each of the numbered items or incomplete statements in this section is negatively phrased, as indicated by a capitalized word such as NOT, LEAST, or EXCEPT. Select the ONE lettered answer or completion that is BEST in each case.

3. Basic principles to follow when prescribing medications include the following EXCEPT

(A) individualization of treatment
(B) informing the patient of potential side effects
(C) noting potential interactions with other drugs the patient is taking
(D) providing multiple refills for convenience
(E) considering the likelihood of nonspecific placebo effects

4. Psychotropic medications affect the following steps in neurotransmission EXCEPT

(A) neurotransmitter reuptake
(B) postsynaptic receptor blockade
(C) induction of liver enzymes
(D) presynaptic receptor blockade
(E) neurotransmitter release

5. In a 30-year-old man with chronic schizophrenia, treatment is changed from administration of haloperidol to administration of the atypical antipsychotic drug clozapine. Which of the following side effects will probably NOT occur with clozapine?

(A) Extrapyramidal symptoms
(B) Constipation
(C) Weight gain
(D) Sedation
(E) Agranulocytosis

6. Which of the following drugs is NOT effective in the treatment of anxiety disorders?

(A) Trifluoperazine
(B) Buspirone
(C) Propranolol
(D) Alprazolam
(E) Imipramine

7. The following psychotropic medications require regular blood monitoring EXCEPT

(A) clozapine
(B) lorazepam
(C) lithium
(D) valproate
(E) carbamazepine

8. A 75-year-old woman living in a nursing home exhibits profound deterioration in mental status over 3 days. Her current mental status is characterized by somnolence alternating with agitation, rambling incoherent speech, disorientation, and inability to focus attention. Which of the following medications is LEAST likely to be responsible for the patient's mental deterioration?

(A) Amitryptyline
(B) Temazepam
(C) Quinidine
(D) Oxybutynin
(E) Buspirone

9. Common side effects in a patient who has bipolar disorder and a therapeutic blood concentration of lithium include the following EXCEPT

(A) diarrhea
(B) tremor
(C) drowsiness
(D) polydipsia
(E) weight gain

10. Important factors to consider when prescribing medications to children and adolescents include the following EXCEPT

(A) higher renal clearance
(B) the child's level of psychosocial development
(C) the family's attitude toward the use of medications
(D) higher hepatic metabolism rates
(E) the child's birth order

ANSWERS AND EXPLANATIONS

1. The answer is D [X D 2 a–c]. Typical symptoms of opioid withdrawal include piloerection, or gooseflesh, chilling, sweating, pupillary dilation, diarrhea, nausea and vomiting, muscle aches, lacrimation, rhinorrhea, yawning, and insomnia. The expression "cold turkey" derives from the characteristic skin appearance during abrupt withdrawal. Hypertension is common in withdrawal, and is transient. Seizures are not common in opioid withdrawal, and pinpoint pupils are seen with opioid overdose.

2. The answer is D [VI A 3, D 1–2]. After psychiatric or medical problems that might interfere with sleep are excluded, the patient should be taught the principles of sleep hygiene. These principles include a regular awakening time, physical exercise early rather than late in the day, no food for 2 hours before going to bed, and using the bed for sleep and sex only. Medication should be used only after careful assessment of the patient's status and a good trial of these techniques. Patients often use alcohol to induce sleep, but it tends to disrupt sleep architecture and cause rebound insomnia.

3. The answer is D [XII A–D]. The basic principles that should be followed in prescribing any medication include individualization of treatment, informing the patient of the benefits and risks of the treatment and of withholding treatment, and consideration of drug–drug interactions and the nonspecific placebo effects that any treatment might carry. Although providing multiple refills to the patient once the proper dose and response are established should be considered if the patient is deemed reliable, it should never be done solely for convenience.

4. The answer is C [I B 3]. Psychotropic medications act on one or more of the steps involved in neurotransmission in the central nervous system (CNS). They might act by affecting the neurotransmitter, receptor, or both. Some drugs induce or suppress liver enzymes (e.g., carbamazepine and valproate, respectively) and have an indirect effect on their own, and other, plasma drug concentrations. However, this effect is not a mechanism of action of a drug.

5. The answer is A [II A 2, E 1, 2]. Extrapyramidal side effects are not associated with the atypical antipsychotics. The typical antipsychotics commonly cause parkinsonism, akathisia, and dystonia (hence the name, neuroleptics). Constipation, weight gain, and sedation occur with the use of all antipsychotic medications and are a function of the specific receptor blockade involved. Clozapine, an atypical antipsychotic agent, causes agranulocytosis in a small percentage of patients. This condition necessitates weekly monitoring of leukocyte count.

6. The answer is A [II D 1 c, E 1; V B 3 b, D 1 a (1)–(2)]. Antipsychotic medications (e.g., trifluoperazine) are poor antianxiety medications. They may cause akathisia, which is a severe subjective sense of restlessness. Buspirone, an azaspirone antianxiety agent, has established efficacy in the treatment of generalized anxiety disorder. Propranolol, a β-blocker, is helpful in managing the autonomic manifestations of anxiety. Alprazolam, a benzodiazepine antianxiety agent, and imipramine, a tricyclic antidepressant agent, are effective in the treatment of panic disorder.

7. The answer is B [II E 2; IV E 1–3; V E 3]. The benzodiazepines do not usually cause long-term effects in the liver, kidneys, bone marrow, or thyroid. They also have a wide therapeutic margin and therefore are relatively safe in case of an overdose. If another central nervous system (CNS) depressant is added, however, the combination can be lethal because the respiratory center is suppressed. Clozapine causes agranulocytosis in some patients. This condition necessitates weekly leukocyte counts. Lithium has a narrow therapeutic window; therefore, monitoring serum lithium concentrations is an important safety precaution. Valproate occasionally causes severe hepatic dysfunction and clotting abnormalities. Carbamazepine sometimes causes bone marrow suppression, which necessitates monitoring of blood count.

8. The answer is E [III E 1; V B 2; IX A 1–2; XI A 3, B 1]. The elderly are particularly vulnerable to psychiatric side effects of medications, even at blood concentrations that are therapeutic in young, healthy patients. Agents with anticholinergic properties (e.g., amitriptyline, an antidepressant, and oxybutynin, an anticholinergic drug used to treat incontinence) may cause toxic delirium at therapeutic doses in vulnerable patients. In the elderly, drowsiness and confusion are common side effects of sedating agents, such as the benzodiazepine temazepam. Quinidine and other antiarrhythmic drugs may cause confusion and delirium in vulnerable patients. In the elderly, buspirone, a new antianxiety agent that acts through the serotonin receptor 5-HT$_{1A}$, seems to be safer than similar agents. In general, polypharmacy, or the prescribing of multiple drugs, should be avoided to minimize side effects and drug interactions.

9. The answer is C [IV E 1 a–c]. Common side effects of lithium, even at therapeutic blood concentrations, include nausea and diarrhea, fine tremor, polydipsia, polyuria, weight gain, and edema. Long-term use may cause hypothyroidism, possibly as a result of impaired

synthesis of thyroxine. Toxic blood concentrations may cause coarse tremor, slurred speech, confusion, seizure, and cardiac arrhythmia.

10. The answer is E [VIII A 2 a–c]. Several points should be considered when prescribing medications to children and adolescents. Renal clearance and hepatic metabolism are typically higher in children than in adults. The child's ability to accept and respond to a drug is closely related to the specific level of psychosocial development of that child and to the family's attitude toward the use of the medication. The long-term effects of psychotropic drugs on psychological development as well as the development of enzyme, neurotransmitter, and endocrine systems in children are unknown. Although studies show that birth order affects certain personality traits, no pharmacokinetic effects are known.

Chapter 4

Genetics of Behavioral Disorders

Nancy A. Breslin
Dilip V. Jeste

I. BASIC PRINCIPLES OF HUMAN GENETICS

A. Genes and chromosomes

1. **Genes** are specific **self-reproducing segments of a chromosome that are responsible for a certain trait or function**.
   a. **Structure**
      (1) Genes are composed of **deoxyribonucleic acid (DNA),** which in turn is composed of regularly alternating chains of phosphates and deoxyribose sugars to which pairs of bases are attached. Genes are considered to be specific discrete sequences of nucleotides within the DNA strand in a given chromosome.
      (2) The particular location of a gene on a chromosome is known as that gene's **locus**. Different forms of a gene that can be found at the same locus are called **alleles**.
   b. **Functional types.** Genes may be subdivided into three functionally different types.
      (1) **Structural genes** code for the specific amino acid sequence in peptides and proteins.
      (2) **Operator genes** interact with substances known as **repressors,** and this interaction controls the activity of structural genes.
      (3) **Regulator genes** modulate the synthesis of repressor substances.

2. **Chromosomes** are structures visible under light microscopy that carry the genes arranged in a characteristic order.
   a. **Structure.** Chromosomes consist of linear strands of DNA and proteins called **histones**.
   b. **Normal human karyotype**
      (1) In humans, there are **23 pairs of chromosomes,** including **22 pairs of autosomes** and **1 pair of sex chromosomes**. The two chromosomes in each pair are similar in structure and position and are termed **homologous**.
      (2) The **sex chromosomes** in males include one X and one Y chromosome, whereas in females, there are two X chromosomes. The **Lyon hypothesis** states that one X chromosome in the female condenses in the embryonic stage of development and appears as a **Barr body** or **sex chromatin**.

3. **Chromosomal disorders.** Some diseases have been shown to be associated with specific chromosomal abnormalities.
   a. **Types**
      (1) In some cases an extra chromosome exists, usually the result of **nondisjunction,** in which the paired chromosomes fail to separate during meiosis.
      (2) In other cases, there is a **deletion,** resulting in the absence of a whole chromosome or part of it.
      (3) Abnormalities also can occur through the process of **translocation,** in which a part of one chromosome becomes attached to another, so that gene replication occurs without an increase in chromosomal number.
   b. **Examples**
      (1) **Down syndrome** is characterized by short stature, mental retardation, and facial abnormalities. Two different types of Down syndrome exist and appear to be identical clinically.

       (a) Usually, Down syndrome results from the presence of three copies of chromosome 21 (**trisomy 21**). This type of Down syndrome is more common in the offspring of older mothers.

       (b) In some cases, Down syndrome is associated with a **translocation of chromosome 21,** which is then attached to chromosome 15. This type of Down syndrome occurs independent of the mother's age.

   (2) **Other trisomy conditions,** including trisomies 8, 13, 14, 15, 18, and 22, also are associated with facial abnormalities and mental retardation.

   (3) **Klinefelter syndrome** is characterized by a male phenotype with infertility, small testes, behavioral disturbances, and a eunuchoid appearance. This syndrome is associated with an **XXY configuration of sex chromosomes**. The autosomes are normal. A Barr body is present.

   (4) **Turner syndrome** is associated with a female phenotype, short stature, webbed neck, gonadal dysgenesis, and sterility. It is associated with a missing X chromosome (an **XO genotype**) and no Barr body.

   (5) **Cri-du-chat syndrome** is characterized by severe mental retardation, hypertelorism (widely separated eyes), microcephaly, and a cat-like cry. This syndrome results from a deletion of the short arm of chromosome 5.

B. **Terminology used in clinical genetics**

  1. Genotype and phenotype
    a. Genotype refers to the **genetic makeup** of a particular individual, usually at a specific locus.
    b. Phenotype refers to the **observable structural and functional characteristics** resulting from the interaction of the individual's genetic constitution with environmental influences.

  2. Genocopy and phenocopy are terms used in reference to individuals who phenotypically resemble one another.
    a. The resemblance in **genocopy** is due to having the same genes.
    b. In the case of **phenocopy,** an individual has the features of a genetic disorder without any evidence that genes are responsible (e.g., there is no family history of the disorder, or genetic markers are not present).

  3. Heritability is a measure of the degree of influence of the genotype on the phenotype. Thus, the heritability of a given disease is the extent (usually expressed as a percentage) to which the individual risk of acquiring that disease is due to inherited factors.
    a. Heritable versus congenital conditions
      (1) **Not all congenital** (present at birth) **conditions are heritable**. For example, congenital hydrocephalus results from a variety of causes, only some of which are genetic.
      (2) **Not all heritable conditions are congenital.** For instance, signs of Huntington disease (an autosomal dominant disorder) usually do not appear until the third or fourth decade of life.
    b. Familial refers to conditions that aggregate in families. The fact that a condition is familial **suggests but does not confirm** that the cause is genetic. This is because families share many things in addition to genes (e.g., diet, level of stress, child-rearing practices).

  4. Penetrance is a measure of the frequency (usually expressed as a percentage) with which a specific genetic trait appears in the phenotype of individuals carrying the responsible gene. For example, it appears that everyone carrying the gene for Huntington disease eventually manifests the disorder; therefore, the gene for Huntington disease has complete (100%) penetrance.

  5. Expressivity is the degree of expression of a given penetrant gene in a particular individual. The expressivity of some genes varies widely among individuals (i.e., some people are mildly affected whereas others have severe manifestations).

6. Homozygosity and heterozygosity
   a. The term **homozygosity** describes the state in which an individual has inherited from both the parents identical alleles in the corresponding loci of a homologous chromosome pair.
   b. In contrast, the term **heterozygosity** describes the state in which an individual has inherited two different alleles in the corresponding loci.

7. Dominance and recessivity
   a. Dominant genes code for traits that can appear in heterozygotes. In other words, only one copy of the gene is necessary for the traits to be expressed.
      (1) Disorders with **autosomal dominant** transmission include some conditions associated with mental retardation or dementia.
         (a) Von Recklinghausen disease (generalized neurofibromatosis) is marked by multiple soft tumors covering the body along with areas of hyperpigmentation.
         (b) Tuberous sclerosis is characterized by tumors on the surfaces of the ventricles of the brain and patchy sclerosis of the brain surface. There are visceral tumors as well.
         (c) Huntington disease causes progressive dementia and choreiform movements, usually beginning in middle adulthood. Psychiatric disturbances, such as depression, and sometimes psychosis, may be present at some stage of the illness. The gene for this disorder is on **chromosome 4**.
      (2) Sex chromosome–linked dominant transmission of diseases is extremely rare.
   b. Recessive genes manifest only in homozygotes (i.e., when both alleles are the same).
      (1) Disorders with **autosomal recessive** transmission include:
         (a) Wilson disease (hepatolenticular degeneration)
         (b) Many inborn errors of metabolism, such as **phenylketonuria (PKU)** [see III D 3 a]
      (2) Most **sex chromosome–linked diseases** are recessive and transmitted on the X chromosome (i.e., X-linked). Women are the carriers in such cases; however, the disease is evident mostly in men. Examples include:
         (a) Duchenne muscular dystrophy, which is characterized by progressive muscular atrophy in childhood
         (b) Hunter mucopolysaccharidosis, which is marked by mental retardation, hypertelorism, dwarfism, deafness, optic atrophy, and skin lesions
         (c) Lesch-Nyhan syndrome, which is characterized by hyperuricemia, self-mutilation, choreoathetosis, cerebral palsy, and impaired renal function

8. Intermediate inheritance. The degree of phenotypic expression depends on whether an individual is homozygous or heterozygous for particular genes. This is called intermediate inheritance.
   a. The classic example of intermediate inheritance is the gene that manifests as **sickle cell disease** in the homozygote and as **sickle cell trait** in the heterozygote.
   b. The importance of intermediate inheritance in behavioral disorders is unclear.

C. | **Terminology used in molecular behavioral genetics**

1. Restriction fragment length polymorphisms (RFLPs) and other polymorphisms. A recent critical advance in genetics was the discovery of a method by which small differences in an individual's DNA can be identified. Because sites where such differences occur have been found all along the genome, an investigator who is pursuing a gene related to a particular condition can first look for **linkage** between a genetic marker (e.g., an RFLP) and the condition.
   a. Restriction endonucleases are enzymes that cause strands of DNA to break at a site that contains a particular base sequence. For example, the enzyme EcoRI always cleaves the nucleotide sequence GAATTC. If one person has that sequence in the middle of a DNA fragment, two fragments will be created when the enzyme is added. A person who has a different sequence at the same site (e.g., AAATTC) will continue to have one long fragment. Thus, **polymorphism** is said to occur at this locus.

    b. Southern blot procedure. DNA fragments are separated using **gel electrophoresis.** The fragments from the locus of interest are then detected with small segments of radioactive DNA called **probes.** The probes **anneal** to specific fragments of the DNA. Two small fragments will present as two bands on the resulting **autoradiogram,** whereas one larger fragment will present as one band, allowing detection of the individual who carries the specific gene sequence. This genetic variability, or DNA polymorphism, is referred to as **RFLP.**

    c. Polymerase chain reaction (PCR) technique. This recently developed, powerful technique allows a small segment of DNA to be directly and specifically amplified more than 1 million times.

2. LOD scores. When an investigator studies one or more families for a link between an illness and a particular gene locus, the data are often presented by means of a LOD (log of the odds) score. For instance, a LOD score of 3 (considered by many to be evidence of linkage) means that the odds of linkage being present (based on various statistical assumptions) are 1000:1 (the $\log_{10}$ of 1000 being 3).

3. Genome. The total collection of DNA in an organism (e.g., the 23 pairs of chromosomes and approximately 3 billion base pairs of DNA in a human) is referred to as the genome.

II. METHODS OF STUDYING GENETICS.
Family studies, twin studies, and adoption studies assess the genetic components and possible modes of inheritance of traits and diseases.

A. Clinical family studies

1. Assessment. Family studies assess the pattern of affliction in the relatives of an affected individual, who is called the **index case, propositus,** or **proband**.

    a. Family studies require the creation of a **pedigree,** which is a family tree that carefully notes the relationships between family members and identifies those who manifest the disorder in question.

    b. The quality of **clinical assessment** is very important. Conducting structured interviews of all family members is preferable to other methods such as looking at records or asking one family member to describe the symptoms of others.

2. Application. Through the study of the pedigree, the likely mode of inheritance may be inferred.

    a. It is likely, for example, that a disease has an **autosomal dominant** pattern of inheritance in a family in which the disease is manifested in one parent and in approximately 50% of the offspring (both male and female).

    b. In the case of **autosomal recessive** transmission, neither parent of the proband may have the disease (although both must be carriers), whereas approximately 25% of offspring (regardless of gender) suffer from the disease, 50% are carriers, and 25% do not have the responsible gene.

    c. In the case of **X-linked recessive** transmission, females are carriers and usually do not show the disease, whereas approximately 50% of the males manifest the illness. It is possible for a female to inherit the disorder if her mother is a carrier and her father has the disorder.

    d. For disorders that follow a **non-mendelian** pattern (not strictly dominant or recessive), one expects to see a correlation between the likelihood that the relative of a proband shares the disorder and the number of genes that the patient and relative have in common. For example, identical twins (sharing 100% of genes) should show higher **concordance** (i.e., both share the disorder) than siblings (who share 50% of genes), who should show higher concordance than half-siblings (who share, on average, 25% of genes).

e. In any disorder with an important genetic component, the incidence of that condition is significantly higher in relatives than in the general population and is **highest in first-degree relatives** (i.e., the parents, siblings, and children of the proband).

B. Molecular family studies

1. Assessment. To establish linkage between a clinical disorder and a particular gene, an investigator first needs a family that includes members with and without the illness. A careful pedigree is created, and blood samples are taken from affected and unaffected members. The work then proceeds in one of two ways.

a. Suspect gene. If a known gene is suspected to cause or relate to an illness (e.g., a dopamine receptor gene and schizophrenia), a link is sought between one allele of the gene and the illness.

b. Shotgun approach. When suspect genes have been found to lack linkage to the disorder being studied, there remains the option of looking for linkage by **systematically moving through the genome** (i.e., selecting several RFLP markers on chromosome 1 to see if any of them demonstrate linkage within the available pedigrees; if no linkage is found, markers on chromosome 2 can be analyzed, and so on).

2. Application. Performing such studies requires making a number of assumptions that can drastically affect the results.

a. Defining the disorder. The investigator must decide who is ill and who is well. For instance, in a linkage study of major depressive disorder, the investigator must decide whether family members with dysthymia (a milder but chronic depressive syndrome) should be considered to be ill or well. **Placing individuals in the wrong category may result in a true linkage being missed.**

b. Premature categorization. When a disorder has a late or variable age of onset, some individuals may be classified as unaffected when, in fact, they will become ill at a later time. The conclusions drawn from the study may be incorrect.

C. Twin studies

1. Assessment. Twin studies assess the degree to which both members of a pair of twins manifest a given trait or disease. If both twins have a certain trait, they are termed **concordant** for that trait; if only one twin of the pair has the trait, the pair is said to be **discordant**.

2. Application

a. Twin studies often compare concordance rates for **monozygotic (identical) twins** (who derive from the splitting of a fertilized ovum) with those for **dizygotic (fraternal) twins** (who derive from two separate fertilized ova). The concordance rate for monozygotic twins is significantly higher than that for dizygotic twins in disorders with a strong genetic contribution.

b. It may be difficult to determine whether such twin studies indicate **genetic transmission of the illness itself** or of an **inherited vulnerability** (i.e., the predisposition to develop schizophrenia or schizophrenia spectrum disorders in certain environmental situations) to develop the illness. For example, both tuberculosis and alcoholism show greater concordance in monozygotic twins than in dizygotic twins, yet in both cases it is a vulnerability, rather than the illness itself, that is inherited.

D. Adoption studies

Adoption studies offer an opportunity to **distinguish between genetic and environmental influences** on behavior. If a condition has a genetic basis, the prevalence of the condition should be significantly greater among biologic relatives than among adoptive relatives. Such studies can be designed two ways, as seen in the following example of studies performed on schizophrenia.

1. An investigator can **start with a group of schizophrenic adults who were raised by adoptive families** and then clinically evaluate the parents and siblings in both the adoptive and biologic families for the presence of schizophrenia or related disorders. Increased prevalence of schizophrenia in the biologic family members is evidence for genetic transmission.

2. An investigator can **start with a group of schizophrenic mothers who gave up their children for adoption** and then clinically evaluate their grown children as well as a **control group** of adoptees who were born to mothers without mental illness. Increased schizophrenia in the first group is evidence for genetic transmission.

III. GENETICS OF PSYCHIATRIC DISORDERS.

Although this area of psychiatric research is exciting, there are a number of factors that make genetic studies of behavioral disorders difficult to conduct and to interpret. These include genetic as well as phenomenologic heterogeneity of psychiatric illnesses, non-mendelian modes of transmission, variable (and often age-dependent) penetrance, and tendencies for assortive mating (i.e., a tendency for persons having an illness to marry each other at a greater than random rate).

A. **Schizophrenia** is a psychotic illness that usually has its onset during the late teens or early adulthood. The lifetime prevalence is approximately 1%. Its clinical features are described in Chapter 15 VI.

1. **Family studies.** Schizophrenia has long been known to run in families, but this does not confirm genetic etiology, since cultural factors (such as religion) also run in families. Family studies have found varying risks for different relatives of a patient with schizophrenia, as shown in Table 4-1.

2. **Twin studies.** Current figures for monozygotic twin concordance range from 35% to 58%, whereas figures for dizygotic twin concordance range from 9% to 26%. Recent investigations, which have used more conservative diagnostic criteria, have yielded somewhat lower figures for the concordance rate than did studies performed before 1965.

3. **Adoption studies.** The prevalence of schizophrenia is significantly higher in biologic than in adoptive relatives of patients with the disorder.

4. **Molecular genetics.** Studies have reported linkage between schizophrenia and various gene loci, including sites on chromosomes 5 (site of the dopamine D1 receptor), 11 (site of the gene for tyrosine hydroxylase), 18, and 19. None of these findings has been consistently replicated, however.

5. **Inheritance of schizophrenia**
   a. **Modes of transmission.** Evidence clearly indicates that genetic factors play a role in the development of schizophrenia. The exact mode of transmission is unknown,

TABLE 4-1. Risk Patterns for Mental Illness in the General Population and in Relatives of Affected Individuals

	Schizophrenia	MDD	Bipolar Disorder
Lifetime prevalence in the general population	1%	15%	1%
Approximate risk for relatives of a patient with the disorder:			
Identical twin	50%	50%	33%–90%
Full sibling or dizygotic twin	10%	15%	25%
Stepsibling (no genes shared)	1%	NA	NA
Parent of patient	5%	13%	22%
Child of parent with mood disorder	NA	21%	NA
Child of one affected parent	12%	NA	25%
Child of two affected parents	40%	NA	> 50%

MDD = Major depressive disorder; NA = not available.

however, and it is apparent that there are **important environmental contributions** to the etiology.

- **(1)** Different investigators have proposed monogenic, digenic, and polygenic **models of transmission,** but none of the proposals is consistent with all of the available data. A **multifactorial etiology** is often assumed.
- **(2)** It is likely that schizophrenia is not a single disease but rather a **syndrome** with several subtypes; genetic factors may be more crucial in some subtypes than in others.
- **(3)** Some investigators apply the term **schizophrenia spectrum disorders** to conditions that are genetically related but do not show the full symptom complex. Schizophrenia spectrum disorders include schizoid, paranoid, and schizotypal personality disorders.

b. What is inherited?
- **(1)** Some investigators have hypothesized that **specific biochemical defects** or **specific symptoms** (e.g., delusions, apathy), "soft" neurologic signs (e.g., grasp reflex), eye movement disturbances, and certain psychophysiologic abnormalities may be transmitted.
- **(2)** Alternatively, other investigators believe that only a **vulnerability** is transmitted.

B. **Mood disorders** are conditions marked by pervasive pathologic changes in mood and include two major forms: **unipolar disorders** (including major depressive disorder) and **bipolar disorders** (including mania). These disorders are discussed in Chapter 15 VII.

1. Family studies
a. Major depressive disorder
- **(1)** The lifetime prevalence of major depression is 15% to 20%, and approximately **50% of affected individuals have a first-degree relative with mood disorder** of one form or the other. The morbidity risk for a mood disorder in the relatives of probands with major depression is shown in Table 4-1.
- **(2)** The relatives of depressed patients are much more likely to develop depression than bipolar illness.

b. Bipolar disorder
- **(1)** The lifetime prevalence of bipolar disorder in the general population is approximately 1%; however, **80% to 90% of individuals with bipolar disorder will have a first-degree relative with a mood disorder**. This very high familial incidence of bipolar disorder can be helpful in the diagnosis of a patient with confusing psychotic symptoms. The morbidity risk for relatives is provided in Table 4-1.
- **(2)** It is likely that there is **more than one pattern of inheritance** for bipolar disorder. In some families of bipolar patients, a higher prevalence of certain X-linked markers [e.g., deuteranopia (a type of color blindness), or glucose-6-phosphate dehydrogenase (G6PD) deficiency] indicates a **possible X-linked pattern of inheritance**. A 1987 study reported an association with **chromosome 11** in an Amish pedigree. However, a problem occurred when some well individuals later developed the disorder (see II B 2 b). Re-analysis with this new information revealed no evidence for linkage. A linkage with **chromosome 18** in a series of pedigrees has recently been reported but remains to be replicated.

2. Twin studies. Morbidity risks for twins with mood disorders are listed in Table 4-1. Twin studies also reveal that **twins of unipolar probands are much more likely to be unipolar than bipolar.** By contrast, **twins of bipolar probands may be either bipolar or unipolar** (although the risk for bipolar disorder is greater). This could be related to the fact that some bipolar patients may not have a manic episode until much later in life.

3. Adoption studies. As is true with schizophrenia, the results of adoption studies of mood (particularly bipolar) disorder reveal a **higher prevalence in the biologic relatives** than in the adoptive relatives of an affected individual.

4. Inheritance of mood disorders. Studies strongly suggest that **genetic factors** contribute to the etiology of mood disorders.

    a. Family and twin studies of **bipolar disorder** indicate a strong genetic component with **phenotypic heterogeneity** (i.e., relatives who have mood disorders may have either bipolar or unipolar disorder), whereas family and twin studies of **major depressive disorder** reveal a similarly strong genetic component but with much **less phenotypic heterogeneity** (i.e., relatives who have mood disorders usually have unipolar disorder).

    b. The exact modes of transmission are unclear. In some families of bipolar patients, there is suggestion of an X-linked mode of inheritance, but no such pattern has been observed in families of unipolar patients.

    c. Some researchers have proposed the existence of **depressive spectrum disease** on the basis of a high prevalence of **alcoholism and sociopathy** in male members of families of probands with major depression.

C. **Alzheimer's disease** causes progressive dementia in older individuals. Postmortem studies show a **loss of cholinergic neurons, frontal atrophy,** and microscopic findings of **senile plaques** (derived from β-amyloid precursor protein) and **neurofibrillary tangles** (derived from **tau proteins**). This disease has been challenging to study genetically because there is rarely more than one generation afflicted within a family at a given time (i.e., the patient's parents are usually deceased and the children have not yet developed the disease). Also, many individuals die before clinical evidence of the disorder becomes apparent. Still, there have been major recent strides in understanding the genetic basis of Alzheimer's disease.

1. In certain families, particularly those in which the disease has an early onset, there appears to be an **autosomal dominant** pattern of inheritance.

2. In most cases, the genetic pattern of Alzheimer's disease is not clear. The concordance rate for Alzheimer's disease in both monozygotic and dizygotic twin pairs is less than 50%, suggesting the influence of **environmental factors** in the etiology.

3. Molecular genetics. Linkage studies have found associations between Alzheimer's disease and several chromosomes, including 14, 19, and 21.

    a. Chromosome 21 has been of interest in part because plaques and tangles are also found in Down syndrome (trisomy 21). This chromosome is the site of the β-amyloid protein precursor gene, and mutations to this gene have been found in several familial Alzheimer's disease pedigrees.

    b. Recent work has shown the gene for **apolipoprotein E (ApoE),** located on **chromosome 19,** to have a strong effect on **susceptibility** to the illness.

        (1) Individuals who are **homozygous for the ApoE4 allele develop Alzheimer's disease much earlier** (on average) than individuals who carry only one E4 gene. Individuals with only the E2 or E3 alleles have the latest onset (approximately age 90).

        (2) One **hypothesis** is that ApoE **binds tau proteins,** which prevents or delays the formation of neurofibrillary tangles in vulnerable individuals. The E4 protein, however, binds tau much less effectively, allowing the damage to proceed.

    c. Many cases of familial, early-onset Alzheimer's disease have been linked to **chromosome 14**.

4. Genetic heterogeneity. The evidence stated previously supports genetic heterogeneity in the etiology of this dementing disorder. It also supports the hypothesis that the various genetic etiologic factors interact with environmental factors. There is some evidence suggesting that presenile Alzheimer's disease (i.e., with onset before age 65) may have a stronger genetic component than later-onset dementia.

D. **Mental retardation.** Some forms of mental retardation are associated with **chromosomal abnormalities. Autosomal dominant, autosomal recessive,** and **X-linked** patterns of transmission are seen. Most cases of mental retardation, however, have an unclear pattern of inheritance in which a number of different genes may be involved. **Environmental factors,** such as anoxia, severe malnutrition, and fetal exposure to excessive alcohol, are also responsible in many cases.

1. **Chromosomal abnormalities** associated with mental retardation include Down syndrome, Klinefelter syndrome, Turner syndrome, and cri-du-chat syndrome.

2. **Autosomal dominant conditions** associated with mental retardation include tuberous sclerosis, von Recklinghausen neurofibromatosis, congenital myotonia, and some forms of muscular dystrophy.

3. **Autosomal recessive conditions** associated with mental retardation include inherited metabolic disorders such as PKU and Hartnup disease.
   a. **PKU** is characterized by mental retardation, fair skin, blue eyes, mild microcephaly, hyperactivity, and movement disorders. It is the result of a deficiency of hepatic phenylalanine hydroxylase. PKU is the most common aminoaciduria associated with mental retardation.
   b. **Hartnup disease** is a condition marked by a pellagra-like rash, emotional lability, psychotic episodes, and mental retardation. It is caused by a dysfunction in the transport of neutral amino acids.

4. **X-linked recessive conditions** associated with mental retardation include Duchenne muscular dystrophy, Lesch-Nyhan syndrome, and adrenoleukodystrophy.

E. Alcohol abuse

1. **Family, twin, and adoption studies** have indicated a **genetic component** to alcoholism.
   a. Twenty percent of adopted children born to alcoholic parents, and only 5% of adopted children born to nonalcoholic parents, were found to be alcoholic before the age of 30 years.
   b. Some studies have reported links between alcoholism, antisocial personality disorder, and certain forms of depressive illness, although the nature of those links is uncertain.

2. **Genetic factors.** There appear to be multiple genetically influenced factors that increase or decrease the susceptibility to alcoholism. One such factor is a **sensitivity to alcohol**.
   a. Evidence suggests that **sons of alcoholic parents** have a higher tolerance for alcohol, so they tend to drink more before feeling inebriated.
   b. Subjects with a **positive family history** of alcoholism tend to have decreased subjective feelings of intoxication, a smaller decrement in psychomotor performance, and less intense hormonal (cortisol and prolactin) responses to ethanol than subjects with a negative family history of alcoholism, despite identical blood alcohol concentrations, comparable drinking histories, and similar responses to placebo.
   c. There have been conflicting reports about a possible association between alcoholism and the A1 allele of an RFLP at the dopamine D2 receptor locus.

F. Other disorders

1. **Personality disorders** are conditions characterized by chronic patterns of maladaptive behavior, wherein the patient usually is unaware of his or her role in the continuing difficulties that arise.
   a. Personality disorders in general have a **concordance rate** that is several times **higher in monozygotic than in dizygotic twins**.
   b. Although it appears that a number of pathologic character traits are inherited, the **most conclusive evidence of genetic transmission exists for antisocial, histrionic, schizoid, schizotypal, and obsessive-compulsive personality disorders**.
   c. In recent years, genetic investigations have revealed a **probable link between schizophrenia and schizoid and schizotypal personality disorders**.
      (1) **Antisocial personality disorder** has also been linked to **somatization disorder and substance abuse**.
      (2) Family members of patients with **borderline personality disorder** are at increased risk for **substance abuse, antisocial personality disorder, and depression**.

2. **Obsessive-compulsive disorder** is seen in association with Tourette syndrome (multiple motor and vocal tics). It is unclear, however, if the obsessive-compulsive disorder noted in the families of patients with Tourette syndrome is identical to that which occurs spontaneously.

3. **Attention deficit disorder. Twin studies** have revealed a higher concordance rate among monozygotic twins than among dizygotic twins, and **adoption studies** have confirmed that there is likely to be a stronger genetic than environmental component to attention deficit disorder.

IV. THERAPEUTIC IMPLICATIONS

A. **Genetic counseling.** Kessler[1] and Tsuang[2] described the following basic steps in the genetic counseling of individuals with behavioral disorders.

1. **Making an accurate diagnosis** is particularly important in psychiatric disorders such as schizophrenia and mood disorders.

2. **Obtaining a family history** involves taking statements from family members. Unfortunately, these statements can often be inaccurate, especially where behavioral disorders are involved.
   a. **Written documentation** and medical records should be obtained if possible.
   b. **Define terms.** Vague terms such as "nervous breakdown" and "depression" should be questioned.

3. **Estimating recurrence risk**
   a. In some disorders, in which the pattern of genetic transmission is clear, the risk of recurrence may be readily estimated.
   b. In other disorders, in which the mode of inheritance is less clear (e.g., schizophrenia), it is usually better to avoid definitive statements.

4. **Psychosocial evaluation of the patient.** It is important to assess the motivation, psychological state, and needs of the patient to determine what information to present and how that information is best presented.

5. **Assessing the risk and burden.** The counselor works with the patient in weighing the likely effects of the risk (i.e., probability of recurrence of a given disorder in the relatives) and the burden (i.e., the expected financial, physical, and psychosocial cost to the family) of the recurrence of the disorder.

6. **Formulating a plan of action.** Although the counselor needs to be relatively authoritative in formulating a plan of action, he or she must exercise special care to take into account the wishes of the patient.

7. **Follow-up** is very important. It involves reassessing the accuracy of information obtained earlier, determining necessary changes in the plan of action, and considering the wishes of the patient.

B. **Prenatal diagnosis**

1. It is now possible to determine not only the gender of the child but also the presence or absence of many pathologic conditions early in gestation. This is done through **amniocentesis** or **chorionic villus sampling,** both of which allow for the growth of fetal cells for chromosomal analysis. Many physicians advocate such testing routinely for pregnant women over the age of 35 years.

2. Pathologic conditions that can be detected with amniocentesis include various **chromosomal abnormalities,** such as Down syndrome, as well as **genetic illnesses** such as Tay-Sachs disease (a sphingolipidosis characterized by progressive dementia, blindness, and paralysis).

3. Research into genetic markers for mental illness will lead to better understanding and new treatments, but it also raises **ethical issues** regarding the use of such markers in prenatal diagnosis.

REFERENCES

1. Kessler S: The genetics of schizophrenia: a review. *Schizophr Bull* 6:404–416, 1980.

2. Tsuang MT: Genetic counseling for psychiatry patients and their families. *Am J Psychiatry* 135:1465–1475, 1978.

BIBLIOGRAPHY

Baron M, Risch N, Hamburger R, et al: Genetic linkage between X-chromosome and bipolar affective illness. *Nature* 326:289–292, 1987.

Bender L: Schizophrenic spectrum disorders in the families of schizophrenic children. In: *Genetic Research in Psychiatry*. Edited by Fieve RR, Rosenthal D, Brill H. Baltimore, The Johns Hopkins University Press, 1975, pp 125–134.

Gusella JF, Wexler NS, Conneally PM et al: A polymorphic DNA marker genetically linked to Huntington's disease. *Nature* 306:234–238, 1983.

Harris MJ, Jeste DV: Late-onset schizophrenia: an overview. *Schizophr Bull* 14:39–55, 1988.

Kaplan AR: *Human Behavior Genetics*. Springfield, Illinois, Charles C. Thomas, 1976.

Kaplan HI, Sadock BJ, Grebb JA (eds): *Synopsis of Psychiatry*, 7th ed. Baltimore, Williams & Wilkins, 1994.

Kay DWK: Genetics, Alzheimer's disease and senile dementia. *Br J Psychiatry* 154:311–320, 1989.

Kelsoe JR: Molecular genetics and psychiatry. In: *Psychiatry*. Edited by Michels R, Cooper AM, Guze SB, et al. Philadelphia, JB Lippincott, 1992, 63:1-20.

Kessler S: The genetics of schizophrenia: a review. *Schizophr Bull* 6:404–416, 1980.

Pardes H, Kaufmann CA, Pincus HA, et al: Genetics and psychiatry: past discoveries, current dilemmas, and future directions. *Am J Psychiatry* 146:435–443, 1989.

Rieder RO, Gershon ES: Genetic strategies in biological psychiatry. *Arch Gen Psychiatry* 35:866–873, 1978.

Robertson MM: The Gilles de la Tourette syndrome: the current status. *Br J Psychiatry* 154:147–169, 1989.

Roses AD: Apolipoprotein E is a genetic locus that affects the rate of Alzheimer disease expression. *Neuropsychopharmacology* 10, 3S/part 1:5S–7S, 1994.

Schlesser MA, Altshuler KZ: The genetics of affective disorder: data, theory, and clinical applications. *Hosp Community Psychiatry* 34:415–422, 1983.

Schukit MA: Biomedical and genetic markers of alcoholism. In: *Alcoholism: Biomedical and Genetic Aspects*. Edited by Goedde HW, Argawal DP. New York, Pergamon Press, 1989, pp 290–302.

Singer S: *Human Genetics: An Introduction to the Principles of Heredity*. San Francisco, WH Freeman, 1978.

Tsuang MT: Genetic counseling for psychiatry patients and their families. *Am J Psychiatry* 135:1465–1475, 1978.

Van Valkenberg C, Lowry M, Winokur G, et al: Depression spectrum disease versus pure depressive disease: clinical, personality and course differences. *J Nerv Ment Dis* 16:341–347, 1977.

Ward CD, Duvoisin RC, Ince SE, et al: Parkinson's disease in 65 pairs of twins and in a set of quadruplets. *Neurology* 33:815–824, 1983.

STUDY QUESTIONS

DIRECTIONS: Each of the numbered items or incomplete statements in this section is followed by answers or by completions of the statement. Select the ONE lettered answer or completion that is BEST in each case.

1. What percentage of offspring of a mother with Huntington disease and an unaffected father is at risk for developing Huntington disease?

(A) 100%
(B) 75%
(C) 50%
(D) 50% (sons only)
(E) 50% (daughters only)

2. Which of the following statements regarding the inheritance of Alzheimer's disease is true?

(A) The apolipoprotein E4 allele protects against the early onset of the disease
(B) For most cases, there is an established family history
(C) Environmental factors play a minimal role in the development of the disease
(D) Linkage studies have found associations between the disease and chromosomes 14, 19, and 21
(E) Early-onset Alzheimer's disease is largely caused by environmental factors

3. What percentage of female offspring would be expected to demonstrate a trait with a Y-linked pattern of inheritance?

(A) 0%
(B) 5%
(C) 25%
(D) 50%
(E) 100%

4. Compared with people without a family history of alcoholism, sons of alcoholics tend to have which of the following responses to ethanol (despite comparable blood alcohol levels)?

(A) Greater prolactin response
(B) Higher cortisol response
(C) Greater psychomotor impairment
(D) Lesser feeling of intoxication

5. Twin studies of schizophrenia have revealed which of the following information?

(A) There is linkage to chromosome 5
(B) There is linkage to chromosome 11
(C) There is higher concordance for monozygotic than for dizygotic twins
(D) There is similar concordance for monozygotic and dizygotic twins
(E) There is little evidence for environmental factors in the etiology of schizophrenia

DIRECTIONS: Each set of matching questions in this section consists of a list of three to twenty-six lettered options (some of which may be in figures) followed by several numbered items. For each numbered item, select the ONE lettered option that is most closely associated with it. To avoid spending too much time on matching sets with large numbers of options, it is generally advisable to begin each set by reading the list of options. Then, for each item in the set, try to generate the correct answer and locate it in the option list, rather than evaluating each option individually. Each lettered option may be selected once, more than once, or not at all.

Questions 6–8

Match the following descriptions of genes with the correct type of gene.

(A) Structural genes
(B) Operator genes
(C) Regulator genes

6. These genes interact with repressors to control the activity of genes that code for specific amino acid sequences in proteins

7. These genes code for specific amino acid sequences in peptide chains and proteins

8. These genes modulate the synthesis of repressors

Questions 9–12

Match each finding from a genetic study with the disorder to which it pertains.

(A) Schizophrenia
(B) Major depressive disorder
(C) Bipolar mood disorder
(D) Alcohol abuse
(E) Obsessive-compulsive disorder

9. Family members of patients with this disorder show an increased incidence of Tourette syndrome

10. Twenty percent of adopted children whose natural parents have this disorder will develop the disorder before age 30

11. Between 80% and 90% of patients with this disorder have a first-degree relative with a mood disorder

12. Various linkage studies have reported associations between this disorder and chromosomes 5, 11, 18, and 19

ANSWERS AND EXPLANATIONS

1. The answer is C [I B 7 a (1)]. Huntington disease is transmitted through an autosomal dominant gene. This means that 50% of all children born to an affected mother and an unaffected father will have the gene for the disease and be at risk of developing it. Because the transmission is autosomal rather than sex-linked, the child's gender is not a determinant of the risk for the disease. In the case of X-linked transmission, 50% of sons are at risk. Dominant transmission suggests that a child with the abnormal gene will have the disease (if he or she lives long enough), whereas a child without that gene will not have the disease. When the transmission is recessive, 25% of the children will be at risk, 50% will be carriers, and 25% will be unaffected.

2. The answer is D [III C]. Most cases of Alzheimer's disease are sporadic; that is, there is not a clear family history of the illness. In a number of pedigrees, however, linkage analysis has revealed associations between Alzheimer's disease and chromosomes 14, 19, and 21. Chromosome 14 has been linked to familial, early-onset cases, which appear to have a stronger genetic component than other cases. Chromosome 19 is the site of the apolipoprotein E (ApoE) gene, and it is the E2 and E3 forms of this gene that appear to delay the onset of dementia. Chromosome 21 contains the β-amyloid protein precursor gene. Although this genetic evidence is strong, it appears that environmental factors are important as well. This conclusion is based in part on the finding that the concordance rate for monozygotic twins is less than 50%.

3. The answer is A [I A 2]. The Y chromosome is the determinant of maleness, and no female carries it. No matter how many X chromosomes are present, the presence of a Y chromosome determines a male phenotype.

4. The answer is D [III E 2 b]. Sons of alcoholic fathers tend to have a reduced response to ethanol in terms of subjective feelings of intoxication, psychomotor impairment, and cortisol and prolactin responses, when compared with people without a family history of alcoholism who have similar blood alcohol concentrations and comparable histories of drinking.

5. The answer is C [III A 2]. Twin studies have shown the concordance rate for schizophrenia in monozygotic twins to be approximately 50%, whereas the concordance rate for dizygotic twins is approximately 25%. Although the higher rate in monozygotic twins is strong evidence for a genetic etiology, the fact that half of the identical twins of affected individuals do *not* become ill is also strong evidence that environmental factors are important. Twin studies alone have not yielded linkage data. Large family pedigrees are of the most help in finding associations between genes and disorders.

6–8. The answers are: 6-B, 7-A, 8-C [I A 1 b (1)–(3)]. Genes may be subdivided into three functionally different types. Structural genes code for the specific amino acid sequences, which produce peptides and proteins. Operator genes interact with repressors, thus controlling the activity of structural genes. Regulator genes modulate the formation of the repressors.

9–12. The answers are: 9-E [III F 2], **10-D** [III E], **11-C** [III B 1 b (1)], **12-A** [III A 4]. Tourette syndrome and obsessive-compulsive disorder run in the same families. Adoption studies have found that 20% of children born to alcoholic parents, then adopted out, will still develop alcoholism by age 30, compared with only 5% of adopted children born to nonalcoholic parents. Family studies have found that 80% to 90% of patients with bipolar mood disorder have a first-degree relative with a mood disorder, compared with only approximately 50% of the relatives of patients with major depressive (unipolar) disorder. Linkage studies have reported associations between schizophrenia and chromosomes 5, 11, 18, and 19. It remains unknown whether the etiology is polygenic, whether there are a number of different genetic subtypes of the disorder, or whether some of these reported findings are wrong.

Chapter 5

Animal Models and Human Behavior

William J. Freed
Lois M. Freed
Magda Giordano

I. EVOLUTION. The question of heritability of behavior arose from the darwinian theory of evolution by natural selection: If physical characteristics are inherited, could behavioral patterns be inherited as well? Certain behaviors appear to be independent of the experience of the animal and thus appear to be inherited. However, many other behaviors are dependent on experience and are learned over time.

A. Inherited behavioral patterns. Ethologists, scientists who study the behavior of animals in their natural habitats, describe patterns of behavior that appear at a specific time in the life of an organism and are triggered by a specific stimulus. These behavioral patterns are expessed in their entirety the first time they appear, without practice or experience, and thus seem to be inherited. In some instances, the behavioral patterns are maintained even without their functional consequences. Ethologists refer to these behaviors as **fixed action patterns.** Some inherited behaviors are further modified by experience (i.e., practice) or physical development.

1. **Lovebirds** provide a clear example of an inherited behavior. Some species of lovebirds transport nesting material by grasping it with their beaks, raising their back feathers, then clamping the strips of nesting material beneath their feathers. Other species carry the nesting material in their beaks. Hybrids grasp the nesting material with their beaks and raise their feathers, but do not transfer the material to their feathers; instead, they carry it in their beaks. Thus, the feather-tucking movements are maintained in the hybrid animals even though they serve no functional purpose.

2. The study of inherited, or innate, behaviors is challenging in higher mammals, including humans, because it is **difficult to exclude the effects of experience on behavior.** Isolation experiments, in which animals are raised in isolation from birth, are the only way to determine whether a behavior is innate or learned. Of course, this type of experiment would be impossible to conduct in humans.

3. In **mammals,** some behaviors appear to be inherited. Certain brood-rearing and display behaviors of squirrels are apparent even in animals that are reared in isolation.

4. In **humans,** certain movements are independent of experience. These movements include lateral head movements and **Moro's reflex,** which is caused by vestibular stimulation or stimulation of the muscles in the neck. Moro's reflex is apparently a phylogenetic remnant of the movements used by subhuman primate infants to cling to their mothers. Other examples are smiling accompanied by a direct gaze, which occurs even in blind infants, and locomotion. Locomotion is an innate behavior that is modified by both practice and physical development.

B. Learned behavioral patterns. In phylogenetically higher animals, particularly mammals, an increasingly larger part of the behaviorial repertoire is learned.

1. The **disadvantages** of a learned behavioral repertoire include an increased period of dependency of the infant while the behavioral repertoire is acquired, a greater amount of time spent by the parents in rearing of offspring, and a smaller number of offspring. These factors result in a lower reproductive rate.

2. The **value** of a learned or acquired behavioral repertoire is a greater ability to adapt to changing environmental conditions and novel situations.

II. **MOTIVATION AND CONSUMMATORY BEHAVIORS.** These behaviors are directly related to the survival of the individual and the species. For this reason, these behaviors are likely to be examples of fixed action patterns and are likely to be inherited in phylogenetically lower animals.

A. **Eating** is important in the behavioral repertoire of animals because a large part of the behavior of many animal species is devoted to finding, acquiring, and ingesting food.

1. **Animal models.** Rats are a good animal model for the study of eating behavior because their omnivorous diet is similar to that of humans. The following eating behaviors occur in rats.

   a. **Neophobia.** When rats encounter a novel food, they sample a small amount before eating a substantial quantity. This behavior limits the ingestion of poisonous substances.

   b. **Conditioned taste aversion (CTA).** Rats avoid substances that cause illness. In experimental situations, CTA occurs when an animal is offered a novel food that does not cause illness. A second, unrelated substance is injected, and causes illness. Therefore, the properties of the illness can be manipulated independently of the food stimulus. CTA is strongest when the illness closely follows the food ingestion. However, these aversions can be established even when the illness is delayed for many hours.

   c. **Selecting a nutritious diet.** Rats that have access to a variety of foods self-select a balanced diet. Learning similar to that seen with CTA plays an important role in this behavior. Children also self-select an adequate diet under appropriate conditions. These conditions do not include the availability of highly palatable foods (e.g., sweets).

   d. **Dietary obesity.** When rats are given a highly palatable diet containing typical human foods and sweets (e.g., cookies), they become obese because of excess food consumption. This condition is known as dietary obesity.

   e. **Specific hunger.** Rats that are deprived of specific nutrients attempt to obtain and ingest foods that contain these nutrients. This behavior is known as specific hunger. Animals show specific hunger for many nutrients, such as calcium, thiamine, and sodium. Most specific hungers appear to be learned. Sodium-specific hunger, however, is not acquired because there are specific taste receptors for sodium. The presence of these receptors attests to the importance of sodium as a nutrient.

2. **Physiologic control of eating behavior.** In humans, hunger is an internally perceived state that is associated with an increased propensity to ingest food. In animals, the internally perceived state cannot be measured, nor can it be shown to exist. Thus, in animals, the term "hunger" is used to describe the propensity to ingest food, not the internal state.

   a. **Peripheral signals.** Early theories of hunger suggested the importance of peripheral signals (e.g., oropharyngeal and gastric sensations). These signals are now known to have little importance. However, gastric distention and entry of food into the intestine contribute to satiety.

   b. **Chemical signals.** A variety of chemical signals may regulate hunger and satiety. These chemical signals include glucose, insulin, free fatty acids, ketone bodies, glucagon, cholecystokinin, calcitonin, and glycerol.

   c. **Central mechanisms** located primarily in the **hypothalamus** and mediated by a variety of factors are important in controlling hunger. Thus, in addition to its role in other physiologic regulatory functions, the hypothalamus has an important role in the control of hunger and eating behavior. The evidence that supports the role of the hypothalamus in feeding behavior comes from biochemical and pharmacologic studies and from results of lesion and electric stimulation studies in animals.

      (1) The hypothalamus responds to chemical signals and regulates feeding behavior in response to those signals. Cells in the lateral hypothalamus and glucoreceptors in the ventromedial hypothalamus respond to changes in glucose use and to levels of insulin and free fatty acids. In animals, the injection of epinephrine and norepinephrine into several hypothalamic nuclei increases eating behavior.

The infusion of 3-hydroxybutyrate into the third ventricle decreases body weight. These findings show that eating behavior and body weight are regulated in part by central mechanisms located in the hypothalamus.

(2) **Lesions of the ventromedial hypothalamus** cause a syndrome of overeating and extreme obesity. This syndrome is characterized by an increase in fat deposition or an altered body weight **set point** that leads to a compensatory increase in eating.

 (a) In these animals, eating behavior is greatly affected by the palatability of food. This alteration in reactivity to the palatability of food is believed to be only one aspect of an overall increase in sensitivity to external stimuli that accompanies obesity. Under certain conditions, overweight subjects eat considerably more when food is immediately accessible or highly palatable, whereas subjects of normal weight tend to eat similar amounts, regardless of the accessibility or palatability of food.

 (b) In rare cases, obesity in humans occurs as a result of lesions caused by viral infection or tumor.

 (c) The effects of hypothalamic lesions are mimicked by injections of gold thioglucose, a neurotoxin that is specifically taken up into glucose-sensitive cells in the hypothalamus. The neurotoxin destroys the glucose-sensitive cells, which leads to obesity.

 (d) **Electric stimulation of the ventromedial hypothalamus suppresses feeding** behavior in animals.

(3) A milder form of obesity is caused by specific **lesions of the ventral noradrenergic bundle**. This norepinephrine-containing system passes through the medial hypothalamus.

(4) **Bilateral lesions of the lateral hypothalamus** cause **aphagia,** as well as impairments in grooming and general activity and a syndrome of sensory neglect. Animals with sensory neglect do not exhibit normal orienting responses to sensory stimuli. These changes are usually caused by interruption of ascending dopaminergic pathways that pass through the lateral hypothalamus.

 (a) **Electric stimulation of the lateral hypothalamus** produces immediate **vigorous eating** behavior. Similar stimulation also induces drinking and other behaviors. It is not known whether this stimulation-induced eating is caused by specific activation of an "eating circuit."

 (b) Nonspecific arousal produced by mild tail-pinch (administered by a metal clamp) induces similar eating responses. This finding suggests that general arousal is involved in the response to lateral hypothalamic stimulation.

B. **Drinking behavior** is categorized into two types on the basis of its relation to physiologic need.

1. **Primary drinking** occurs in response to physiologic need caused by either **dehydration** or **decrease in blood volume (hypovolemia)**. Primary drinking may occur in response to water deprivation, ingestion of a hypertonic solution, sweating, diuresis, substantial blood loss, or fluid redistribution through edema.

 a. **Dehydration-induced drinking, or osmometric thirst,** occurs after an increase in sodium intake causes water to leave the cells. The hypothalamus contains specialized receptors known as **osmoreceptors**. They are sensitive to cellular dehydration.

 b. **Hypovolemic drinking, or volumetric thirst,** occurs after blood volume decreases because of sweating, diarrhea, or blood loss. The amount of extracellular fluid decreases, and changes occur in blood pressure. The decrease in blood volume activates **baroreceptors** in the great veins, and several reflexes occur.

 (1) The result is an increase in water reabsorption from the urine (caused by arginine) and an increase in blood pressure (caused by the release of vasopressin by the pituitary).

 (2) Activation of the sympathetic nerves causes the release of norepinephrine and epinephrine and an increase in heart rate and vasoconstriction.

    (3) The release of **renin** from specialized kidney cells leads to the formation of **angiotensin II**. Angiotensin II acts on the **hypothalamus and subfornical organ** and induces drinking.

2. Secondary drinking is not motivated by actual physiologic need. It occurs when the animal does not have a water deficit. Secondary drinking may be associated with the ingestion of dry food or may occur because the fluid is palatable. Both animals and humans drink in advance of dehydration that is caused by the ingestion of food. In humans, social habits play an important role in drinking behavior. People often drink if other people are drinking or because of social convention (e.g., coffee breaks, teatime).

    a. The importance of primary and secondary drinking differs among species. Both rats and humans ingest water in excess of minimal physiologic needs when they eat. They compensate for a water deficit slowly. Rats also ingest excessive amounts of palatable solutions (e.g., a combination of saccharin and sucrose). On the other hand, dogs compensate for a water deficit rapidly and accurately by ingesting a large quantity of water in a single drinking session.

    b. Rats and several other animal species can be induced to drink large amounts of water through a paradigm known as **schedule-induced polydipsia**. When an animal is deprived of food and is given a small morsel of food once every 60 seconds to 3 minutes, it will drink large amounts of water, sometimes as much as 50% of its body weight in 3 hours. This abnormal behavior is a potential animal model for obsessive-compulsive disorder in humans.

3. Oral metering. How do animals and humans know how much to drink? Factors that determine how much an animal or human will drink include cooling of the mouth and ingested volume. In experimental situations, if oral feedback from water ingestion is bypassed, or if ingested water is prevented from being absorbed, animals still **drink in proportion to water deficit**.

4. Drinking behavior in humans

    a. Abnormal conditions. Adipsia (absence of drinking behavior) is rare. However, **polydipsia (drinking too much)** or **hypodipsia (drinking too little)** occurs with some conditions.

        (1) Tumors and other lesions of the anterior wall of the third ventricle can cause a decrease in drinking and impaired release of vasopressin.

        (2) A case report describes a man born without salivary glands.[1] He drank frequently, but ingested normal quantities of water. This finding is consistent with experiments in desalivated rats that show that a dry mouth may affect the timing of drinking behavior, but not the total amount of water consumed.

        (3) Polydipsia occurs in many schizophrenic patients. The cause of this disorder is not known. In extreme cases, polydipsia causes hyponatremia, decreased level of consciousness, seizure, and even death.

        (4) Alcoholism is the most common form of abnormal drinking behavior in humans. Alcoholism is associated with the pharmacologic effects of alcohol rather than with drinking behavior itself. Some animals ingest large amounts of alcohol voluntarily. For example, mice of the C57 strain will voluntarily consume approximately 90% of their fluid intake as 10% alcohol in preference to tap water.

    b. Secondary drinking is common in humans, especially the ingestion of alcoholic and caffeine-containing beverages. Even in primitive societies, water often is not the primary beverage.

C. **Sexual and reproductive behavior.** Reproductive success determines the survival of the species, so this behavior is important. In general, species that are low on the phylogenetic scale have more rigid and stereotypical mating behaviors. Sexual behavior becomes more reflexive and stereotyped as it progresses from approach and courtship through copulation. In humans, sexual behavior is strongly influenced by sociocultural factors, and it serves purposes other than reproduction. For example, sexual behavior in humans is used for recreation and as a means to express emotion between individuals.

1. **Sexual development**
   a. **Before birth.** In the early stages of development, genetically determined male and female animals are outwardly similar. Gonadal sex is determined by chromosomal sex, and in most cases, they are identical. However, genital sex and secondary sexual characteristics are determined by hormonal messages, and they may differ from chromosomal sex because of exposure to sex hormones. Both sexes pass through a stage during which they are sensitive to **hormonal stimulation**. In rats, this stage occurs at birth and shortly thereafter. In humans, this stage occurs from the seventh week to the third month of gestation. During this time, the internal and external genital organs develop in response to hormonal signals. Animal studies show that exposure to testosterone during this stage causes the development of male characteristics and masculine behavioral patterns. An animal that is not exposed to testosterone will develop in a female direction. **The direction of sexual behavior is determined early in development.**
      (1) The presence of inappropriate sex hormones during this period may produce abnormal individuals. For example, **androgen insensitivity syndrome** is a condition in which the cells of a genetic male do not respond to androgen. The individual is born with feminized external genitalia. Such individuals are usually raised as females and as adults behave as females.
      (2) Only external sex characteristics and behavior are influenced by sex hormones during this stage of differentiation. For example, the presence of androgens during the development of a female may cause male external sex organs and male behavior patterns to develop, but the animal will still have the internal reproductive organs of a female. In a disorder known as **congenital adrenal hypertrophy,** the fetus is exposed to excess levels of androgen. In a genetic female, this condition results in the masculinization of the external genitalia. However, if the animal is raised and treated as a female, it exhibits female gender identity and behavior.
      (3) This differentiating effect is seen not only for sexual behavior, but also for other gender-specific behavioral patterns. For example, although testosterone normally stimulates fighting in male mice, it does not do so in animals that are castrated at birth (i.e., animals that are not differentiated males).
   b. **Puberty.** In rats, puberty occurs at approximately 2 months (about 1/20 of the life span). In humans, puberty occurs at approximately 13 years (about 1/6 of the life span). Although the direction of sexual behavior patterns is determined earlier, the expression of these patterns is stimulated at puberty.
      (1) At puberty, sex hormones (testosterone in the male, estrogen in the female) are produced and stimulate the development of secondary sexual characteristics (e.g., deepening of the voice and development of body hair in males, enlargement of the breasts in females). Sex hormones also may stimulate or inhibit sexual behavior. If sex hormones are absent during puberty, secondary sex characteristics and sexual behavior patterns are not expressed. Other hormones, such as growth hormone (GH), are involved in the somatic changes that occur during puberty.
      (2) The role of sex hormones during puberty is exemplified by a disorder known as **5α-reductase deficiency**. This is a condition in which a genetic male lacks the enzyme that is necessary to convert testosterone to **dihydrotestosterone (DHT)**. DHT causes the development of male external genitalia. Individuals that do not have this enzyme are born with ambiguous or feminized genitalia, and are raised as females. At puberty, however, testosterone causes the development of secondary male characteristics. Therefore, at puberty, these individuals experience growth of the penis, lowering of the voice, and descending of the testes. These individuals usually adopt a male gender identity and eventually make an adequate adjustment.

2. **Sexual behavior**
   a. In rats, male and female sexual behavior, including maternal behavior (e.g., nest building), is caused by the stimulation of parts of the preoptic area of the hypothalamus. **The control of sexual behavior by hormones is direct and pronounced in**

lower animals. In higher animals, hormones play a less important role, and neuronal, social, and environmental factors are more important. However, in higher animals, the presence of sex hormones during development influences the connections of neurons in the preoptic area of the hypothalamus, which can have lasting effects on sexual behavior.

    b. In prairie voles, the posterior pituitary hormones, vasopressin and oxytocin, may be associated with the formation of characteristic pair (female–male) bonding. Oxytocin levels increase during the mating period, and injection of oxytocin into the brain induces pair bonding in female voles. In contrast, no pair bonding occurs when an oxytocin receptor antagonist is administered. In male voles, vasopressin plays a similar role. Other species of voles, meadow and montane voles, are polygamous. In these voles, the distribution of oxytocin receptors differs from that of prairie voles.

    c. Monkeys that are deprived of social contact during infancy do not show normal sexual behavior as adults. **Normal sexual and maternal behavior in humans is probably** also **dependent on environmental and social interactions during infancy.**

D. **Aggression.** Aggression in animals is divided into several types, depending on the stimulus. For example, aggression elicited by pain may differ from aggression exhibited by a predator in search of prey. Aggression shown by a mother protecting her young may have still different properties.

    1. **Role of the hypothalamus.** In cats, two types of aggression are caused by stimulation of the hypothalamus.

        a. **Stimulation of the medial hypothalamus produces an affective attack,** a rage-like syndrome characterized by hissing, snarling, unsheathing of claws, and piloerection.

        b. **Stimulation of the lateral hypothalamus produces a stalking, or quiet biting, attack,** which is a predatory response without rage-like features. The quiet biting attack is specifically directed toward natural prey.

    2. **Other limbic structures.** In rats, lesions of the **septal area** of the brain produce a rage-like syndrome that subsides over several weeks. The effects of these lesions vary among species. For example, the rage syndrome does not appear in mice, but a permanent flight reaction occurs. Consistent rage-like syndromes are not seen in other species, such as cats and monkeys. Thus, **the septal area does not appear to have a primary role in controlling aggression.** On the other hand, **the amygdala appears to have an important role in aggression and emotional response.**

        a. **Animal models**

            (1) Bilateral removal of the amygdala of rhesus monkeys causes **Klüver-Bucy syndrome.** This syndrome is characterized by taming of the animal, lack of fear of natural enemies (e.g., snakes), inability to recognize common objects, hyperactive and abnormal sexual behavior, and a tendency to place all objects in the mouth.

            (2) Similar changes, particularly the taming effect, can be produced in several other species, such as the wild Norway rat, which is normally aggressive. Although friendliness toward human experimenters increases with exposure, animals with amygdala lesions may become more or less aggressive toward members of their own species. Inappropriate social responses are also observed.

        b. **Human behavior. The role of the amygdala in human aggression is controversial.**

            (1) Some violent patients have tumors or other abnormalities of the amygdala. Damage to the amygdala and surrounding areas is shown by noninvasive neuroimaging [computed tomography (CT) and magnetic resonance imaging (MRI)] procedures in some violent patients. The amygdala has been removed in some extremely violent patients, although this surgery produces changes in addition to the reduction in violent behavior.

            (2) One case of Klüver-Bucy syndrome is reported in a human.[2] A man had bilateral damage to the temporal lobes as the result of a viral infection. His behavior was normal before the infection, but afterward, he showed flat affect, emotional indifference, increased oral exploration, bulimia, inability to recognize objects and people, altered sexual preference, and socially inappropriate behavior.

(3) Clinically, there appears to be some **correlation between temporal lobe seizures and aggressive behavior.** Bilateral temporal lobectomy results in less aggressive behavior in some patients. Neurosurgical treatment of violent epileptic patients was also attempted at one time, with variable results and limited success.

3. Other areas involved in the regulation of aggressive behavior are the prefrontal cortex and the cerebellum. In humans, lesions of the orbital prefrontal cortex may cause aggressive behavior and disregard for societal rules. In monkeys, lesions of the vermis, flocculonodular lobe, lobulus implex, and paramedia lobule diminish aggressive tendencies.

E. **Self-stimulation of the brain.** The behaviors described in earlier sections are involved in the maintenance of a stable internal environment (homeostasis), needed for the survival of the individual. Sexual behavior is involved in the survival of the species. The ability to perform behaviors that maintain homeostasis can lead the individual to perform additional behaviors. In some cases, behavior is motivated by artificial rewards or reinforcers, such as electric stimulation of the brain, although electric brain stimulation and natural rewards appear to have similarities. In 1954, it was discovered that rats return to the part of a chamber in which they receive stimulation of the hypothalamus, and that rats press a lever rapidly and vigorously to obtain stimulation of the lateral hypothalamus. This behavior is called **intracranial self-stimulation.**

1. Brain areas that support self-stimulation. The most vigorous intracranial self-stimulation is obtained from areas with connections to the medial forebrain bundle, including the lateral hypothalamus. Reinforcing effects are obtained from a number of other brain areas, particularly the **ventral tegmental area (VTA),** the **septal area,** and the **prefrontal cortex.**

2. The effects of intracranial self-stimulation are dramatic. In one well-known example, a rat stimulated itself 2000 times per hour for 26 hours, slept continuously for almost 1 day, and then resumed the self-stimulation at the previous rate. However, the degree of pleasure involved in the stimulation cannot be determined from the rate alone. The rapidity and persistence of the response might occur because the stimulation does not satiate, as do natural rewards.

3. A stimulus that supports self-stimulation often induces eating or drinking responses. Under certain conditions, animals will work to obtain the stimulus only if food is also present. Brain stimulation that produces rewards does not necessarily cause the sensation of eating, but rather, seems to cause a motivation to eat.

4. In human subjects, pleasurable sensations are elicited mainly from stimulation of the septal area of the brain. Although they are pleasurable, these sensations are not overwhelming and do not seem to exceed the pleasurable sensations obtained by natural rewards.

5. Intracranial self-stimulation is used to study drugs of abuse. By determining the effects of drugs of abuse on self-stimulation in animals, scientists can begin to understand substance abuse behavior in humans.

F. **Animal models of substance abuse**

1. In addition to the primary reinforcers, substances other than food and water may sustain behavioral responses in animals and humans. Animals are willing to work to self-administer substances such as **opiates, stimulants,** and **nicotine.** These drugs seem to possess intrinsic hedonic properties for the animals. Human substance abusers can verbalize their desire for a drug as well as the pleasure they derive from it. In addition, they may engage in a variety of behaviors, including criminal acts, to ensure access to their drug of choice. Several animal models are used to test drugs for their abuse potential and to learn more about substance abuse behavior in humans.

   a. **Self-administration.** Animals learn to press a lever or nose-poke (a behavior exhibited by rats in their normal environment) to receive an infusion of a drug. The work required to obtain an infusion can be increased over time to determine how much the animals will work for a reward. Drugs for which animals of various species (nonhuman primates, dogs, rats) will work include opiates, stimulants, and nicotine.
   b. **Choice paradigms.** A variety of choice paradigms exist. In one case, the animal is given a choice between going into a chamber associated with a test substance (e.g., amphetamine) and another chamber associated with a control substance (e.g., saline). This paradigm is known as **conditioned place preference**. In other models, animals are given a choice between administration of a drug or a primary reinforcer, such as food.
   c. **Conditioned reinforcement paradigm.** The animals are trained in an operant box with two levers. Responses on one lever produce a brief stimulus followed by a drug injection. Responses on the other lever have no effect. After the animals learn to self-administer the drug, pressing the active lever produces the stimulus followed by a saline injection (testing phase). Responses on the levers during the testing phase are compared with responses before drug administration. The number of responses on the active lever provides a measure of the incentive properties of the neutral stimulus. These properties are developed through pairing with the drug infusion.
   d. **Self-stimulation paradigm.** The animals are trained to self-stimulate by pressing a lever or by nose-poking. The experimenter controls the intensity (current) and duration of the stimulus. In one paradigm, the minimum duration required to maintain the behavior (threshold duration) is determined. After administration of a stimulant, such as cocaine, the threshold diminishes, whereas the administration of dopamine antagonists increases the threshold duration. This method is also useful for testing the time course of the effects of drugs.

  2. Animal models of drug abuse are useful in identifying psychoactive drugs with low potential for abuse, in developing treatment strategies, and in understanding the environmental and biologic factors involved in human substance abuse. Laboratory studies with psychomotor stimulants (e.g., cocaine, amphetamine) show that the reinforcing properties of a drug are caused by an interaction between the drug and the environmental circumstances under which it is administered.[3] Behavioral pharmacologic studies of opioids (e.g., morphine) can identify drugs that can be used as analgesics and have limited potential for abuse.

III. **LEARNING.** It is difficult to compare learning across species because motivation and performance cannot be equated. The most useful studies examine differences in types of learning among species. Some forms of learning, such as habituation, are seen in all species, from invertebrates to humans. However, different mechanisms of learning may be involved. Other forms of learning, such as imprinting, only occur in some species. Most animals can learn only tasks that are consistent with their species-specific behavioral repertoire. For example, birds are easily conditioned to perform pecking movements, but do not easily learn to manipulate bars and levers. Rats are more easily conditioned to nose-poke than to press levers.

A. **Primitive forms of learning.** Some forms of learning are observed in animals at all levels of the phylogenetic scale. For example, habituation and sensitization were studied extensively in the marine snail *Aplysia*.

  1. **Imprinting** is a specialized form of learning that occurs primarily in birds, and only during a short period after hatching. If it does not occur within approximately 1 day after birth, it will not occur at all. Studies by **Lorenz** show that birds learn to follow the first large, moving object that they see.[4] Normally, birds are imprinted to follow their mothers, although they can also be imprinted to follow almost any animal, human, or object (e.g., a box containing a ticking clock). Some mammals exhibit a form of imprinting (e.g., voles).

2. **Nonassociative forms of learning.** In nonassociative learning, an animal learns about the properties of a stimulus, such as whether it is noxious or rewarding.
   a. **Habituation is a progressive decrease in the behavioral response to a nonnoxious repeated stimulus.** Decrements in responses during habituation are not caused by fatigue. Habituation may occur for simple elicited responses, such as orientation toward a sound or withdrawal of the foot in response to a tactile stimulation. Habituation may also occur in more complex situations, such as the progressive decline in exploratory behavior that occurs when animals are continuously exposed to unfamiliar environments. In this case, habituation involves a complex interaction between multiple stimuli and behavioral responses.
   b. **Exploration.** Large changes in the environment cause fear, whereas small changes lead to curiosity and exploration. If large changes do not produce overly threatening or painful stimuli, the animal becomes habituated to the fear and begins to explore. Exploration does not satiate, as do eating, drinking, and sexual behavior. Thus, every time a change occurs in the environment, exploration takes place.

3. **Sensitization** is a heightened response to a wide array of stimuli after exposure to an intense, threatening, or noxious stimulus. A sensitizing stimulus may override the effects of habituation. For example, after a person is habituated to a repetitive noise, a strong pinch can restore the response to the noise.

B. **Associative learning.** An animal incorporates meaningful information about its environment into its behavioral repertoire through conditioning. There are two types of conditioning: classic and instrumental.

1. **Classical conditioning** involves relations between environmental events and the responses that they cause. These responses are usually autonomic. The concept of classical conditioning is derived from a paradigm devised by the Russian physiologist **Pavlov.** In his experiments, a dog was restrained and salivation was elicited by blowing meat powder into its mouth. The sound of a bell was repeatedly associated with the administration of the meat powder. The bell alone did not elicit salivation until after many associations between the bell and the meat powder. This paradigm involves several stimuli and responses, or reflexes.
   a. An **unconditioned stimulus** is the stimulus that elicits the response without conditioning (e.g., meat powder).
   b. An **unconditioned reflex** is the reflex elicited by the unconditioned stimulus directly, without conditioning (e.g., salivation).
   c. A **conditioned stimulus** is the initially neutral stimulus that is associated with the unconditioned stimulus during the experiment (e.g., a bell).
   d. A **conditioned reflex** is the reflex caused by the conditioned stimulus alone, without the unconditioned stimulus. Although the conditioned reflex is always superficially similar to the unconditioned reflex, the two are never identical. For example, the conditioned reflex is usually weaker than the unconditioned reflex.

2. **Instrumental conditioning** involves the relations among specific types of stimuli; behavioral responses, usually skeletomotor responses, of the animal; and environmental events. Behavior that is directly caused by environmental events is called **respondent behavior.** Behavior that is not caused by a known environmental stimulus before conditioning occurs is called **operant behavior.** Instrumental conditioning is **trial-and-error learning.** In simple terms, **behaviors that are rewarded will increase,** and **behaviors that are punished will decrease.**
   a. **Principles of instrumental conditioning**
      (1) The scientific study of instrumental conditioning was initiated by **Thorndike** and **Skinner.** They defined instrumental conditioning, and emphasized that **behavior is controlled by its consequences.** The behavior of an animal is not characterized in terms of the subjective experience of the animal, which cannot be measured objectively. Stimuli are characterized as reinforcing rather than as rewarding.

(2) In a specific situation, without previous experience, an animal shows a random sequence of behaviors. Some of these behaviors are followed by **positive reinforcement** (i.e., reward). These behaviors are reinforced, and therefore **increase in frequency**. Behaviors that cause **avoidance or escape from noxious stimuli are also reinforced (negative reinforcement),** and the probability of their occurrences also **increases.** Behaviors that are followed by **punishment usually decrease in frequency**. Through many conditioning experiences involving the acquisition of food, avoidance of threatening situations, or other benefits, enduring changes in the behavioral repertoire of an animal or human may occur.

(3) Types of reinforcers

    (a) In animal experiments, reinforcement usually involves **primary reinforcers** (e.g., food, water, escape from a noxious stimulus).

    (b) In humans, reinforcement is more subjective. Praise and other social stimuli as well as **secondary reinforcers** are important. Secondary reinforcers have no intrinsic value, but reinforce behavior through their association with a primary reinforcer. For example, patients in a behavioral modification program are given tokens for completing choices. These tokens may be exchanged for candy or soda.

    (c) Discriminative stimuli also control behavior through their association with reinforcers. These stimuli signal the availability of a reinforcer. For example, animals can be trained to press a lever when they see a light that signals the availability of the reinforcer, and not to press the lever when they hear a sound that has never been associated with a reinforcer. Discriminative stimuli are used to learn more about the sensory systems of animals. An example of a discriminative stimulus is the light in a vending machine that indicates that a selection is not available.

b. Two types of experimental paradigms are used to study instrumental conditioning.

  (1) In maze-learning paradigms, animals learn complex behavioral responses that involve locomotion and spatial relations.

    (a) Early mazes (e.g., **Lashley type 3 maze, Warner and Warden multiple T-maze**) used successive left–right choices or successive choices between alternative alleyways.

    (b) A newer type of maze is the **radial arm maze** that was devised by Olton. This maze consists of a central hub with a number of radiating alleyways (usually eight). Food reinforcements are located at the end of each alleyway. Animals are allowed to make eight trips down the alleyways. To obtain the maximal amount of food, they must remember which alleyways they have already visited.

    (c) Another commonly used maze is the **Morris water maze**. Rats must swim to find a submerged platform on which to rest. The platform is placed just below the surface of the water in a large tank, and powdered milk or latex powder is added to make the water opaque. The platform may be moved to test spatial learning. Spatial cues are distributed around the room to allow the animals to orient themselves.

  (2) Operant conditioning involves a simple behavioral response (e.g., pressing a bar by a rat, pecking a disk by a pigeon, nose-poking by a rat or mouse). The rate of the behavior is modulated according to a **schedule of reinforcement**. Two types of schedule are used.

    (a) Ratio schedules

      (i) In ratio schedules, **the number of responses is the key to the reinforcement**. The simplest type of ratio schedule is **continuous reinforcement** (CRF) in which every response is followed by a reinforcement. CRF is an example of a **fixed-ratio (FR) schedule,** in which every response is followed by a reinforcement. For example, on a fixed ratio of 40 (FR 40) a rat receives a reinforcement after every 40 responses.

        (ii) With a **variable-ratio (VR) schedule,** the number of responses needed to obtain a reinforcement varies and is calculated as an average over the entire session.

    (b) Interval schedules

        (i) On a **fixed-interval (FI) schedule,** a reinforcement follows the first response after a given interval (e.g., every 5 seconds). Responses at other times are not followed by a reinforcement. This type of schedule leads to a particular response pattern: Responses increase as the end of the interval approaches and decrease after the reinforcer is received.

        (ii) In **variable-interval (VI) schedules,** the period preceding the reinforcement varies. The length of the interval is varied randomly around a mean length of time. Thus, the first response after a variable interval is reinforced so that the animal cannot predict when reinforcement will occur. The VI schedules are the **most resistant to extinction**.

    (c) Differential reinforcement of low rates (DRL) is another type of schedule. With this schedule, the animals are reinforced after a fixed interval if no responses have occurred in the interim.

    (d) In **extinction,** no responses are reinforced.

3. Special types of conditioning. Classical conditioning typically involves autonomic responses, or responses that are reflexively elicited by the environment. **Instrumental conditioning** typically involves skeletomotor responses, or responses that are not elicited reflexively by an environmental stimulus. However, some forms of conditioning do not fit into either category.

    a. Autoshaping. Some skeletomotor responses are caused by reinforcement. Therefore, they are susceptible to conditioning by classic paradigms.

        (1) An experiment with pigeons shows that if the availability of food is signaled by a key that is illuminated just before the food is available, lighting the key will cause pecking, even though the pecking does not cause the food to be delivered.

        (2) Autoshaping occurs for responses that are closely associated with the reinforcement. For example, the delivery of food reinforces pecking in pigeons and rooting in pigs.

    b. Biofeedback. Some autonomic responses can be controlled if they are monitored mechanically and the subject is given feedback about the responses.

        (1) Biofeedback can be used to help a patient learn to modulate the temperature of his middle finger. When the capillaries at the extremities constrict, the temperature of the extremities drops. Relaxation causes the capillaries to dilate, and the extremities become warmer. With biofeedback, a device is attached to the finger and the temperature of the finger is displayed on a meter to show the patient his response.

        (2) Evidence of biofeedback conditioning in animals is inconclusive. However, such conditioning occurs in humans, and patients can control various autonomic processes to a certain extent. These procedures can be useful for patients with **migraine headaches, hypertension, or stress**. In a patient who has tension headaches, electrodes are placed over the surface of the cervical or scalp muscles. Contraction of these muscles is assumed to cause the headaches. The patient receives feedback about contraction of the muscles, and she may use relaxation techniques to diminish both the contraction and the pain. When some patients with migraine headaches are trained to control their finger temperatures, they report a concomitant decrease in the frequency of headaches.

IV.   **CONFLICT SITUATIONS. In their natural environment, animals select food, water, and sexual partners, and encounter fear- and pain-provoking stimuli. Conflict occurs when alternatives exist;** stress occurs as a result of unresolved conflict.

A. **Classification of conflict situations.** Conflict situations are classified as approach–approach, approach–avoidance, or avoidance–avoidance, depending on the behavioral alternatives.

1. **Approach–approach conflict** occurs when incompatible approach responses are present. For example, an animal has access to more than one food source or sexual partner.

2. **Approach–avoidance conflict** occurs in the presence of incompatible approach and avoidance responses. For example, an animal finds a food source that is in an open area and is susceptible to predators.

3. **Avoidance–avoidance conflict** occurs when two incompatible avoidance responses are present. For example, an animal must choose between an uncomfortably cold area and an area that is open to predators.

B. **Behaviors exhibited in conflict situations**

1. **Suppression of lower-priority responses.** In most conflict situations, one alternative has a low priority. That alternative is usually suppressed to allow expression of the higher-priority response. For example, some birds spend approximately 30% of the day grooming and resting in the summer. However, in the winter, when food is less plentiful, the birds spend 90% of the day feeding, so less time is available for other activities.

2. In conflict situations, animals show **preparatory movements** (i.e., components of the alternative behaviors that are in conflict). They may alternate between preparatory movements for each behavior, or they may compromise by incorporating components of several alternative behaviors.

3. **Displacement behavior** occurs in birds and other animals in conflict situations. This behavior occurs when animals are prevented from continuing or executing a prominent behavior, such as aggression, sexual behavior, or feeding. For example, the behavior may be suppressed by the sudden appearance of a competitor. In this situation, an animal may suddenly exhibit apparently irrelevant behaviors, such as grooming or pecking at the ground. In humans, due to societal constraints, other behaviors, such as vigorous exercise, substitute for aggressive behavior. This substitution may be considered a form of displacement behavior.

4. **Humans** address unresolved conflict differently. One approach is direct action aimed at changing a person's perception of a stressful event. (e.g., practicing before giving a speech). Another method is palliation, or addressing the symptoms of stress instead of the source of stress (e.g., taking a tranquilizer before giving a speech). In addition, humans use a variety of intrapsychic techniques to cope with stress. **Freud described defense mechanisms,** which are unconscious mental techniques that are used to protect the ego (a division of the mind) from anxiety. Common defense mechanisms include denial, rationalization, displacement, and repression. For example, the person giving the speech may dismiss the importance of the situation by rationalization. In addition to Freud's theory, a number of cognitive theories, including the cognitive dissonance theory, attempt to predict how a person will behave in a conflict situation.

C. **Schedule-induced behavior**

1. Schedule-induced polydipsia (see II B 2 b) is an experimental analogy of displacement behavior that may provide a model for obsessive-compulsive disorder in humans.

2. Behaviors other than drinking, such as aggression, may also be elicited by intermittent delivery of small food pellets (schedule-induced aggression).

D. **Inhibitory avoidance.** In this type of paradigm, animals learn to inhibit a natural response to avoid receiving a mild electric shock.

1. **Passive avoidance.** Mice or rats, which usually avoid brightly lit areas, are trained in a two-chamber box. One chamber is dark, and the other is brightly lit. The animals are placed in the light chamber. They receive a shock when they enter the dark compartment. During the retention trial, the animals are placed in the light chamber. The time that it takes them to enter the dark compartment is the retention score. Animals learn to stay in the light chamber in one trial.

2. **Two-way active avoidance.** A modification of this paradigm involves the presentation of a stimulus before the shock is activated. The animals learn to leave the chamber when the stimulus is present to avoid receiving a shock.

V. ANIMAL MODELS OF PSYCHIATRIC DISORDERS

A. **Conditioned (experimental) neuroses.** When an animal is evaluated with discrimination tests (e.g., an animal must discriminate between two different, but similar, tones) and the discrimination is gradually made more difficult, at some point, the animal may show inappropriate behavior. These responses are known as **experimentally conditioned neuroses.** Conditioned neuroses are most likely to develop when strong motivators, such as shock, are used; positive and negative stimuli are alternated without repetition; and stimuli are presented rapidly. These behaviors were originally observed in an experiment by a student of Pavlov. In the experiment, dogs were trained to discriminate between a circle and an ellipse. The ellipse was gradually made more and more like a circle. When the ratio between the length of the axes was 9:8, dogs could no longer discriminate between the shapes. They began to show violent and emotional behaviors in a testing situation. The inappropriate responses persisted during continuing testing. Similar responses are observed in sheep, goats, cats, rats, and monkeys.

B. **Response–suppression paradigms.** These experiments use a motivator, such as food, but require the animal to endure a threatening or painful situation to obtain the food.

1. In the **Geller-Seifter conflict test,** animals are trained to press a lever to obtain food, but only some of the lever presses are rewarded with food. During some periods, all levers pressed are rewarded, but the animals are also shocked each time they press the lever. A light signals the shock periods, and lever pressing is normally suppressed. This test is a useful method of **testing antianxiety agents.** Drugs such as benzodiazepines, which reduce anxiety in humans, increase lever pressing during the shock periods of this test.

2. Based on this principle, several other tests for antianxiety agents were developed. In these tests, animals must enter a large, brightly lit area to obtain food, or they are allowed to explore a brightly lit section of a testing enclosure. Another test uses an elevated X-maze that has some arms open to the environment and others with side and end walls. Antianxiety agents reduce the reluctance of animals to enter the open arms, which are usually threatening. Such situations are, at least at face value, analogous to anxiety-provoking situations that affect humans (e.g., agoraphobia, or fear of open spaces).

C. **Obsessive-compulsive disorder.** Some species have naturally occurring behavioral disorders of grooming. These disorders have been argued to resemble obsessive-compulsive disorder in humans, and share similar ethological and physiologic bases.

1. **Canine acral lick dermititis** occurs in some breeds of dogs (e.g., setters, German shepherds). Dogs with this disorder lick their paws excessively. This licking leads to hair loss and ulceration of the skin.

2. Some avian species engage in excessive preening and feather plucking. Some nonhuman primates show excessive autogrooming and trichotillomania (hair pulling).

D. **Dementia**

1. Experimentally induced lesions of the **nucleus basalis magnocellularis** and the **medial septal area** are used to reproduce some of the pathologic changes observed in **Alzheimer's disease**. These areas are the anatomic analogues of the nucleus basalis of Meynert, the origin of the basal forebrain cholinergic system. This area is severely affected in patients with Alzheimer's disease.

2. Animals with lesions are tested in a variety of learning tasks (see III B 2). Animals with lesions of the basal forebrain cholinergic system perform poorly in maze-learning tasks designed to measure cognitive function and attentional processes.

E. **Depression**

1. **Maternal separation** in nonhuman primates is a possible model of depression. Under experimental conditions, young animals are separated from their mothers at various stages of development.
   a. Initially, **protest behavior** is observed. The animals show increased vocalizations and increased activity, and they attempt to return to the mother. Later, despair, or depression, occurs. The animals are socially withdrawn and hypoactive. They reduce their food and water intake and spend more time engaged in self-directed behaviors.
   b. **Neurobiologic changes** are also observed, including changes in heart rate, body temperature, sleep behavior, and adrenocortical responses.
   c. Similar symptoms are observed in children who are neglected or abandoned for long periods.

2. **Learned helplessness** is a term used to describe a paradigm developed in dogs by Seligman.[5] In this paradigm, the **avoidance of shock becomes impaired** in animals because of prior **exposure to unavoidable shock**. Dogs are given inescapable shock and are compared with dogs that received shock from which they could escape or received no shock at all. In a new testing situation, in which the animals can escape shock, animals that previously received inescapable shock passively accepted the shock and do not learn to escape.
   a. This behavior is attributed to the formation of an **expectation that the outcome of subsequent situations cannot be controlled.**
   b. Learned helplessness occurs in fish, rats, cats, dogs, monkeys, and humans in laboratory situations. In experiments with humans, subjects are given problem-solving tasks, but the experiment is structured so that the subjects cannot succeed. After the subjects realize that they cannot control the outcome, they typically stop attempting to solve subsequent problems.
   c. Such animals show reduced aggression, weight loss and anorexia, and deficits in social and sexual behavior in addition to the deficits in shock avoidance. These behaviors resemble the symptoms of major depressive disorder (see Chapter 15 VII A).
   d. **The syndrome can be prevented by prior exposure to escapable shock,** particularly when the exposure occurs in infancy. **Learned helplessness is a possible animal model of depression.** Antidepressants and electroconvulsive therapy (ECT) reverse learned helplessness in rats.

F. **Schizophrenia**

1. Behavioral changes induced in animals by stimulant drugs, such as phencyclidine (PCP) and amphetamine, are used as models of schizophrenia. These models are useful for testing antipsychotic drugs.

2. Studies in which hippocampal lesions are used to augment the effects of stimulant drugs or to produce behavioral abnormalities may provide models of schizophrenia.[6] In one model, lesions were induced in the ventral hippocampal area of newborn rats. These rats showed behavioral abnormalities only after puberty. This observation is analogous to the pubertal onset of schizophrenia.

REFERENCES

1. Becker JB, Breedlove SM, Crews D (eds): *Behavioral Endocrinology.* Cambridge, MA, MIT Press, 1992.
2. Moyer KE (ed): *Physiology of Aggression.* New York, Raven Press, 1976.
3. Markou A, Weiss F, Gold L, et al: Animal models of drug craving. *Psychopharmacology* 112:163–182, 1993.
4. Roediger HL II, Capaldi ED, Paris SG, et al: *Psychology.* New York, HarperCollins, 1991.
5. Roediger HL II, Capaldi ED, Paris SG, et al: *Psychology.* New York, HarperCollins, 1991.
6. Lipska BK, Jaskiw GE, Weinberger DR: Postpubertal emergence of hyperresponsiveness to stress and to amphetamine after neonatal excitotoxic hippocampal damage: a potential animal model of schizophrenia. *Neuropsychopharmacology* 9:67–75, 1993.

BIBLIOGRAPHY

Becker JB, Breedlove SM, Crews D (eds): *Behavioral Endocrinology.* Cambridge, MA, MIT Press, 1992.

Brobeck JR (ed): *Best & Taylor's Physiological Basis of Medical Practice.* Baltimore, Williams & Wilkins, 1982.

Cooper JR, Bloom FE, Roth RH: *The Biochemical Basis of Neuropharmacology,* 6th ed. New York, Oxford University Press, 1991.

Hinde RA: *Animal Behavior. New York, McGraw-Hill, 1970.*

Kandel ER, Schwartz JH, Jessell TM (eds): *Principles of Neural Science.* Amsterdam, Elsevier North Holland, 1991.

Kaplan HI, Sadock BJ (eds): *Comprehensive Textbook of Psychiatry,* 5th ed. Baltimore, Williams & Wilkins, 1989.

Lipska BK, Jaskiw GE, Weinberger DR: Postpubertal emergence of hyperresponsiveness to stress and to amphetamine after neonatal excitotoxic hippocampal damage: a potential animal model of schizophrenia. *Neuropsychopharmacology* 9:67–75, 1993.

Markou A, Weiss F, Gold L, et al: Animal models of drug craving. *Psychopharmacology* 112:163–182, 1993.

Meltzer HY (ed): *Psychopharmacology: The Third Generation of Progress.* New York, Raven Press, 1987.

Moyer KE (ed): *Physiology of Aggression.* New York, Raven Press, 1976.

National Institutes of Health: Vole mates, vasopressin keeps the home fires burning. Research brief, *JNIH Res* 6:41–46, 1994.

Rapoport JL: Recent advances in obsessive-compulsive disorder. *Neuropsychopharmacology* 5:1–10, 1991.

Roediger HL II, Capaldi ED, Paris SG, et al: *Psychology.* New York, HarperCollins, 1991.

Rosenberg RN (ed): *Comprehensive Neurology.* New York, Raven Press, 1991.

Tinbergen N: *The Study of Instinct.* New York, Oxford University Press, 1974.

STUDY QUESTIONS

DIRECTIONS: Each of the numbered items or incomplete statements in this section is followed by answers or by completions of the statement. Select the ONE lettered answer or completion that is BEST in each case.

1. The lowest degree of inherited behavior is exhibited by

(A) invertebrates
(B) birds
(C) mammals
(D) humans

2. The experimental study of conditioned taste aversion (CTA) requires

(A) a novel substance that causes illness immediately after ingestion
(B) a novel substance that causes illness either immediately after ingestion or later
(C) a novel substance that does not cause illness
(D) a poison that produces obvious signs of illness
(E) an antimetabolite (i.e., substance that interferes with the use of an essential metabolite)

3. Displacement behavior is an example of

(A) conflict behavior
(B) schedule-induced behavior
(C) conditioned neuroses
(D) classical conditioning
(E) primitive learning

4. The area of the brain that is involved in the regulation of feeding and drinking is the

(A) hypothalamus
(B) amygdala
(C) hippocampus
(D) cerebellum
(E) septum

5. Exploration is closely associated with what form of learning?

(A) Operant conditioning
(B) Classical conditioning
(C) Autoshaping
(D) Imprinting
(E) Habituation

6. Which of the following methods is used to test antianxiety agents?

(A) Radial arm maze
(B) Ventromedial hypothalamic lesions
(C) Elevated X-maze
(D) Biofeedback
(E) Oral metering

7. Which type of brain lesion is used to create an animal model of dementia?

(A) Cerebellum
(B) Amygdala lesions
(C) Hypothalamic lesions
(D) Nucleus basalis magnocellularis

DIRECTIONS: Each of the numbered items or incomplete statements in this section is negatively phrased, as indicated by a capitalized word such as NOT, LEAST, or EXCEPT. Select the ONE lettered answer or completion that is BEST in each case.

8. The following mechanisms are involved in hypovolemic drinking EXCEPT

(A) activation of osmoreceptors
(B) activation of baroreceptors
(C) release of renin from the kidney
(D) increase in heart rate and vasoconstriction

9. All of the following statements regarding Klüver-Bucy syndrome are true EXCEPT

(A) it results from the removal of or damage to the temporal lobes
(B) it is characterized by hyperactivity and a decreased fear of natural enemies
(C) it is characterized by increased oral manipulation, heightened sexual behavior, placidity, and inappropriate social behavior
(D) it is observed in humans with damage to the hypothalamus
(E) it is characterized by the inability to recognize common objects

10. Nonassociative forms of learning include all of the following EXCEPT

(A) exploration
(B) sensitization
(C) conditioning
(D) habituation

DIRECTIONS: Each set of matching questions in this section consists of a list of three to twenty-six lettered options (some of which may be in figures) followed by several numbered items. For each numbered item, select the ONE lettered option that is most closely associated with it. To avoid spending too much time on matching sets with large numbers of options, it is generally advisable to begin each set by reading the list of options. Then, for each item in the set, try to generate the correct answer and locate it in the option list, rather than evaluating each option individually. Each lettered option may be selected once, more than once, or not at all.

Questions 11–13

Match the schedule of reinforcement-controlling behavior with the corresponding situation.

(A) A carpenter being paid by the piece
(B) A gambler in a casino
(C) A customer receiving a daily newspaper delivery

11. Fixed-ratio schedule

12. Fixed-interval schedule

13. Variable-interval schedule

ANSWERS AND EXPLANATIONS

1. The answer is D [I A]. The lowest degree of inherited behavior is exhibited by humans. Clearly, the behavioral repertoire of higher organisms is primarily learned. However, even human infants exhibit a few inherited patterns, such as smiling, rooting, and lateral head movements.

2. The answer is C [II A 1 b]. The purpose of the conditioned taste aversion (CTA) paradigm is to create an aversion to an initially neutral stimulus by pairing it with a substance that produces illness. The animal is offered a novel food that does not cause illness. A second, unrelated illness-producing substance is then injected. The illness does not necessarily have to produce overt signs. In addition, not all poisonous substances produce CTA.

3. The answer is A [IV B 3]. Displacement behavior is irrelevant behavior that is exhibited in response to an approach–avoidance conflict. The clearest examples of displacement behavior are seen in birds, although similar behaviors are observed in other species.

4. The answer is A [II A 2 c, B 1 a]. Various areas of the hypothalamus, including the lateral and ventromedial areas, have important roles in the regulation of feeding and drinking. The amygdala, hippocampus, cerebellum, and septum are primarily involved in the control of other behaviors, including learning and aggressive behavior.

5. The answer is E [III A 2 a–b]. Habituation and exploration are closely related. Exploration continues until the animal habituates to novel stimuli. The animal does not explore excessively novel stimuli until it habituates to these stimuli.

6. The answer is C [V B 2]. Tests of antianxiety agents involve exposing the animals to a stressful situation, such as shock or elevated open spaces. The radial arm maze is a test for memory. Biofeedback is a technique that is successfully used mainly in humans. This technique trains subjects to regulate autonomic responses by providing them with immediate information about these responses. Ventromedial hypothalamic lesions induce a syndrome of overeating and obesity. Oral metering is used to study drinking behavior.

7. The answer is D [V D]. In Alzheimer's disease, the major site of degeneration is found in the basal forebrain cholinergic system. Experimental lesions in animals are placed in analogous anatomic areas, including the medial septal area and the nucleus basalis magnocellularis.

8. The answer is A [II B 1 a]. Osmoreceptors in the hypothalamus are activated in response to cellular dehydration, which results in dehydration-induced drinking. Hypovolemic drinking occurs after decreases in blood volume cause activation of baroreceptors in the great veins. Activation of the baroreceptors leads to increases in water absorption, increases in heart rate and vasoconstriction, release of renin by the kidney, and formation of angiotensin II. Angiotensin II acts on the hypothalamus and subfornical organ to induce drinking.

9. The answer is D [II D 2 a–b]. Klüver-Bucy syndrome is reported in humans, but it results from damage to the temporal lobes, not the hypothalamus. In animals, the syndrome is characterized by such diverse features as hyperactivity, increased sexual behavior, inappropriate social behavior, placidity, decreased fear of natural enemies, and inability to recognize common objects.

10. The answer is C [III A 1–3]. Through exploration, sensitization, and habituation, animals learn about the properties of a stimulus. Conditioning, whether classical or instrumental, involves the association between neutral and meaningful stimuli. By means of conditioning, a previously neutral stimuli, such as the ringing of a bell, can acquire significance, such as signaling the delivery of food.

11–13. The answers are: 11-A, 12-C, 13-B [III B 2 b (2) (a)–(b)]. The carpenter is paid a certain amount of money for every piece finished, so every response is rewarded on a 1:1 ratio. The customer receiving the newspaper obtains his reward at a fixed interval. As long as the customer pays for the newspaper delivery, he receives the reinforcer after a fixed period. In contrast, the gambler at the casino sometimes will win and sometimes will lose. The gambler cannot predict when the reinforcement will come, so he must continue to play. This situation is an example of a variable-interval schedule of reinforcement.

Chapter 6

Statistics and Research Design

Madeline M. Gladis
Robert C. Alexander

I. **INTRODUCTION.** Many aspects of brain function, mental life, and behavior are unknown. Scientific inquiry is one approach that can advance knowledge in the behavioral sciences and provide a basis for rational decision making.

A. **The aim of science is to explain natural phenomena.** Critical elements of scientific inquiry are theories and hypotheses.

1. **Theories are sets of definitions, propositions, and facts** that are arranged systematically to provide general explanations of phenomena. Theories specify **relations among variables and allow the prediction of certain variables** from other variables. An example of a theory in the behavioral sciences is that schizophrenia is caused by a viral infection that occurs during the second trimester of pregnancy.

2. **Hypotheses are conjectural statements** that link two or more variables. Hypotheses should use variables that can be clearly defined and tested. An example of a hypothesis is that children whose parents are alcoholics will have higher rates of depression as adults.

B. **Scientific research is the systematic and empirical investigation of hypotheses.**

1. When possible, **observations are controlled** so that only one of the possible explanations for the proposed relation between variables is examined.

2. Scientific beliefs are based on **data**. Theories are constructed and confirmed or discarded based on the results of empirical inquiry.

C. **Types of research in the behavioral sciences.** Research can be **experimental or correlational,** depending on whether the investigator has control over and can manipulate any of the variables. Conclusions based on correlational research are not as firm as conclusions based on experimental research.

1. In **experimental research,** direct control of a variable permits measurement of the effect of the variable on another variable (e.g., subjects with memory loss are randomly assigned to receive drug or placebo, and the effect of the drug on memory is measured).

2. In **correlational research,** variables cannot be controlled directly. Variables are observed, and correlations between them are determined (e.g., a researcher interviews the mothers of retarded and normal children to determine whether the mothers of the retarded children drank more alcohol during pregnancy).

II. **MEASUREMENT AND STATISTICS. Statistics is the mathematics of the collection, organization, and interpretation of data.** To conduct research that generates meaningful results, it is important to design the statistical analysis before collecting the data. Almost all research in the behavioral sciences uses some type of statistical analysis. To understand published scientific research, the reader must be familiar with statistics.

A. **Types of variables. A variable is anything that can be measured or manipulated** in a study. In a true experiment, the **independent variable** is controlled by the experimenter and is presumed to have an effect on the **dependent variable**. Even in studies in which experimental manipulation is not possible (i.e., correlational studies), one variable is often hypothesized to be an antecedent or cause of the other. An important distinction is made between **qualitative and quantitative variables** based on their underlying scale of measurement. These types of variables are treated differently in the analysis of data.

1. **Qualitative variables**
   a. A **nominal scale** names observations and classifies them into mutually exclusive categories. Medical diagnoses are nominal variables, as are demographic characteristics, such as sex, ethnicity, and religion.
   b. An **ordinal scale** is a ranking of observations according to some criterion. The ranking orders the data from lowest to highest (e.g., a patient's status after a medication trial can be ranked from "much worse" to "much better"). The rankings are based on subjective criteria because the magnitude of difference between any two rankings cannot be measured.

2. **Quantitative variables**
   a. In an **interval scale,** observations also are ranked, but the differences between any two points of measurement are known and are equal. Temperature and other physiologic variables are measured on interval scales.
   b. A **ratio scale** has equivalent intervals between points. The ratios are also equivalent because a true zero point exists. Height and weight are ratio variables because the zero point is not arbitrary. Both interval and ratio scales have actual numeric values.

3. Most behavioral researchers assume that they are working with interval scales, and they analyze the data accordingly. However, the same variable can be used differently in different analyses. For example, age can be considered a nominal (18–30 years versus older than 30 years) or an interval variable (age in years).

B. **Descriptive statistics. The goal of descriptive statistics is to organize and summarize data** so that they are accessible and useful. Descriptive methods provide a clear picture of the data in a particular sample. No inferences are made about the characteristics of the population from which the sample was drawn. A number of standard methods are used to describe data.

1. **Frequency distributions.** Raw scores can be summarized in a **table of frequencies and cumulative frequencies**. These tables show the distribution of data among categories (for qualitative data) or over all of the possible values (for numeric, or quantitative, data). These numbers can be used to generate a **histogram plot,** with scores marked along the x-axis and frequencies marked along the y-axis (Figure 6-1). Plotting large numbers of data typically produces a **bell-shaped curve**. This curve is called a **normal, or Gaussian, distribution**. The normal distribution is theoretical because its properties are defined mathematically. The population distribution of many variables is assumed to be normal, and the sample distribution is often assumed to be normal if the sample is large. More efficient ways to summarize data are based on the properties of this normal distribution.

2. **Measures of central tendency.** The average score in a distribution can be described in three ways: **mean, median,** and **mode**.
   a. The **mean** is the sum of the scores divided by the number of scores. It is a useful measure for statistical analysis because it considers all scores. It is most consistent with the true population mean when several samples are drawn from a population. However, it is sensitive to extreme scores, causing the distribution to be positively or negatively skewed. For example, if four subjects have scores of 4, 5, 6, and 8 on a test, the mean score for the group is 5.75. The addition of one subject with a score of 20 would change the mean to 8.6. Use of the mean is restricted to interval and ratio variables, in which the distance between scores is meaningful.
   b. The **median** is the point that divides the distribution into two groups of equal size. Half of the scores fall below this value; half fall above it. It is computed as the fiftieth percentile. The median is not as sensitive as the mean to extreme scores, and is less useful for analyzing data.

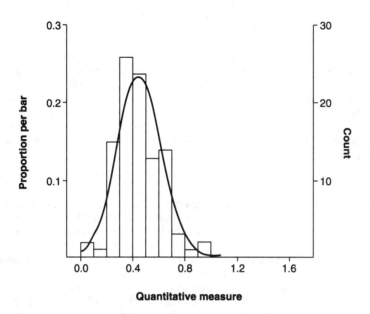

Quantitative measure

FIGURE 6-1. Histogram plot of data. Scores are marked on the x-axis, and frequencies are marked on the y-axis. A curve showing a normal distribution is superimposed.

   c. The **mode** is the most common score in the distribution. It is a crude measure that is most appropriate for describing nominal data. When two values occur frequently, the distribution is **bimodal**. In a normal (**symmetric**) distribution, the mean, median, and mode values will be similar. Distributions that are not normal (**skewed**) have dissimilar measures of central tendency.

3. **Measures of dispersion or variability** indicate how much the scores deviate from the typical score (the average). There are several measures of dispersion (variation) of scores around the mean.

   a. The **range** is the simplest, most obvious measure of variation. It is the difference between the highest and the lowest scores. It is not considered an adequate measure of variability because it is distorted by extreme scores.

   b. The **variance** is more informative than the range because all of the scores are used to calculate it. The variance indicates how much the individual scores deviate from the mean. In computing the variance, the mean is subtracted from each score, the differences are squared and then summed, and this sum is divided by $N - 1$, where N is the sample size. The variance is high when scores are widely scattered, and low when scores cluster around the mean.

   c. The **standard deviation (SD)** provides a measure of dispersion that is expressed in original (unsquared) units. It is the square root of the variance. In a normal distribution, 68% of the scores fall within 1 SD of the mean, 95% fall within 2 SDs, and 2.5% fall within each tail. When an original score is **standardized** (transformed to a **Z score** by subtracting the mean and dividing the remainder by the original SD), its numeric value indicates its distance from the mean in terms of SDs. For example, a Z score of $+1$ indicates that the original score lies 1 SD above the mean, and a Z score of -2 indicates that the original score lies 2 SDs below the mean.

   d. The **standard error of the mean** is a related measure that is frequently used in statistical tests. The standard error is the SD divided by the square root of the sample size; thus, the larger the sample size, the smaller the error. Use of the standard error is based on the assumption that if a number of samples were drawn from the population (**sampling distribution**), the variability of the means of the samples would be less than the variability of the raw scores from a single sample. The standard error is this measure of variability of sample means. It is therefore a better approximation of the true population value, which cannot be measured directly.

C. **Inferential statistics.** Whereas descriptive statistics are used to describe the data, **inferential statistics are used to make inferences about the characteristics of a population** based on a small sample from the population. Inferential statistics are frequently used to determine whether groups **differ significantly** in some variable. Because their function is to show whether the observed differences could have occurred by chance alone, inferential statistics are based on **probability theory**. Types of inferential statistics include **parametric and nonparametric tests**. The choice of statistical test depends on the type and number of variables being studied.

1. **Hypothesis testing.** When groups are compared, hypotheses that involve true population differences are posed.
   a. The first step is to specify a **null hypothesis (H_0:** that no differences exist between groups). If statistical calculations show that it is unlikely that the observed differences were caused by chance alone, **the null hypothesis can be rejected** and the **alternative hypothesis (H_1:** that differences exist between groups) accepted. If the likelihood that a difference occurred by chance alone is less than one in twenty, the difference is **statistically significant** at the .05 level.
   b. Two types of errors can occur in the interpretation of results.
      (1) A **type I error** is the incorrect rejection of the null hypothesis (e.g., concluding that there are group differences when the differences occurred by chance). The likelihood of a type I error is equal to alpha, a significance level that is usually set at .05.
      (2) A **type II error** is the incorrect acceptance of the null hypothesis when the alternative hypothesis is true (e.g., concluding that there are no group differences when such differences exist). The likelihood of a type II error can also be calculated and is symbolized by the Greek letter beta. The risks of type I and type II errors have practical implications. Decisions about the level of significance that must be reached to reject the null hypothesis (traditionally .05 or .01) are often based on methodological considerations that are specific to each experiment.
   c. **Confidence intervals** provide some degree of certainty about the accuracy of population estimates. For example, if the mean and variance are known for the scores of a sample of $N = 30$, the range of scores that has a 95% probability of including the true population mean can be calculated. This range is the 95% confidence interval. It can be used to determine the probable value of a single population mean and the probable value of the difference between two population means.
   d. A **one-tailed test** is used if the differences are hypothesized to occur in one direction only (e.g., test scores are predicted to increase). A **two-tailed test** is used when no predictions have been made about the direction of results (e.g., an experimental treatment could lead to improvement or worsening of symptoms). Because the significance level of a two-tailed test is halved (e.g., from .05 to .025), larger differences are necessary to reject the null hypothesis. Most behavioral research uses two-tailed tests.
   e. The **power of a test** is defined as the probability that the null hypothesis will be rejected if it is false. It is the complement of a type II error. Power is computed with the significance criterion alpha, estimates of the magnitude of the true effect in the population, and the sample size.[1] In practice, power is used to determine whether a sample is large enough to show statistically significant effects.

2. **Parametric tests** are used when at least one of the variables being analyzed is interval or ratio.
   a. A **t test** is used to compare the means of two samples to show how often the difference between means would occur by chance. A t test consists of one independent variable that is nominal or categorical (e.g., presence or absence of treatment) and a dependent variable that is quantitative or continuous (e.g., improvement in score).

The null hypothesis is that the population values of the two groups are not different. The null hypothesis is rejected if the computed value of *t* is greater than the critical value of *t* in a *t* table.

    (1) An **unpaired *t* test** compares independent samples. The difference between the sample means is divided by the estimated standard error of the difference. For example, if the mean achievement test score of all first graders from school A were compared with the mean achievement test score of all first graders from school B, an unpaired *t* test would be used.

    (2) A **paired *t* test** compares sample means from the same group (e.g., pretest and posttest scores) or a matched group of subjects. Difference scores for each pair are computed, and the mean of these scores is divided by the square root of the variance of the difference scores over the number of pairs.

b. An **analysis of variance (ANOVA)** is used to compare the means of multiple groups. It is called **one-way ANOVA** if there is just one independent variable (e.g., active drug versus placebo) and **two-way ANOVA** if there are two independent grouping variables, or factors (e.g., drug versus placebo and sex). A **repeated measures ANOVA** is used when the same measure is used on multiple occasions. Both main and interaction effects can be studied in a two-way procedure. The formula for ANOVA involves calculating the ratio of the variation between groups to the variation within groups. This measure is called the **F ratio**.

c. Simple correlation and regression

    (1) A **correlation statistic** indicates the degree to which two quantitative variables are related. Two variables can be **uncorrelated** (no relation), **positively correlated** (as the value of one increases, the other also increases), or **negatively correlated** (as the value of one increases, the other decreases). Correlations range from -1.00 to $+1.00$. The value indicates the strength of the relation, and the sign indicates the direction of correlation. **Pearson's correlation coefficient (r)** is the most commonly used correlation statistic for quantitative data. Its statistical significance can be tested. Correlation does not show or even suggest causation.

    (2) A graphic depiction (called a **scatter plot or scattergram**) is often used to show the relation between two variables. If a straight line can be drawn through the scores plotted along the x- and y-axes, the variables have a **linear relation**. The line is computed with a **least squares approximation procedure,** which minimizes the sum of the squared horizontal distances between the points and the line (Figure 6-2).

    (3) In **regression statistics,** the line can be used to predict a probable Y score from a known X score with the use of the **slope** (the ratio of change in X to change in Y) and the **intercept** (the point at which the line crosses the vertical axis). In **multiple regression analysis,** several independent variables (X_1 to X_n) are used to predict a single dependent variable (Y).

3. Nonparametric tests are used when both independent and dependent variables are nominal or ordinal. This situation arises frequently in behavioral and medical research. For example, an investigator might be interested in the relation between the presence and absence of a disease and the levels of a risk factor for the disease.

a. The **chi-square test** is a common nonparametric test. The first step in using this test is to construct a **contingency table** in which the rows represent various levels of the first criterion of classification and the columns represent levels of the second criterion of classification. The **ratio of observed to expected frequencies** in the cells of the table is called **chi-square**. This ratio indicates whether the numbers differ from those that would be expected if no association was present. A **Fisher exact test** is used as an alternative to chi-square when expected cell frequencies are small (< 5).

b. Other nonparametric tests have been developed for one-sample tests (e.g., binomial test), for ranked (ordinal) data (e.g., Mann-Whitney U test), and for measures of association similar to the correlation coefficient [e.g., Spearman's rank correlation coefficient (rho), Kendall's rank correlation coefficient (tau), and Cohen's kappa].

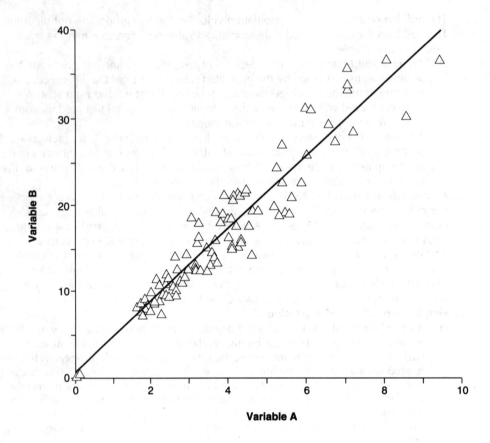

FIGURE 6-2. Scatter plot of the relationship between variable A and variable B. The regression line computed with the least squares approximation procedure is superimposed.

4. **Multivariate techniques** involve more than one dependent variable. They were developed to circumvent statistical problems that arise when multiple univariate tests are performed on a set of dependent variables. Hotteling's T^2 test is used to compare two groups and the multivariate analysis of variance (MANOVA) is used when more than two groups are compared. Other multivariate methods yield information that aids in the classification of variables or subjects. These methods include discriminant function analysis, factor analysis, and cluster analysis.

5. **Meta-analysis** refers to the quantitative combination of data from independent trials. Specific statistical techniques are used to detect effects and examine trends in pooled data.

III. RESEARCH DESIGN. Research design encompasses all of the steps taken to plan and execute a study, from the formulation of hypotheses to the analysis of data.

A. **Validity and reliability.** The meaningfulness of an experiment depends on the validity and reliability of its design and of its measurements.

1. **Design.** Careful attention to experimental design ensures that validity and reliability have been addressed.
   a. Research has **internal validity** to the extent that conclusions about cause and effect can be drawn. Did the experimental treatment or manipulation have an effect?

Internal validity is threatened when extraneous variables are not controlled. The effects can be confused (confounded) with the effects of the independent variable that is being studied. Differences between groups may influence the outcome of a study. For example, if patients are allowed to volunteer for either a treatment group or a group receiving no active treatment (waiting list condition) in a study of psychotherapy, the group volunteering for the waiting list condition might do better than their treated counterparts if they were less depressed at the start of the experiment.

b. **Construct validity** is the correct conceptual interpretation of the independent and dependent variables and the relation between them. For example, a study of cognitive therapy must include a conceptually relevant outcome measure, such as ratings of patient cognitions, to show the effectiveness of the cognitive component. Otherwise, the therapeutic effects could be seen as nonspecific and open to different theoretical interpretations.

c. A study has **external validity** if the causal relation that it identifies can be generalized to other times, places, and subjects. Studies performed with college students are sometimes criticized because the findings might not extend to other groups or settings. Findings from studies of a particular diagnostic group (e.g., brain abnormalities in schizophrenic patients) in one country are usually thought to be generalizable to patients in another country, assuming that identical diagnostic criteria are used.

d. **Reliability** in research means that the findings are replicable. Exact replications of methods and results show reliability, whereas replications in different settings and with different procedures show external validity.[2] Without adequate reliability, a measure is not interpretable. High reliability, however, does not guarantee good scientific results.

2. **Measures.** Research measures are chosen for their ability to **operationalize** (define in terms of operations) the construct of interest. Examples of constructs in the behavioral sciences include clinical disorders (psychiatric diagnoses), behaviors (hyperactivity), mood states (depression), and cognitive abilities (memory). Validity and reliability are also required at the measurement level.

a. **Validity** is the extent to which an instrument measures what it purports to measure. Is the scholastic aptitude test (SAT) a measure of intelligence? Is pulse rate a good measure of anxiety? Several types of validity are relevant to measurement.

(1) **Face validity** involves a subjective process of deciding whether the test or instrument appears to measure the construct of interest. It is evaluated informally by the investigator or formally by a group of experts. An example of a measure with face validity is the widely used Hamilton Rating Scale for Depression. This scale provides a means of assessing the severity of patients' depression and contains straightforward items (e.g., depressed mood, loss of interest in work and activities, thoughts of suicide) that all clinicians treating depressed patients would agree are key components of the depressive syndrome.

(2) **Concurrent validity** is the ability of a test to distinguish between subjects that are known to differ through other indicators. For example, children who score low on a measure of attention should also do poorly in school.

(3) **Predictive validity** is the ability of a test to predict future differences between groups (e.g., college performance predicted by SAT scores).

(4) **Construct validity** is the extent to which a measure captures the construct of interest. It is evaluated through convergent validity and discriminant validity. **Convergent validity** is agreement between instruments that attempt to measure the same construct. **Discriminant validity** is disagreement between instruments that attempt to measure different constructs. For example, the validity of a new measure of depression could be assessed by testing whether patients identified as "depressed" by this scale are also found to be depressed using evidence from other sources, such as clinicians' assessments, self-report, and other rating scales of depression.

b. A **reliable measure** produces findings that do not fluctuate randomly from one administration to the next or when alternative forms of assessment are used. Reliability is assessed in many ways.

(1) Test–retest correlation is computed when an instrument is administered twice to the same sample. A small amount of error is expected, but relative positions on a scale should be similar from one administration to the next.

(2) Cronbach's alpha is a measure of the **internal consistency** of a test or scale. It is computed by correlating each item with the total score and averaging the correlation coefficients.

(3) The **split-half reliability model** is based on splitting the scale into two parts and examining the correlation between the parts.

(4) Inter-rater reliability refers to the degree that two or more raters using the same instrument will obtain the same result. For dichotomous data (absence or presence of one category or another), the **intraclass correlation coefficient** is a suitable measure. For more than two categories, a **kappa** or **weighted kappa** statistic is used. For ratings on a quantitative scale, an analysis of variance intraclass correlation coefficient can be used.

B. Types of studies

1. True experiments. In a true experiment, the experimenter has control over the treatment or condition (the independent variable), and subjects are randomly assigned to two or more study groups. At least one group receives the intervention, and one group does not. This classic paradigm is used to test a theory (specifically, hypotheses about group differences) rather than to describe the world as it exists. Most laboratory studies and clinical trials are true experiments. Some of the elements of a true experiment are described below.

a. Random assignment is a method of assigning subjects to treatment groups to ensure that the groups are equivalent. All subjects have an equal chance of being assigned to any one of the study conditions. This method controls for (eliminates) the influence of extraneous subject variables that might mask the true effect of the variable of interest. Differences observed between the groups at the conclusion of the study can then be attributed with greater confidence to the experimental manipulation. For example, if an experimenter wanted to assess the effects of a mathematics review course on test scores, natural variations in the mathematical aptitude of students would require that students be randomly assigned to the experimental and control groups.

b. Double-blind random assignment is designed to reduce bias stemming from subject and experimenter awareness. The subject may become aware of the study hypothesis, and this knowledge may cause changes in behavior, or the experimenter may inadvertently communicate how the subject is expected to behave. With double-blind random assignment, neither the subject nor the experimenter knows the group assignment of subjects.

c. A **placebo,** which is an inert substance or sham treatment delivered to members of a control group, is used to reduce bias stemming from awareness of research conditions.

d. Outcome measures can include:

(1) Direct observation by experimenters (e.g., nurses' ratings of manic behavior of patients on an inpatient unit). **Interobserver agreement** must be shown (reliability), and the behaviors must reflect what they are assumed to reflect and not something else (validity).

(2) Questionnaires and self-report rating scales that tap attitudes, emotions, or behaviors. Questionnaires are inexpensive to administer. They are also believed to increase the validity of self-report because they offer subjects anonymity and minimize interviewer bias. A disadvantage is that subjects may not take a questionnaire seriously, and may give little thought to their responses. Some may not respond at all. Therefore, the findings may not be reliable. Scales that are designed to measure a particular construct (e.g., self-esteem) must be pretested for reliability and validity.

(3) Interviews of subjects. Interviews are believed to yield a better response rate than questionnaires and rating scales, and they are more effective than questionnaires for obtaining complex or emotionally oriented information. Misunderstandings can be corrected, and interviewers can encourage subjects to elaborate on specific topics and to talk about sensitive issues. A combination of the interview and questionnaire methods is frequently used in behavioral research (e.g., to measure improvement in a trial of psychotropic medication).

2. **Quasiexperiments.** Variations on the classic experimental designs are often implemented outside the laboratory because random assignment to treatment conditions often is not possible. Quasiexperimental designs used in field settings usually can control timing of the interventions and the selection of subjects being evaluated, but the baseline characteristics of these subjects cannot be controlled.[3] Because the study groups are not equivalent, the researcher must be aware of extraneous variables that may affect outcome. Many public health studies are quasiexperiments because random assignment of community members to a preventive intervention (e.g., an antismoking campaign) would not be feasible. **Self-selection** of subjects into study groups is a significant problem for field studies.

3. **Correlational studies.** In correlational studies, no attempt is made to manipulate a variable and observe its effect on a second variable. Instead, two variables are measured, usually simultaneously, and their relation is assessed.
    a. The **disadvantage of a correlational study** is that it does not permit conclusions to be drawn about cause and effect. This problem occurs because experimenters cannot be certain whether X causes Y, Y causes X, or a third variable (measured or unmeasured) causes both X and Y. For example, people who abuse alcohol have high scores on measures of depression. However, it is not clear whether depression leads people to drink, whether alcoholism induces depressed mood, or whether some underlying factor (e.g., a common genetic susceptibility) causes both tendencies.
    b. The **advantage of a correlational study** is that it permits the investigation of naturally occurring characteristics and phenomena that cannot be studied experimentally. **Surveys** are the best example of correlational studies. Surveys attempt to measure the prevalence or distribution of characteristics (e.g., attitudes, behaviors, psychiatric disorders) in the population and to assess the relation between these characteristics.
        (1) Survey research depends on **random sampling** to ensure that the individuals studied are representative of the population to which results will be generalized. In a random sample, each subject in the larger population has an equal chance of being surveyed. Several variants of random sampling techniques are used.
        (2) Statistical methods are used in survey research to define the relation among variables and to generate and test causal hypotheses. Cause cannot be proven in correlational designs, but causal relations can be supported, often through the elimination of alternative explanations.

4. **Retrospective and prospective studies.** In epidemiology, the distinction is made between **retrospective and prospective designs**. Both are observational (nonexperimental) studies because no attempt is made to study the effect of a factor that is under the control of the experimenter.
    a. In a **retrospective** design (also called a **case–control study**), individuals with a certain disease and individuals without that disease are compared, and their risk factors for that disease are evaluated. Those with the disease are called **cases** and those without the disease are called **controls**. An **odds ratio** is computed to determine whether there is a statistically significant difference in the proportion of cases and controls exposed to the risk factors.
    b. In a **prospective** study, disease-free individuals with varying levels of exposure to certain risk factors are studied for an extended period of time to determine which subjects will subsequently have the disease. Odds ratios are also used in prospective studies to establish associations between risk factors and incidence of disease.

C. **Ethics in research.** The manner in which research is conducted has consequences for the study subject, the academic community, and society. In some instances, moral standards have been violated. Ethical issues are involved in all aspects of research, from the selection of the study topic to the way in which results are reported. Ethical concerns are not limited to experimental situations that include deception or aversive techniques.

1. **The problem.** Kidder[2] described questionable practices that are encountered in behavioral research. These practices include lack of informed consent, coercion, deception, exposure to physical and mental stress, and withholding of benefits.

2. **The solution.** The conduct of research is subject to the approval of institutional review boards. Funding sources also consider the ethical aspects of experimental procedures. Organizations whose members conduct research have developed guidelines that describe the responsibilities of the researcher. Informed consent, protection from harm, and confidentiality are emphasized. Ultimately, however, the responsibility for the ethical conduct of research rests with each investigator.

IV. EXAMPLES OF RESEARCH DESIGN

A. **Experimental study.** Many individuals with chronic psychosis consume excessive amounts of fluid. Water intoxication develops in some patients, and it may result in death. Subjects with chronic psychosis and documented water intoxication underwent a double-blind, placebo-controlled trial of an experimental medication. The study consisted of a 2-week observation period, a 3-week active treatment period, and a 3-week placebo treatment period. The order of treatment was randomly assigned. Each subject was weighed three times daily to determine daily weight gain. Serum sodium levels were obtained daily to measure water intoxication.

1. This example is an **experimental study** because the investigators controlled the **independent variable,** drug or placebo. The experiment was also **double-blind** because neither the subjects nor the investigator knew whether a subject was taking the experimental drug or placebo until after the study was completed.

2. The **hypothesis** is that the experimental medication will decrease the amount of water consumed daily and the occurrence of water intoxication (**dependent variables**).

3. The **dependent variables** are measured by determining serum sodium level and weight gain over the course of each day. These measures do not precisely operationalize the constructs being studied.

4. The data can be analyzed in a number of ways. The average weight gain or average serum sodium level in the third week in each study period (active drug or placebo) can be compared with a **paired *t* test**. The daily weight gain and sodium level from each of the 3 weeks in each study period can be compared with a **repeated measures ANOVA**. In addition, the number of sodium levels in each study period that are lower than a predetermined level can be compared with a **chi-square test**.

B. **Correlational study.** Despite objective evidence to the contrary, many adolescents who live in urban areas that have a high incidence of acquired immune deficiency syndrome (AIDS) may not perceive the threat of AIDS as real or immediate. High school students from a large urban area were surveyed about their perceived risk of AIDS, risk behaviors, knowledge about AIDS, and a measure of style of coping with threatening information (degree of repression–sensitization).

1. This example is a **correlational study** because the investigators do not control any of the variables.

2. The main **hypothesis** is that adolescents who have a predisposition to deny threat will minimize their perceived risk of AIDS.

3. The **outcome variable** is the perceived risk of AIDS. This variable was measured through direct questioning (i.e., "What are your chances of getting AIDS?") The **predictor variables** are demographics, risk behaviors, knowledge about AIDS, and degree of repression–sensitization. These variables are also measured through carefully chosen questions.

4. The data can be analyzed using hierarchic **multiple regression**. Multiple regression allows the investigators to examine the linear relation between perceived risk (Y) and the variables degree of repression–sensitization (X_1), demographics (X_2), knowledge about AIDS (X_3), and risk behaviors (X_4). The contribution of each variable can also be assessed by controlling for the effects of all of the other variables.

REFERENCES

1. Cohen J: *Statistical Power Analysis for the Behavioral Sciences.* New York, Academic Press, 1977.

2. Kidder LH: *Research Methods in Social Relations.* New York, Holt, Rinehart, & Winston, 1981.

3. Campbell DT, Stanley JC: *Experimental and Quasi-experimental Designs for Research.* Boston, Houghton Mifflin, 1963.

BIBLIOGRAPHY

Campbell DT, Stanley JC: *Experimental and Quasi-experimental Designs for Research.* Boston, Houghton Mifflin, 1963.

Cohen J: *Statistical Power Analysis for the Behavioral Sciences.* New York, Academic Press, 1977.

Hamilton M: Development of a rating scale for primary depressive illness. *Br J Soc Clin Psychol* 6:278–279, 1967.

Kidder LH: *Research Methods in Social Relations.* New York, Holt, Rinehart, & Winston, 1981.

Streiner N: *PDQ Statistics.* Philadelphia, BC Decker, 1986.

Welkowitz J, Ewen RB, Cohen J: *Introductory Statistics for the Behavioral Sciences,* 4th ed. New York, Harcourt, Brace, Jovanovich, 1991.

STUDY QUESTIONS

DIRECTIONS: Each of the numbered items or incomplete statements in this section is followed by answers or by completions of the statement. Select the ONE lettered answer or completion that is BEST in each case.

1. Scores on a test that measures attention are normally distributed, with a mean of 50 and a standard deviation (SD) of 10. What percentage of the population will have a score higher than 60?

(A) 10%
(B) 16%
(C) 25%
(D) 35%
(E) 50%

2. A variable X is found to correlate with another variable Y with a Pearson's correlation coefficient (r) of 0.87 ($P < .05$). Which of the following is true?

(A) X causes Y
(B) Y causes X
(C) Increases in X are associated with increases in Y
(D) Decreases in X are associated with increases in Y
(E) X is not significantly correlated with Y

Questions 3–5

An investigator wants to study the effectiveness of a new type of group therapy for smoking cessation. She recruits 40 smokers and asks 20 of them to volunteer for the therapy. Three months later, she measures the number of cigarettes smoked daily by all 40 smokers.

3. What key component is missing in this experiment?

(A) Random assignment
(B) Hypothesis
(C) Independent variable
(D) Operationalized outcome measure
(E) Dependent variable

4. A possible source of bias is self-selection. It is an example of a threat to

(A) reliability
(B) external validity
(C) internal validity
(D) generalizability
(E) predictive validity

5. The outcome measure (number of cigarettes smoked daily) is an example of a

(A) qualitative variable
(B) nominal variable
(C) quantitative variable
(D) nonparametric variable
(E) ordinal variable

DIRECTIONS: Each of the numbered items or incomplete statements in this section is negatively phrased, as indicated by a capitalized word such as NOT, LEAST, or EXCEPT. Select the ONE lettered answer or completion that is BEST in each case.

6. Each of the following is an example of an ordinal variable EXCEPT

(A) cancer pain rating
(B) socioeconomic status
(C) marital status
(D) improvement with medication graded from "much worse" to "much better"
(E) degree of drug addiction

7. Interval variable data can be analyzed with all of the following techniques EXCEPT

(A) linear regression
(B) *t* test
(C) chi-square
(D) Hotteling's T^2
(E) analysis of variance (ANOVA)

DIRECTIONS: Each set of matching questions in this section consists of a list of four to twenty-six lettered options (some of which may be in figures) followed by several numbered items. For each numbered item, select the ONE lettered option that is most closely associated with it. To avoid spending too much time on matching sets with large numbers of options, it is generally advisable to begin each set by reading the list of options. Then, for each item in the set, try to generate the correct answer and locate it in the option list, rather than evaluating each option individually. Each lettered option may be selected once, more than once, or not at all.

Questions 8–9

For each statement, select the most appropriate statistical term.

(A) Mean
(B) Mode
(C) Median
(D) Variance
(E) Standard error

8. The measure of central tendency that is most sensitive to extreme scores

9. The most informative measure of dispersion of scores

ANSWERS AND EXPLANATIONS

1. The answer is B [II B 3 c]. Sixty-eight percent of the scores will fall within 1 standard deviation (SD) of the mean (34% on either side of the mean). One-half of the remaining scores will be more than 1 SD from the mean (16% on either side of the distribution).

2. The answer is C [II C 2 c (1)]. X and Y are positively correlated, and the correlation reaches statistical significance. Correlation does not imply causation; therefore, it cannot be concluded that either X causes Y or that Y causes X. Because the correlation coefficient is positive and statistically significant, increases in X are associated with increases in Y.

3. The answer is A [III B 1]. The hallmark of a true experiment is random assignment to ensure equivalency of groups. The smokers in this study were not randomly assigned. The group that volunteered for therapy may be more motivated to quit smoking and therefore may not be equivalent to the group that did not volunteer.

4. The answer is C [III A 1 a]. Threats to internal validity are caused by uncontrolled variables that may influence the outcome of the study. In this case, the volunteers for the experimental condition may have been more motivated at the outset to discontinue smoking. It would therefore be difficult to draw the conclusion that the therapy caused any difference in outcome between the groups.

5. The answer is C [II A 2 b]. The number of cigarettes smoked daily is an example of a quantitative variable because it has an actual meaningful numeric value. Nominal and ordinal variables are examples of qualitative variables that represent categories.

6. The answer is C [II A 1 a–b]. Marital status is a category and an example of a nominal variable. Ordinal variables represent sets of ordered categories; sometimes these categories are devised by the researcher.

7. The answer is C [II C 2 a–c]. Interval variable data cannot be analyzed with chi-square unless they are first converted into categorical data. The chi-square analysis requires the construction of a contingency table, in which the rows represent categories derived from one variable, and the columns represent categories derived from another variable.

8–9. The answers are: 8-A [II B 2 a], **9-D** [II B 3 b]. Because the mean takes all scores into account, it is most influenced by extreme scores. The variance is the measure of the extent to which individual values differ from the mean. Because the variance is calculated by subtracting the mean from each value, it is the most informative measure of dispersion of scores. Like the mean, the variance takes all scores into account.

Chapter 7

Theories of the Mind

Jerry M. Wiener

I. **INTRODUCTION.** These theories are organized frames of reference for understanding the origins and interactions of thoughts, feelings, and behaviors at the interface between brain function and the environment. Other chapters discuss the basic organization and functions of the brain that underlie all behaviors but do not explain individual human development. This chapter describes the theories that attempt to explain behavior within a biopsychosocial model. Psychoanalytic, learning, cognitive, psychosocial, and biomedical theories are discussed.

II. **PSYCHOANALYTIC (PSYCHODYNAMIC) THEORY** is based on the concept of **conflict among forces within the mind (intrapsychic conflict).** This theory is identified with the work of **Sigmund Freud** (1856–1939) that began in the early 1890s. It is sometimes referred to as Freudian theory, although subsequent work has greatly added to and changed many of Freud's initial concepts. The theory originally developed as an explanation of behavior and symptoms known as **neuroses** (e.g., phobias, obsessions, hysteria) that were understood as the result or solution of an intrapsychic conflict between a revived childhood sexual wish and the force of conscience. The theory gradually expanded to include both normal and abnormal development and personality formation. The term **psychoanalysis** is used to refer to a body of **theoretic concepts,** a method and technique for the **treatment of certain mental disorders** (e.g., personality disorders; see Chapter 11) and a **method for learning about mental process.**

A. **Basic concepts**

1. **Unconscious mental process** is a key concept of psychoanalytic theory that proposes that a great deal of mental activity occurs outside of an individual's awareness, but is influential in determining conscious thought and behavior. Unconscious mental activity includes thoughts, wishes, urges, feelings, and fantasies that would be considered **unacceptable or dangerous** if they became conscious or if the individual acted on them. Parts of the personality that are also considered unconscious, or functioning outside of the individual's awareness, include:
   a. The **conscience (superego),** which provides judgment associated with feelings of guilt or shame
   b. **Defenses,** such as denial and projection (see II A 5)
   c. **Automatic behavior,** such as driving home from work without thinking about it

2. **Psychic determinism** proposes that all mental activity, conscious and unconscious, is meaningful and purposeful and is connected with previous life experiences. Consequently, no mental activity or behavior is random, accidental, or meaningless unless it is caused by abnormal brain activity, such as a seizure.

3. **Instincts, or drives,** are the motivating forces behind thoughts and behaviors. They originate from biosomatic processes and are experienced as **urges, wishes, and fantasies.**
   a. The two major **categories of drives** are sexual (libido) and aggressive. Drives press for discharge and the associated feeling of release and gratification.
   b. The drives and the methods available for discharge are in stages, known as **psychosexual stages.**

4. **Psychosexual stages** are the gradual, sequential emergence of the sexual drive (instinct) from infancy (infantile sexuality) to adulthood (genital sexuality). These stages reflect the interaction between physical and nervous system **maturation** and individual experience (**development**).

   a. The **oral stage** encompasses the period from birth to 1½ years. During this period, the primary means of drive discharge and gratification is through sucking (innate behavior), chewing, and feeding.

   b. The **anal stage** spans the period from 1½ to 3 years. During this stage, sphincter control is achieved and the primary focus shifts to the anal zone and the behaviors associated with expulsion and retention.

   c. The **phallic (oedipal) stage** extends from 3 to 6 years of age. During this period, the genitals become the primary source of interest, discharge, and organization of urges into wishes and fantasies. Characteristic behaviors include curiosity, exhibition, and masturbation. The **Oedipus complex** is both the central theme of this stage and a core concept of early psychoanalytic theory.

      (1) The **Oedipus complex** includes the wish of the child for an exclusive and quasiadult libidinal relationship with the parent of the opposite sex. This wish includes a desire to exclude and replace the same-sex parent, who is perceived as a rival.

      (2) **Conflict** results from the fear of parental displeasure and retaliation and from attachment to the same-sex parent. Boys experience this fear of retaliation as **castration anxiety,** whereas girls fear the **loss of the mother's love** and approval.

      (3) These issues are considered the most important organizing forces behind the formation of conscience and the development of personality. The child relinquishes the rivalous sexual wishes and maintains the relationship by identifying with, or becoming like, the same-sex parent.

   d. The **latency stage** extends from the resolution of the oedipal conflict at approximately 6 years of age to the onset of puberty. During this period, drive interests are invested in peer relationships, socialization, and acquisition of knowledge and skills (e.g., athletics).

   e. The **genital stage** begins with the onset of puberty. It is the only stage that is associated with explicit neuroendocrine and biosomatic maturational components. **Ideally, the drives, aims, and objectives of the earlier stages are integrated** as components of foreplay **into primary genital sexuality**. In some cases, they determine or distort the primary sexual organization (e.g., sexual perversion).

5. **Defenses** are mental operations that develop and function outside of awareness. They can help people to **ward off anxiety (danger) and maintain a sense of safety, well-being, and self-esteem**. With the maturation of perception and cognition, defenses emerge and develop. They may be thought of as less or more mature. Defenses may emerge episodically, as in reaction to a traumatic event; may become habitual as a part of an individual's personality; or may become fixed as a part of a neurotic symptom, as in the avoidance component of a phobia. Defenses are defined and classified in order from the earliest and most primitive to later and more complex.

   a. **Denial,** or turning away, is blocking perceptual information from awareness or conscious acceptance (e.g., a woman refuses to believe that her father is seriously ill).

   b. **Projection** is the attribution of an unacceptable inner wish, feeling, or thought to another person or entity. It is a core component of **paranoia** (e.g., a man experiences anger toward his wife as her anger toward him). Projection is common in individuals who believe that their angry or sexual wishes are unacceptable.

   c. **Splitting** is the perception of individuals as all good or all bad, (e.g., a woman sees herself as virtuous and views a rival at work as evil).

   d. **Repression** is a core organizing process by which urges, thoughts, wishes, or feelings that the individual considers unacceptable or dangerous are maintained at an unconscious level (e.g., a man feels tense around a coworker but is unaware he feels competitive and views him as a rival).

e. Reaction formation is exaggerated recognition of only one side of an attitude or relationship (e.g., a woman is aware only of loving her younger sister, never of any resentment or rivalry).

f. Isolation of affect is the separation of a thought or event from a difficult or painful **feeling** (e.g., a seriously injured accident victim calmly describes the incident, but experiences no emotion).

g. Rationalization is substituting an acceptable motive for all attitude or behavior that otherwise might be self-serving or unacceptable (e.g., "The reason I did that was for your own good").

h. Undoing is a thought or action that the individual believes neutralizes the consequences of another thought or action. This defense is often unconscious and is associated with rituals and superstition (e.g., a person knocks on wood to ward off danger).

i. Regression is as much a process as a defense. It is the return to an earlier form of thought or behavior, often in response to a current stress or threat. Regression is common in young children (e.g., a child begins to suck his thumb after a new sibling is born).

j. Intellectualization is a common defense that involves mastery of a painful or threatening issue with knowledge and explanations (e.g., a woman learns everything she can about her recently diagnosed illness).

6. The **structural model** of mental functioning is an elaboration of psychoanalytic theory from which it developed into a general **theory of human development**. Mental processes and behavior are organized into related groups of functions that are referred to as the structures of id, ego, and superego.

   a. The **id** is the **psychic representation of drives** (wishes). These drives are largely unconscious, particularly sexual and aggressive infantile and childhood drives (e.g., sucking drives, anal-retentive drives, sadistic and destructive drives).

   b. The **ego** is a group of functions that permit **adaptation** to the demands of the drives and to the requirements of external reality. They allow for drive discharge and gratification and take safety and feelings into account. Functions are classified as primarily maturational (i.e., biologic, genetic) or developmental in origin.

   (1) Maturational functions include motor activity, sensory function, language, and cognition and memory.

   (2) Developmental functions include defenses and signal anxiety, reality testing, object relationships, sexual development, identity, and overall integration of personality.

   c. The **superego** encompasses **conscience and the ego-ideal**.

   (1) Conscience. Judgment and self-criticism are affectively **regulated by guilt** (an individual's sense of what he should and should not think, feel, or do).

   (2) Ego-ideal. Aspirations and values are affectively **regulated by shame**.

   (3) The conscience and the ego-ideal develop through the transfer of prohibitions, permissions, expectations, and values from **external authority figures** (usually parents) to an internal agency.

B. **The five perspectives of psychoanalytic theory** refer to approaches to viewing and organizing thoughts, feelings, and behavior.

1. The **genetic perspective** proposes that all types of mental activity, conscious and unconscious, and behavior are related to earlier development and experience. Therefore, earlier forms of thinking, wishing, and behavior may reemerge (e.g., regression).

2. The **dynamic perspective** views all behavior as a compromise among internal intrapsychic forces. These largely unconscious forces include biologic drives, defenses, affects, conscience, values, and perceptions of self and others.

3. The **economic perspective** focuses on psychological energies that are analogous to physical energy and originate in biologic instinctual drives. Energies that are derived from sexual and aggressive drives are subject to blockage, transformation, and discharge. For example, biting may be the direct discharge of an oral aggressive drive.

Biting, or the wish to bite, may be inhibited by fear of punishment. Therefore, the energy is blocked and transformed, resulting perhaps in a symptom such as tooth grinding or an aversion to certain foods.

4. The **structural perspective** organizes mental activity and behavior according to function into stable and enduring structures. These structures are the id, ego, and superego (see II A 6).

5. The **adaptive perspective** views psychological processes and mental development as rooted in behavior that is genetically programmed to provide for adaptation to the environment (e.g., grasping, sucking, head turning, eye following). Therefore, all behavior represents some aspect of adaptation to reality.

C. **Psychoanalysis** is characterized by the encouragement of **free association** as a method of observing the derivatives of the unconscious process, the associated defenses, and the resultant behaviors. The frequency of treatment is variable, but it is usually **four or five times per week** to permit a focus on intrapsychic rather than external events and to allow **full development and resolution of transference**. The length of treatment is open ended, but is usually 3 to 5 years.

1. **Transference and countertransference** are important components of treatment. **Transference** refers to attitudes, feelings, thoughts, and wishes that originate with important figures in the past (e.g., parents) and are **unconsciously reenacted** with individuals in the present. In analysis, this process in the patient progressively focuses on the analyst and is then subject to analysis. **Countertransference** is transference on the part of the analyst toward the patient. To minimize the role of countertransference, personal analysis is essential in an individual who is considering becoming an analyst.

2. **Techniques of psychoanalysis**
   a. **Clarification** involves obtaining further associations and information about past issues and relationships (e.g., connecting the present to the past).
   b. **Confrontation** is identifying defenses, resistance, and other unconscious influences on behavior by noting connections, continuities, and inconsistencies.
   c. **Interpretation** is identifying the patient's unconscious wishes and thoughts and their associated affects as they emerge through clarification and confrontation.

3. **Defense analysis and working through** are based on the understanding that intrapsychic conflict is most apparent through the operation of the defenses of the ego. As the nature and operation of these defenses are identified, the conflicts and unconscious wishes emerge. The process of working through requires repeated examination of all connections and ramifications of the personality structure.

III. **LEARNING THEORY (BEHAVIORISM)** is based on the assumption that all types of behavior and personality development represent the acquisition and organization (i.e., learning) of reactions, responses, and patterns. These functions originate in and are governed by principles of learning and are subject primarily to environmental influences. Learning theory is particularly associated with the work of **Pavlov (conditioned reflex or classic conditioning),** Watson (**behaviorism**), and Thorndike and Skinner (reward and punishment paradigms, or **operant conditioning**) [see III B 2; Chapter 5 III B 2 b (2)]. Although internal motivations (e.g., hunger, thirst) are acknowledged, the focus is on **external events** in eliciting, maintaining, or eliminating a behavior. Learning theory considers unimportant anything that cannot be observed, described, and measured. Such concepts as the unconscious, intrapsychic conflict, and the disease, or medical, model are considered unnecessary or inappropriate. According to this theory, maladaptive behaviors such as phobias and aggression are learned in the same way as adaptive, or normal, behaviors.

A. **Basic concepts**

1. **Learning** is the acquisition, modification, and elimination of behaviors and response patterns that occur in association with environmental conditions. Learning establishes a connection between a stimulus and a response.

2. A **stimulus** is a cue. Any internal or external event may act as a stimulus.

3. A **response** is behavior that occurs in association with a stimulus. Responses may be motoric, cognitive, affective, or imaginal.

4. **Motivation** is provided by **innate, or primary, needs** (e.g., hunger) that prompt the organism to act, or it may result from **learned motives**. Learned motives are behaviors that are **rewarded by a reduction in painful tension** and are repeated and refined throughout the life cycle. They may include the need for praise and approval as well as dependent behavior.

5. **Reward, reinforcement, and punishment**
   a. A **reward** may be either primary or learned. **Primary rewards satisfy the primary needs** for food, drink, and shelter. The classification of sexual and social needs is not clear, but these needs are usually considered primary as well. **Learned rewards satisfy** a **motive** rather than a primary need. Learned rewards include dependency, power, control, and praise.
   b. **Reinforcement** is similar to reward. When a primary need or learned motive is satisfied, an association is established between a stimulus and a response. For example, when a child indicates that he is hungry and is given food, a primary need is satisfied with a primary reward. **The reward reinforces the behavior** that is used to communicate the need. If the child is praised for eating, the praise becomes a learned reward and a secondary reinforcer.
      (1) **Continuous reinforcement** (presented after every response) eventually loses its reward value, and the **behavior is extinguished**.
      (2) **Fixed-ratio reinforcement** (given after every second or every third response) is more effective than continuous reinforcement.
      (3) **Variable, intermittent, and unpredictable reinforcement** establishes the strongest, most effective type of learning (i.e., repetition of the behavior). The Las Vegas slot machine is the classic example.
   c. **Punishment** is an aversive, painful, or frustrating event **as defined by the subject**. It may involve withholding a positive response or reward. Disapproval or criticism may be painful or may be reinforcing by providing attention. Punishment may eliminate or simply suppress the behavior.

6. **Stimulus generalization** is the application of a response that is learned in one situation (e.g., fear of a particular dog) to similar situations (e.g., fear of all dogs or all four-footed animals). The similarity may be determined by a concrete resemblance in size (e.g., all small animals), color (e.g., all brown animals), shape, and so forth. Generalizations of this type are common in young children. Similarity may be established by **language,** which is the most common basis for generalization in humans. For example, the term "dog" might at first represent a specific four-footed animal, then all four-footed animals, and finally one class of four-footed animals. This last step is known as **discriminated generalization**.

7. **Extinction.** A previously learned behavior disappears if the reward is withheld so that the behavior is not reinforced or if the reward is continuous and thereby loses its reinforcing quality.

B. **Types of learning** include classic conditioning, operant conditioning, cognitive behavioral learning, and observational and imitational learning.

1. **Classic conditioning** elicits an inherent (reflex) nonlearned behavior (e.g., salivation) in response to a **learned stimulus** (e.g., bell, buzzer). The **unconditioned stimulus** for the

inherent behavior of salivation is food (e.g., if a buzzer sounds each time food is presented, the animal begins to salivate at the sound of the buzzer). Any inherent behavior, including fear or anxiety, can be conditioned to appear in response to a learned stimulus.

2. **Operant conditioning** elicits a new, noninherent (nonreflex) behavior in response to a stimulus that acts as a reward or a punishment.
   a. Operant conditioning is used to elicit a desired behavior or extinguish an undesired behavior by using the principle that **behavior is a function of its consequences**. If a behavior is followed by a rewarding consequence (e.g., attention, praise, success), the behavior will be reinforced and therefore repeated. If the consequence is unpleasant or nonrewarding, the behavior will not be repeated and will be extinguished.
   b. Classic operant conditioning focuses on **observable behavior**. Intervening variables (e.g., motivational state, ideation, fantasy) are largely ignored. For example, a child's temper tantrum (stimulus) is followed by parental attention or gratification (response). This behavior is rewarding to the child and therefore reinforces the behavior. Ignoring the tantrum or isolating the child briefly is a change in the response that removes the reinforcement and extinguishes the behavior.

3. **Cognitive behavioral learning** (Bandura) recognizes the existence of **intervening variables between stimulus and response** and the complexity of important behaviors. According to this theory, ideation, imagery, and meaning must be considered in any attempt to understand, predict, or influence behavior.

4. **Observational and imitational learning** recognizes that behavioral changes can occur as a result of **observing or imitating another's behavior** without any external, observable reward. This theory introduces the clearly nonoperant (i.e., nonobservable) concept of increased self-esteem or an enhanced sense of mastery as the reward or reinforcer.

C. **Treatment techniques** related to learning theory are discussed in order from the behaviorally most objective to the most subjective.

1. **Aversive conditioning** is linking an unwanted behavior (e.g., drinking alcohol) with a noxious or painful stimulus (e.g., electric shock), leading to aversion for alcohol. This conditioning can be extended to the thought of alcohol, the smell of alcohol, and so on.

2. **Positive reinforcement and extinction** links a desired behavior (either spontaneously occurring or taught) with an immediate reward, at first consistently and then intermittently. Conversely, this technique links an undesirable behavior with the absence of response.

3. **Systematic desensitization** (Wolpe) is used to eliminate phobic behaviors (e.g., irrational fear, avoidance). Avoidance reduces or eliminates anxiety and therefore is positively reinforcing in a self-defeating way. The goal of this technique is to desensitize the individual to the situation.
   a. The individual is taught how to relax completely.
   b. The sensitized (anxiety-provoking) stimulus is gradually introduced so that the link between the stimulus and the anxiety is gradually weakened.
   c. The sensitized stimulus is introduced by asking the patient to imagine the anxiety-provoking situation while she is relaxed.

4. **Modeling** is learning new behaviors and overcoming inhibitions to desired behavior. The patient observes someone else performing the desired action or imagines himself or others performing the behavior. This technique is similar to desensitization. Assertiveness training is a variant of this approach.

IV. **COGNITIVE THEORY** is a set of propositions for understanding intellectual (cognitive) development from birth through adolescence and maturity. This theory is based primarily on the observations, experiments, and inferences of the Swiss epistemologist

Jean Piaget. It describes a fixed set of stages and sequences, each of which builds on the previous one. Cognitive theory continues to have a profound influence on the understanding of development and on other theories, including psychoanalytic and learning theories.

A. **Basic concepts**

1. The infant is born with **two types of reflex patterns, classic and innate**.
    a. **Classic reflexes** are inherent, fixed stimulus–response patterns that are not significantly affected by learning or experience. Examples include the Babinski, knee jerk, and cranial nerve reflexes.
    b. **Innate reflex patterns (reflex schema)** are present at birth, but they require stimulation for activation and stabilization. Examples include the sucking reflex, the grasping reflex, eye following, and smiling.

2. **Assimilation and accommodation** describe all interactions between the organism and the environment. Together they lead to **adaptation**.
    a. **Assimilation is the incorporation of external stimuli into existing innate reflex patterns**. These stimuli enlarge, but do not fundamentally alter the pattern, or schema.
        (1) At a basic level, the infant assimilates the nipple into the inborn reflex schema of sucking or assimilates an object placed in his palm into the reflex schema of grasping.
        (2) At a higher level, by assimilation, the child retains a preexisting understanding, even in the presence of a new or different perception. For example, if a child identifies flying objects as birds, then he identifies an airplane as a bird as well, and this perception is assimilated into the preexisting schema.
    b. **Accommodation occurs when a reflex, reflex schema, or conceptual understanding is changed by experience** to fit the new perception. Thus, reflex systems are progressively modified to form new behavioral units. Infant behavior provides several examples.
        (1) Sucking behavior is activated and modified into different types, or patterns, of sucking for different objects [e.g., breast (nutritive), pacifier (nonnutritive)].
        (2) Eye-following and smiling reflex patterns are initially activated by a broad range of stimuli. The infant progressively discriminates the meaningful stimuli, especially the mother's voice and face.
    c. **Adaptation is the result of the interaction of assimilation and accommodation.** Each interaction involves varying degrees of assimilation and accommodation that progress to an **equilibrium**. Equilibrium, reestablished by assimilation and accommodation, becomes adaptation.

3. **Motivation,** or the origin of action, may be a **change in the state of the organism** (e.g., hunger activates sucking and crying behaviors), **environment, or both**. This change creates a **disequilibrium in the reflex schema or,** later, in the **cognitive system**. Equilibrium is reestablished by assimilation and accommodation. Reflex systems, or schemata, are activated only by an appropriate stimulus. For example, a nipple does not activate the grasping reflex, and a rattle does not activate the sucking schema.

B. **The stages of cognitive development** are the **sensorimotor stage,** which extends from birth to 2 years, and the **conceptual–representational stage,** which extends from 2 years to maturity.

1. **The sensorimotor stage** is divided into **6 periods** that describe a **relatively fixed sequence** of progressively emerging cognitive abilities.
    a. The time from **birth to 1 month of age** is a period of **reflex operations**. During this stage, the exercise, consolidation, and early differentiation of innate reflex patterns (e.g., sucking, grasping, crying) occur.
    b. The period from **2 to 5 months of age** is the stage of **primary circular reactions**. Reflex patterns are activated and coordinated. For example, if an infant sees both his

hand and an object at the same time, he will grab at the object (**coordinating seeing and grabbing**). The infant does not act on or search for an object that he cannot see. At this stage, the infant does not realize that objects, including persons, have an independent existence.

c. The period from **5 to 9 months of age** is the stage of **secondary circular reactions**. This stage is the beginning of intentional activity and interest in the results of that activity (e.g., causing an object to move or swing and then repeating that action on other objects). The infant gradually learns that objects have a separate existence, and truly **imitative behavior** begins.

d. The time from **9 months to 1 year of age** is a period of **coordination of schemata**. Goal-oriented behavior begins. The infant can **remember objects** that are **out of sight**. The infant realizes that objects, including people, have an independent existence and independent properties.

e. The period from **1 year to 18 months of age** is the stage of **tertiary circular reactions**. The child becomes increasingly aware of objects as independent and therefore **separate from the self**. The capacity for **concept formation,** or thinking about an action and then acting, begins. During this period, **language begins to develop**. Words represent things.

f. The time from **18 months to 2 years of age** is the stage of **invention of new means**. The capacity for true mental representation of objects develops. For example, a child will look for an object where it might be, rather than where it was last seen. The child achieves a clear sense of separation of external events and objects from the self as well as a sense or an image of the self. The stage is set for intelligent, conceptual **thought**.

2. The **conceptual–representational stage** is divided into **four periods**.

a. The time from **2 to 4 years of age** is the **preoperational period**. By maturation and learning, the child's capacity for symbolic and representational thought expands. **Thinking** begins to serve the purpose of direct action on objects in an earlier stage. The child can learn by considering an action and its consequences rather than by performing the action.

b. The period from **4 to 7 years of age** is characterized by **intuitive thought**. The child has an increasing capacity for **symbolic thought**. The child comprehends classes of objects and can classify them according to their **similarities and differences**. For example, at 4 years of age, a child may say that apples and oranges are both round, but by 7 years of age, she may say that they are both fruit. The child can **intuit,** or arrive at a correct answer without being able to explain why or how.

c. The period from **7 to 11 years of age** is the stage of **concrete operations**. During this period, the child acquires **three important capacities for logical thought: reversibility, conservation, and rules of logic**. **Reversibility** involves reciprocal or two-way relations (e.g., between square and square root, between water and vapor). **Conservation** involves changes in dimension, color, or location that do not change the essential nature or identity of an object. **Rules of logic** involve concepts of similarities, differences, and relativity (e.g., greater than, less than).

d. The period from **adolescence to maturity** is characterized by **formal operations**. The individual can reason and arrive at conclusions without the presence of concrete objects and therefore is capable of **purely abstract, symbolic thought**. The adolescent can conceptualize the past, present, and future as a continuum and consider what might be possible. The individual can conceptualize death and the finiteness of existence in final, mature terms. Therefore, the adolescent becomes capable of both logical planning for the future and philosophic thought about values, ideals, and the meaning of life.

V. **PSYCHOSOCIAL THEORY** is a broad systematic framework for understanding patterns and sequences of psychological development in the context of social and cultural factors. This approach is identified with the work of **Erik Erikson,** who originally was trained as a teacher in the Montessori method. Erikson's work describes an underlying

basic developmental plan that unfolds **sequentially,** similar to Freud's concept of psychosexual stages and Piaget's stages of cognitive development. Erikson's approach is significantly influenced by psychoanalytic theory. The basic concepts include **eight stages** that extend from infancy through old age. Each stage is grounded in maturation interacting with experience, and each is characterized by a core **developmental task** that requires active confrontation and successful resolution. Each early stage has a primary **zone,** or part of the body, around which major social interactions occur, and each zone has a primary **mode** by which interactions and transactions occur.

A. In the **oral–sensory stage,** which occurs from **birth to 1 year of age,** the **mouth** is the dominant zone. However, children also obtain information through seeing, hearing, touching, and grasping. The dominant **modes** of behavior are taking in, feeling stimulated, and feeling filled and satisfied. Consistent experience and parental stimulation help the child to achieve the **task** of developing a sense of **basic trust versus a sense of mistrust** by the end of the first year.

B. In the **muscular–anal stage,** which extends from **1 to 3 years of age,** the **anal region** is the dominant zone. Voluntary sphincter control is usually achieved at approximately 18 months of age. More broadly, the child experiences general neuromuscular maturation and increasing motor autonomy, including walking, balance, and language, during this period. The dominant, but not exclusive, **mode** of behavior is holding on and letting go. The child must balance internal drives with external control and authority. The **task** is the achievement of a healthy sense of **autonomy and acceptance of limits versus control by shame and doubt.**

C. In the **locomotor–genital stage,** which extends from **3 to 6 years of age,** the **genital (phallic) area** is the dominant zone. During this stage, active, inquisitive, competitive, and comparing behaviors are seen. The **task** of the child is to be like her parents. The dominant **modes** of behavior during this stage are **intrusive (phallic) and competitive for boys and inclusive and competitive for girls.** The **crisis** of this stage is conflict between aggressive, risk-taking, exuberant, competitive behavior, known as **initiative,** and the fear of punishment and retaliation, which is internalized as an inhibiting sense of **guilt.**

D. During the period from **6 to 12 years of age,** there is no dominant somatic zone or mode. **Development shifts from a predominantly self-centered and intrafamilial focus to the** larger world of **school, other adults, and peers.** During this stage, the acquisition of knowledge and skills by externally, or objectively, measured learning, achievement, and mastery is important. The outcome is either a realistically based and rewarding sense of **industry** (competence) or a sense of **inferiority** (incompetence).

E. **Adolescence,** which extends from **12 to approximately 20 years of age,** is marked by dramatic neuroendocrine and physical changes that are initiated by **puberty.** There is both continuation and upheaval of the previously established sense of self. Adolescents experience intense new feelings and sexual impulses, a new body image, and a striving for independence. During adolescence, the individual must establish a new sense of identity, including sexual identity and preparation for intimacy, vocational identity, and role within the family and peer group. The alternative to **identity consolidation** is **role diffusion, or role confusion,** which may result from failure to master the tasks associated with earlier stages, uncertain sexual identity, or excessive dependency that interferes with healthy independence.

F. **Young adulthood,** which is the period from **20 to 30 years of age,** is associated with the attainment of vocational goals, independence from the parents, and the **capacity for sexual and social intimacy**. The capacity for intimacy is based on a sense of trust, autonomy, initiative, and identity that has developed during previous stages. The alternative is withdrawal, fear of commitment, and an excessive need for control, leading to **emotional isolation.**

G. **Adulthood,** the period from **30 to 65 years of age,** is typically characterized by the establishment of a family. During this stage, the individual assumes the parental role. The individual recognizes that all options are no longer open and that choices are limited, and he strives to achieve a balance between wish and reality and between satisfaction and disappointment. The challenge is to maintain a sense of **generativity,** a continued sense of productivity and satisfaction and a sense of responsibility for guiding the next generation, versus an attempt to preserve the illusion of youth (**self-absorption**), the inability to allow children to become independent, or a sense of emptiness and **stagnation**.

H. **Maturity** is a period of **biologic decline,** although there is great individual variation. There are **gradual decrements** in strength, energy, tolerance to stress, and physical health. For most individuals, maturity involves retirement, a change in economic circumstances, the loss of loved ones, and the **realization of mortality**. Many individuals have physical and emotional reserves that enable them to adapt to change, decline, and especially loss. **Ego integrity** involves an individual's sense of pride or satisfaction in her past and her family (children and grandchildren) and a sense of equanimity about the life cycle. The alternative is **despair,** which is depression, lack of self-regard, and a sense of futility associated with an increase in alcoholism, physical illness, and in men, suicide. This sense of despair is often mistaken for organic mental changes and senility.

VI. **BIOMEDICAL THEORY** proposes that all types of mental activity and behavior are caused by brain function, which is dependent on the maturational stage and neurologic integrity of the brain.

A. **Maturation and development** include factors such as myelinization of the nervous system that occurs well into adolescence, endocrine influences on the brain during adolescence, and the effects of aging on memory, cognition, and behavior.

B. **Neuroanatomic status** includes considerations such as ventricle size (often enlarged in schizophrenia), temporal lobe structures that affect sexual and aggressive behavior, and limbic system damage associated with hallucinations and intense fear and rage.

C. **Circulatory status,** including malformations, obstructions, ruptures, or insufficiency, may affect various areas of the brain and lead to a variety of mental symptoms.

D. **Neuroendocrine and neurochemical function** are explained in Chapters 1, 2, and 3.

E. Biomedical theory of mental illness proposes that most **major psychiatric disorders have a significant biologic component** in their etiology and pathophysiology.

1. In **schizophrenia** (see Chapter 4 III A 5), a genetic predisposition is commonly found, a dysfunction in the dopamine neurotransmission system is assumed, and hypoactivity in the prefrontal cortex frequently is shown on positron emission tomography (PET) scan.

2. In **affective disorders** (manic-depressive and depressive), a strong family history and a genetic predisposition are commonly found, and a dysfunction in the norepinephrine and serotonin neurotransmission systems is the most accepted current hypothesis of pathophysiology.

3. **Attention deficit hyperactivity disorder (ADHD)** in children and adolescents is believed to reflect a dysfunction in serotonin metabolism in the reticular activating system (RAS).

4. **Delirium** is an acute, usually reversible mental disorder that affects orientation, perception, cognition, and reality testing. The etiology is discussed in Chapter 15 III A 2.

5. Dementia is a chronic, usually nonreversible condition that affects memory, cognition, and ability to function independently. Disorders that cause dementia are discussed in Chapter 15 III B 2.

VII. **SUMMARY.** Theories of the mind (e.g., cognition, feeling, fantasy) cannot be separated from the structure and function of the brain and from the theories related to them. Psychiatrists sometimes are referred to as physicians of the mind, but the mind cannot be understood or mental illness clinically approached without an understanding of the theories of the mind and the structure and function of the brain.

BIBLIOGRAPHY

Erikson E: *Identity Youth and Crisis.* New York, WW Norton, 1968.

Piaget J: *The Origins of Intelligence in Children.* New York, International University Press, 1952.

Rothstein A: *Models of the Mind.* New York, International University Press, 1985.

Wiener JM (ed): *Textbook of Child and Adolescent Psychiatry.* Washington, DC, American Psychiatric Press, 1991.

■ STUDY QUESTIONS

DIRECTIONS: Each of the numbered items or incomplete statements in this section is followed by answers or by completions of the statement. Select the ONE lettered answer or completion that is BEST in each case.

1. In psychoanalytic theory, characteristics of unconscious mental process include

(A) the conceptual–representational stage of thought
(B) innate reflex patterns and defenses
(C) thoughts, wishes, and feelings that are considered unacceptable or dangerous
(D) language, cognition, and recall
(E) assimilation and accommodation

2. Unawareness of a perception is

(A) intellectualization
(B) denial
(C) rationalization
(D) isolation of affect
(E) splitting

3. The structural model proposes that

(A) development is divided into four stages of conceptual thought
(B) personality emerges mainly out of maturation of drives
(C) mental functioning is divided into three groups of functions known as id, ego, and superego
(D) the superego includes defenses and signal anxiety in its functions
(E) the maturational functions of the ego include defenses, reality testing, and object relations

4. Learning theory proposes that

(A) there are primary and learned needs and rewards
(B) continuous reinforcement is the most effective reward strategy
(C) classic conditioning associates a learned behavior with an unlearned (reflex) stimulus
(D) the focus of classic operant conditioning is on transference and fantasy
(E) assimilation and accommodation produce adaptation

5. Which example shows assimilation in cognitive theory?

(A) An infant smiles preferentially at the sound of her mother's voice
(B) A child grasps and shakes a pencil as if it were a rattle
(C) A child learns to identify different four-footed animals according to their particular characteristics
(D) A child sees an airplane for the first time and says "that's not a bird!"
(E) An infant sucks on the nipple of a bottle of milk in a steady, rhythmic fashion and on his pacifier with a different pattern

Questions 6–9

A 5-year-old only child is doing well in kindergarten; seems outgoing, competitive, and alert; and seems to have a good relationship with his mother. After his sister is born, he seems subdued, begins to suck his thumb, says he is having bad dreams, and is reluctant to leave his mother's side in the morning. He says that he is afraid that something will happen to her.

6. The thumb sucking and reluctance to leave his mother's side are indications of

(A) a sensorimotor form of thinking
(B) classic conditioning
(C) projection and intellectualization
(D) regression and projection
(E) reaching the formal stage of cognitive development

7. This child's developmental stage is a combination of

(A) oedipal, intuitive, and locomotor–genital
(B) latency, concrete operations, and modeling
(C) representational thought, oral, and phallic
(D) generative, operant conditioning, and innate reflex
(E) sensorimotor, anal, and identity formation

8. At first, the boy's mother agrees to his anxious wish that she not leave right away when taking him to school, expecting his anxiety to diminish. However, each day he insists that she stay longer. This behavior can be explained by the concept of

(A) extinction and imitational learning
(B) reinforcement and operant conditioning
(C) aversive conditioning
(D) modeling
(E) transference

9. After a few days, the teacher tells the boy and his mother that her remaining at the school is not helpful to either of them and that she should reassure her son and leave. After a few days of fearfulness, the boy seems less afraid and is functioning better. This behavior can be understood as the result of

(A) learned generalization
(B) rationalization
(C) extinction
(D) clarification and interpretation
(E) primary reward

DIRECTIONS: Each of the numbered items or incomplete statements in this section is negatively phrased, as indicated by a capitalized word such as NOT, LEAST, or EXCEPT. Select the ONE lettered answer or completion that is BEST in each case.

---

10. According to Erikson's concept of psychosocial development, the period of latency includes all of the following features EXCEPT

(A) a shift in focus from the family to relationships with peers
(B) a dampening of the oedipal conflict
(C) the expanded acquisition of knowledge and skills as a source of mastery and self-esteem
(D) the development of initiative versus an inhibiting sense of guilt
(E) learning to combine competition with cooperation

ANSWERS AND EXPLANATIONS

1. The answer is C. [II A 1]. Unconscious mental process is the theory that mental activity occurs outside of awareness and is unavailable for voluntary recall when the thought would be considered dangerous or unacceptable if it reached conscious awareness.

2. The answer is B [II A 5 a]. Denial is a turning away from an event.

3. The answer is C [II A 6]. The key concept of the structural model is its organization of related groups of functions of mental processes and behavior into three structures: id, ego, and superego.

4. The answer is A [III A 4, 5 a]. Primary needs include hunger and thirst and may include sexual and social needs. Learned needs include dependency, attention, and approval.

5. The answer is B [IV A 2 a]. In this example, the child incorporates an object (pencil) into a preexisting schema (grasping and shaking a rattle), rather than adjusting the behavior (changing the schema) to accommodate two different stimuli.

6. The answer is D [II A 5 b, i]. Projection leads the child to fear danger to his mother from the outside rather than from his unacceptable anger at her for bringing a rival into their relationship. Regression to earlier forms of behavior is evident in the thumb sucking and reluctance to separate from his mother.

7. The answer is A [II A 4 c; IV B 2 b; V C]. At 5 years of age, the child shows evidence of being in the phallic–oedipal psychosexual stage (good relationship with mother, outgoing and competitive), the locomotor–genital psychosocial stage, and the intuitive cognitive stage.

8. The answer is B [III A 5 b, B 2]. Reinforcement establishes a connection between a stimulus (the child's anxiety and wish for his mother to stay) and a response (the mother stays). According to the theory of operant conditioning, the child's behavior is rewarded by a decrease in anxiety as long as the mother is there, so the behavior persists and increases through reinforcement.

9. The answer is C [III A 7]. Extinction is the disappearance of a previously learned behavior (e.g., insisting that the mother stay) if the reward is removed and the behavior is not reinforced.

10. The answer is D [II A 4 d; V C]. The development of initiative versus guilt is the core task of the locomotor–genital stage, which spans the period from 3 to 6 years of age. This stage precedes the latency stage, which occurs after dampening and resolution of the intense intrafamilial oedipal conflict and leads to involvement in school and relationships with peers.

Chapter 8

The Life Cycle

James Egan

I. DEFINITION OF TERMS

A. **The life cycle** is best understood within the context of the **biopsychosocial model**. This model proposes that all behavior can be viewed as an interaction among biologic, psychological, and sociocultural variables.

B. **Growth** is an increase in physical size.

C. **Maturation** is the biologically based, phylogenically determined, sequential evolution of forms and functions (e.g., motor and sensory functions, language, cognition).

D. **Development** is the acquisition of abilities and functions through experience.

II. INFANCY TO TODDLERHOOD

A. **Biologic factors**

1. **Prenatal and postnatal influences**
   a. **Genetic factors** have a significant effect on the biologic potential of a fetus. The process of development is sequential and genetically determined, as are certain disorders and conditions.
      (1) Hereditary factors are responsible for attention deficit hyperactivity disorder in approximately 40% of affected children.
      (2) Other common genetically determined conditions include Down syndrome (trisomy 21), Klinefelter's syndrome (XXY), and fragile X syndrome.
   b. **Response to sensory stimulation in utero** is shown by fetal monitoring. The fetus responds to stimuli with certain reflex patterns, such as sucking and kicking. These responses suggest that conditioned learning may begin in utero.
   c. **Sex and survival factors.** Approximately 160 male conceptions occur for each 100 female conceptions. However, at birth, the ratio is much lower. Thus, one third of male embryos do not survive until birth. The reasons are not known, but certain findings are clear.
      (1) Some boys who survive are at considerable risk for brain dysfunction.
      (2) Approximately 5% of middle-class boys and 10% of lower-class boys have attention deficit hyperactivity disorder. The male–female ratio is approximately 10:1.
   d. **Gestational age and weight at birth** are predictors of outcome. Infants with low birth weight for gestational age fare worse than infants who are the expected weight for gestational age.
   e. **Perinatal factors** (e.g., postmaturity, eclampsia, serious dystocia) also affect biologic potential.

2. **Abilities of the neonate**
   a. **Attachment behaviors** (e.g., crying, clinging) that are present at birth increase the likelihood of maternal care and aid the infant in attaching to the mother.
   b. Neonates have a number of innate, simple **reflexes.**
      (1) **Moro's, or startle, reflex** is flexion of the extremities in response to sudden stimulation. A similar reflex is closing the eyelids in response to light.

      (2) The **palmar grasp reflex** is less adaptive. The infant responds to a finger placed in his palm by contracting, grasping, and clinging.

      (3) The **rooting and sucking reflexes** aid in feeding. When the infant's cheek is stroked, he turns toward the touch (rooting reflex). If an object is placed in the infant's mouth, he responds by sucking it (sucking reflex).

      (4) The **Babinski reflex** is hyperextension and spreading of the toes when the sole of the foot is stroked. Adults normally respond to this stimulus by clenching the toes. In an adult, the Babinski reflex indicates neurologic damage.

   3. The motor, vocal, and sensory development sequences of infants are shown in Table 8-1.

   4. Cognitive maturation. By the age of 18 to 24 months, a child can perform elementary trial-and-error reasoning. For example, the child will attempt to place a square into the square opening of a form box after trying to insert it into the circular or triangular opening.

B. **Psychological and social development**

   1. The **principal psychological task of the first year of life** is the formation of an **intimate differentiated attachment** to the mother or primary care giver. This process is impeded when the child has a wide variety of care givers, as occurs in institutionally reared children, or when the mother is emotionally unavailable (e.g., as a result of depression or serious deficits in her early development). Infants who do not form this early attachment may have an impaired capacity for empathy and for establishing close, warm, reciprocal relationships.

TABLE 8-1. Developmental Sequences in Infants and Young Children

Development	Age	Description
Motor	1 month	Lifting the head up from the prone position
	2 months	Lifting the chest up from the prone position
	4 months	Sitting with support
	7 months	Sitting without support
	8 months	Standing without support
	10 months	Creeping
	11 months	Walking when led by the hand
	13 months	Climbing stairs
	15 months	Adept at independent locomotion
Vocal	At birth	Crying
	6–8 weeks	Cooing, the precursor to later babbling and speech
	2 months	Development of 7 phonemes*
	6 months	Development of 12 phonemes
	12 months	Development of 18 phonemes; words such as "mama" and "dada" emerge
	18 months	50 words
	3 years	More than 1000 words
	4 years	Style of adult language is established
Sensory	At birth	Infant can discriminate sound and visually follow a light; capacity for visual fixation within several hours after birth
	10 days	Infants can differentiate the smell of mother versus nonmother
	4 months	Infants can fully accommodate visually; visual fixation is increased if the pattern is complex and especially if it resembles the human face

*There are 35 phonemes (distinct sounds) in adult American speech.

2. The **smile** is an innate reflex response at birth (i.e., endogenous smiling). Infants smile in response to a face at 8 weeks of age (i.e., exogenous smiling), and they smile specifically in response to the mother's face (i.e., social smiling) at 12 to 16 weeks of age. This social smile is an early marker of the development of a specific, differentiated relationship with the mother. Other markers are the preferential vocalization, visual pursuit, and anticipatory gesturing of the 5-month-old infant in the presence of the mother.

3. **Stranger anxiety** begins when the infant is between 7 and 9 months old. It is another marker of the attachment process, in which the infant becomes distressed when she encounters an individual who is not the mother or primary care giver. The infant is reacting to the presence of someone other than the mother as well as to the mother's absence.
   a. The presence of stranger anxiety suggests that the infant can maintain or recall a mental image, or representation, of the mother, even when she is not present. The ability to maintain representations in the absence of current stimuli is known as **object permanence**.
   b. **Anaclitic depression** is the name given by René Spitz[1] to the reaction of apathy, emotional withdrawal, and diminished developmental quotient that occurs when an infant is separated from the mother between 6 and 12 months of age.

4. Margaret Mahler[2] proposed a description of the sequential development of **object relations** within the framework of psychoanalytic theory.
   a. Between birth and 1 month of age, the infant has little self-aware interaction with the environment. This period is known as the stage of **normal autism**.
   b. Between 2 and 4 months of age, the infant experiences **symbiotic development,** or a sense of oneness with the mother. During this period, the infant is unaware that he and the mother are separate individuals.
   c. Between 5 and 9 months of age, the infant experiences **differentiation,** a gradually increasing awareness that the mother is a separate entity. During this stage, the infant typically performs what is known as a customs inspection of the mother. He explores her eyes, nose, and mouth, and pulls at her hair.
   d. Between 10 and 17 months of age, the child practices locomotion (**practicing phase**). The child moves away from his mother and then returns to her for encouragement and emotional support. During this period, the toddler is unaware of the dangers of physical injury and moves about with exuberance.
   e. Between 18 and 36 months of age, the child experiences the **rapprochement subphase**. During this period, the child's sense of invulnerability and omnipotence is tempered by the increasing realization that the mother is not always available to protect him.
      (1) **Separation anxiety** reaches its peak at 18 months of age. The child manages her anxiety by clinging to the mother, or shadowing, and darting away.
      (2) As the psychological separation of mother and child is accomplished, the child gradually realizes that he is a distinct entity. This realization is known as **individuation**.

5. When a child between 12 and 30 months old is separated from the mother, his behavior follows a predictable pattern.
   a. The child protests (e.g., crying) for 1 to 2 days.
   b. The child then appears subdued and quietly depressed (i.e., demonstrating despair).
   c. If the mother and child are not reunited in 3 to 4 weeks, the child becomes **detached,** is emotionally unrelated to the mother, and fails to respond to the mother's leaving.

6. Other aspects of psychological development between 18 months and 3 years of age
   a. **Play**
      (1) Initially, play has a **compensatory or self-soothing function** that provides pleasure and release of tension. Next, the child plays as **a way to master functions**. For example, a 9-month-old infant plays peekaboo and later hide-and-seek to master the anxiety associated with separation and loss. An 18-month-old child will spend hours practicing going up and down stairs.

    (2) Doll play is common in toddlers. The child feeds and takes care of dolls as his parents take care of him. Toddlers engage in **dramatic play** by dressing in their parents' clothing and pretending to be grown up or by imitating the activities of their parents (e.g., shaving, cooking, cutting the grass).

  b. Autonomy and self-awareness. Between 18 and 36 months of age, the child attempts to separate psychologically from the mother.

    (1) To achieve a greater sense of autonomy, the child often exhibits noncompliant behavior and resists parental authority. Saying "no" or "I'll do it my way" gives the toddler a subjective sense of power and autonomy.

    (2) This behavior affects all aspects of the toddler's life. She may refuse to eat, sleep, or eliminate at parental request. Collectively, these conflicts are known as the "**terrible twos**." When these conflicts are severe, disorders of conduct, sleeping, eating, or eliminating may develop.

C. Sociocultural factors

1. Many powerful economic and sociocultural forces influence the developmental process. For example, the rate of **psychiatric disorders** is approximately twice as high in inner cities as it is in rural areas.

2. Similarly, the frequency of **attention deficit hyperactivity disorder** is twice as high in low-income families as it is in middle-class families. The lower incidence in middle-income families is probably the result of better prenatal nutritional status and obstetric care.

3. The risk of **obstetric complications** is increased in young, poor mothers as well as in the "elderly primigravida," who is often in the upper middle class. The inverse relationship between socioeconomic level and reproductive complications is reported by Pasamaneck and Knoblock.[3]

4. Psychosocial, or sociocultural, retardation is a deficiency in language, speech, or cognitive skills associated with inadequate early stimulation. This deficiency usually occurs in families at lower socioeconomic levels.

5. For a different perspective, it is instructive to consider two significant developmental steps in infancy and early childhood in terms of socioeconomic level. These differing experiences will be reflected in differing personality styles.

  a. The typical middle-class infant is weaned from the breast or bottle to the cup at 1 year of age. Many lower-class children still use bottles at 3 to 4 years of age.

  b. Most middle-class children achieve toilet training between 18 months and 3 years of age. Many children from disadvantaged homes complete bowel training by 14 months of age.

III. CHILDHOOD. The years between 3 years of age and puberty are a period of significant change. Emphasis shifts from the child's relationship with the mother, to her relationship with both parents, to socialization with her peers.

A. Biologic and maturational factors

1. Physical growth

  a. At 3 years of age, the average boy is 38 inches tall and weighs 33 pounds. The average girl is 37 inches tall and weighs 32 pounds.

  b. At 6 years of age, the average child is 46 inches tall and weighs 48 pounds. The brain is 90% of its adult weight.

  c. At 9 years of age, the average child is 55 inches tall.

2. Motor development

  a. At 2 years of age, a child can reproduce a circle; at 3 years, a cross; at 5 years, a square; and at 7 years, a diamond.

  b. At 3 years of age, a child can walk up stairs unaided, stand on one foot, and build a tower of nine or ten cubes.

3. **Speech and language development** proceeds rapidly. Between 3 and 5 years of age, the average child learns two new words daily.

4. **Cognitive maturation** continues from the sensory motor stage, which involves object permanence (see II B 3 a), to two further stages during childhood: the preoperational and concrete operational stages.

    a. **The preoperational stage** (2–7 years of age) is marked by a transition from a focus on action and sensation to a focus on thought. This cognitive stage has several characteristics.

    (1) **Symbolic function** first appears in this stage. The child learns that words and objects are symbols (e.g., the word "doll" is a symbol for the object that is a doll, and the object that is a doll is a symbol for a baby).

    (2) **Egocentrism** is a feature of the preoperational stage whereby the child cannot put himself in the place of someone else. One facet of egocentrism is that a child can conceive of an object as only one class at a time. For example, the child can group objects by color or shape, but not by both characteristics.

    (3) **Animism** is a belief that every object is alive and has feelings and thoughts. This belief includes such objects as feces, and therefore may affect toilet training (e.g., a child may not want to give up something perceived as alive inside).

    (4) **Artificialism** is a belief that all things are made by humans and for humans, and that everything has a specific use. At this stage, children can perform certain types of reasoning only with visual, not verbal, representation. In addition, children believe that all questions have answers, and that adults know the answers.

    (5) At this stage, children do not have any concept of the ability to **conserve;** they can comprehend only one property or dimension of an object at a time. If an object changes shape, as in Piaget's[4] classic example of clay, the child cannot comprehend that the object conserves its original mass or volume.

    (6) The child cannot distinguish between **physical and psychological causality**. For example, a child may believe that an illness is punishment for a thought or an action.

    b. **The concrete operational stage** (7–11 years of age) is marked by the ability of the child to master many of the tasks encountered during the preoperational stage.

    (1) At this stage, a child understands **reversibility**. By learning that processes can be reversed mentally, the child can grasp the concept of **conservation** (e.g., understanding volume and mass).

    (2) During this period, the child learns to put himself in the place of someone else. In addition, he can comprehend multiple classifications as well as the simultaneous occurrence of two or more classes. As a result, he can order objects serially along a dimension (e.g., smallest to largest).

B. Psychological and social development

1. **Psychosexual development**

    a. After the child establishes an emotionally positive attachment, a sense of autonomy, and a sense of self, she enters the **phallic (oedipal) stage** (3–6 years of age) of development. This stage is characterized by the Oedipus complex (see Chapter 7 II A 4 c).

    (1) This stage is marked by a primary interest in the genitals as the focus of pleasure and concern. This interest is manifested by masturbation, exhibitionism, and curiosity.

    (2) The **Oedipus complex** involves the triadic relationship among the father, mother, and child in which the child wishes to have sole possession of the parent of the opposite sex.

    (3) This complex of feelings leads to **oedipal conflict,** in which the child feels intense rivalry with the parent of the same sex and fears retaliation, usually in terms of bodily damage. In boys, this fear is called **castration anxiety**. Girls often fear the loss of love.

    (4) The Oedipus complex passes at approximately 6 years of age. The child relinquishes the desire for the parent of the opposite sex and resolves to grow up to

be like the parent of the same sex. The child also identifies with the authority of the parent, and an **internalized conscience, or superego,** develops.

   b. Latency is the period between the resolution of the oedipal conflict and the onset of puberty.

     (1) This period is characterized by a strict conscience and strong defenses, such as reaction formation (e.g., I hate girls), identification (e.g., superheroes), and displacement (e.g., competition through involvement in Little League instead of with the father).

     (2) Fantasies are common during this stage. In the **"family romance"** fantasy, the child imagines that he is not the product of his own, devalued parents, but that he has "real" parents who are rich and powerful. A child may have an imaginary companion who is an individual (sometimes a twin) or animal that provides companionship, love, and attention.

2. Play is an important part of the young child's world.

   a. At 3 to 4 years of age, **role playing** is common. The child usually pretends to be a powerful adult or, ironically, the feared monster of his nightmares or fantasies. This type of play is a form of mastery.

   b. When young children play in a group, each child functions autonomously. This pattern is called **parallel play**. The capacity for interactional, or reciprocal, activity that is known as **cooperative play** develops later.

   c. The young school-age child usually engages in group games that range from hide-and-seek to board games or participation in organized sports. These activities provide bodily mastery, self-confidence, and an opportunity to establish peer relationships. They also provide an outlet for subliminated competitiveness and opportunities to experience and resolve anxiety about winning and losing.

3. Social development

   a. At 3 years of age, nursery school or day care, play groups, and birthday parties help the child to expand her social sphere.

   b. Entry into school continues this process.

     (1) The child's social world is enlarged as she forms peer relationships (e.g., a best friend) and enters into group relationships, especially with children of the same sex.

     (2) School is the socially prescribed experience that prepares children to fulfill their roles as adults.

IV. ADOLESCENCE

A. Biologic factors

1. Puberty encompasses the biologic changes that occur in early adolescence. These changes include genital enlargement and growth of pubic and axillary hair. Girls also experience breast development and menarche. Semen production begins in boys. Puberty usually occurs between 10½ and 12½ years of age in girls and between 12 and 14½ years of age in boys. Although they are biologically based, these changes have profound psychological consequences.

2. During this period, cognitive development reaches its final stage, the **formal operational stage** (11 years of age and older).

   a. Most adolescents can perform **abstract and propositional thinking** about multiple variables, consider a problem from multiple points of view, and analyze several variables independently and as part of a whole. For example, the adolescent can look at 20 chairs and identify the ways in which they are alike and the ways in which each chair is different.

   b. Adolescents can discuss and analyze **abstract concepts of truth or virtue**.

   c. Egocentrism changes in form. The adolescent typically believes that he is constantly watched by others.

B. **Psychological factors**

1. **Developmental tasks**

a. **Psychological separation from the parents** is a lifelong process, but the struggle for autonomy is a common feature of early adolescence. Parents and adolescents may disagree about many issues, including grooming, household chores, homework, and choice of friends. A serious conflict between dependency and autonomy is seen in patients with anorexia nervosa.

b. **The consolidation of one's sense of self** is a major developmental task during adolescence. Erikson referred to this process as the formation of **ego identity**. As part of this process, the adolescent's sense of the ideal self undergoes considerable modification. This change often reflects values that are acquired from peers and differ from parental ideals. This situation leads to conflict between the adolescent and his parents and helps him to define himself as distinct and thus separate from his parents.

c. Development of the **capacity for love relationships** outside of the family is an important feature of late adolescence. Dating and crushes are common in midadolescence, and more mature love relationships often occur by late adolescence.

d. **Control of impulses,** especially sexual and aggressive impulses, is an important milestone of adolescence. Severe over- or undercontrol of sexual and aggressive impulses usually indicates a developmental disturbance.

2. **Adolescent turmoil.** Extreme behavioral and emotional shifts were once thought to reflect the normal upheaval of adolescence. Within this framework, suicide attempts, sexual promiscuity, substance abuse, and academic failure could be understood as reactions to the stress of adolescence. These disturbances were called **adolescent turmoil** or an **adjustment reaction to adolescence**. However, empirical studies of normal adolescents do not support this view. Normal adolescents usually do not show serious emotional or behavioral changes, and these problems are now viewed as evidence of disorder.

C. **Sociocultural factors**

1. The length of adolescence as a developmental stage is socioculturally determined. In general, the more highly developed, or industrialized, a culture is, the longer the period of adolescence.

2. In unindustrialized cultures, young people nearing puberty join the adults of the same sex in performing their customary tasks. Thus, entry into the adult world begins early. Marriage and procreation usually follow shortly thereafter, so by 14 to 15 years of age, most young people function as adults. Young people in these cultures do not experience adolescence as it is understood in the United States.

3. Socioeconomic level significantly influences the nature of middle and late adolescence. In lower-class families, formal education often ends with high school graduation or earlier. Young people from these backgrounds usually join the workforce by 16, 17, or 18 years of age. Many also marry and bear children during this period. Individuals from the middle and upper socioeconomic groups often pursue formal postsecondary education. For them, adolescence may be prolonged until 25 or 26 years of age. Some authorities call this extended period of dependence on the family of origin the stage of **youth**.

V. ADULTHOOD

A. **Early adulthood** is the period from 20 to 40 years of age.

1. **Biologic factors.** During this period, the body reaches its physical, reproductive, and cognitive peaks. Adult development is less concerned with the acquisition of new capacities than with the application of available capacities.

2. Psychological factors. During this stage, individuals establish families and careers.

    a. Marriage and parenthood. An important task in early adulthood is the development of the capacity for intimacy in a loving, sexually satisfying relationship. This relationship leads to the hallmark of this phase, parenthood. Parenthood is dramatically different at 25 years of age than at 55 or 65 years of age. Parenthood reactivates conflicts and dynamics from the individual's family of origin. Issues of autonomy and dependency as well as triangular oedipal themes reemerge.

        (1) Parenthood permanently alters the life of the individual and the structure of the marital relationship. Having children provides parents with an opportunity to resolve lingering conflicts from their own childhoods. Parenthood also permits people to heal wounds, hurts, and frustrations from the past (e.g., giving the child piano or tennis lessons that the parent wanted, but never received).

        (2) Healthy families are those that can adjust to shifting demands. The shifts are the results of the developmental movements of each member, altering the family equilibrium or dynamic. The children of effective parents develop and emerge from the family with little strife. These parents convey a clear set of expectations to the children and thereby demonstrate that the parents, not the children, are flexibly in charge of the family.

        (3) Separation and divorce occur in many American families. People whose parents divorce are much more likely to divorce than those whose parents do not. It represents another identification with the parents. People who lack psychological flexibility may find the strains of marriage and parenthood overwhelming. These people are likely to divorce.

    b. Career. Adult identity is influenced by occupation. The competing demands for time and energy among the roles of parent, spouse, and worker cause stress at this stage of development.

3. Sociocultural factors. Socioeconomic level plays a pivotal role in the structure of adult development.

    a. Offspring of middle- and upper-class families usually postpone marriage and parenthood while they continue their education for a number of years (e.g., to study medicine).

    b. In lower-class families, formal education often ends with high school. At this point, the adolescent begins his vocational life. The responsibilities of marriage and parenthood may be undertaken shortly thereafter.

B. **Middle adulthood** is the period from 40 to 60 years of age.

1. Biologic factors. The aging process shapes the psychological development of middle adulthood. Aspects of illness and death emerge as inescapable facets of life during this phase of the life cycle.

    a. Menopause, which occurs in women between 40 and 53 years old, marks the end of the reproductive years. Ovarian function is lost, and menstruation ceases.

        (1) Symptoms include irregular bleeding, vasomotor imbalances (i.e., hot flashes), and sweats, with decreases in estrogen secretion and changes in organic and metabolic functions.

        (2) Hormone replacement therapy is controversial in the treatment of postmenopausal women. Its benefits include relief of vaginal atrophy and vasomotor imbalances as well as retardation of bone loss. Its hazards include an increased risk of uterine endometrial carcinoma.

        (3) Menopause is a **biologic event,** but the most common effects are **psychological**. Confronted with the end of their reproductive life, women may experience anxiety and depression as they appraise their lives and examine their choices.

    b. Men have no specific biologic equivalent to menopause. Hormone levels in men decrease only slightly during middle adulthood. Muscle strength and endurance can be preserved with regular exercise.

2. Psychological factors

    a. The **midlife crisis** is a dramatic change in commitment to career and spouse. It is usually accompanied by self-doubt, stress, anxiety, agitation, or depression. Midlife crisis may be caused by debilitating personal illness, the death of a spouse, the responsibility of caring for an elderly parent, job loss or lack of career advancement, or the presence of dependent adult children.

b. A less severe form of this crisis is **midlife transition,** which occurs in 80% of individuals in their forties. Many people experience a discrepancy between their aspirations and their actual lives. In addition, they begin to sense the finiteness of time (Colarusso and Nemiroff).[5]

c. Relationships with children change. As children grow into autonomous adults, parents must relinquish control over them. This change may make the parents feel powerless or resentful.

d. During this stage, many people experience declining health and the death of their parents. For many people, the death of a parent is their first personal contact with death. People often experience fear regarding their own death, and begin to view time in terms of how much remains rather than how much has passed.

e. This stage also brings pleasure. As children become autonomous, parenting responsibilities diminish, allowing more time for the marital relationship and other pursuits. People of this age often have wisdom, experience, rank, and power.

VI. LATER ADULTHOOD AND OLD AGE begin at age 60 years.

A. **Biologic factors.** Gradually diminishing physical and cognitive capacities combine with the increased likelihood of acute and chronic illness as individuals enter late adulthood. The rate of decline varies significantly.

1. The **pathological process of aging** is influenced by many factors (e.g., genetics, nutrition, environmental conditions) that cause physical changes.

a. Loss of tissue elasticity is most commonly manifested as wrinkling of the skin.

b. Postural changes related to loss of elasticity and bone mass may cause shrinking.

c. Deficits in auditory and visual capacities are common because of neural and non-neural changes. Individuals compensate for these losses to varying degrees.

2. Cognitive capacities (e.g., recall, learning new information) may be diminished. However, not every individual experiences an appreciable loss of mental ability. Cognitive decline may be affected by level of intelligence, lack of motivation, disuse, or disease, but not necessarily by diminished brain function.

3. During this period, a **general decline in physical function** occurs, but physical incapacitation is not an inevitable consequence of aging. For example, the frequency and intensity of sexual activity diminish with age, but interest and participation in sexual activity continue in both men and women, even into their nineties.

B. **Psychological factors**

1. Retirement is a critical point in development, a time when an individual may believe that he is of no more use. Many people experience a reduction in income with retirement. This change may lead to increased anxiety about paying for future medical or nursing care.

2. As they face the prospect of dying, many people assess their lives. Individuals who believe that they have lived a good, moral life may experience a reaffirming sense of integrity. However, a negative evaluation may cause despair (Erikson).[6]

3. Improvements in medical care are allowing individuals to live longer, healthier, and more productive lives than in the past. Most older men are married, whereas the majority of older women are widows because of the higher death and remarriage rates for men. Interestingly, only 20% of older individuals require institutional care, although many older adults fear that they will become dependent or senile.

C. **Sociocultural factors.** An increasing percentage of the population is 65 years of age or older. When the postwar baby boom generation reaches retirement, more than 20% of the United States population will be older than 65 years of age.

1. Erikson refers to the last stage of psychosocial development in the life cycle as **ego identity versus despair.** Ego identity is maintained if the individual views his life as satisfying and fulfilling. Individuals who do not achieve a final integration of the choices and events in their lives will experience despair.

2. American society, which is traditionally youth oriented, is becoming increasingly conscious of old age. Senior citizens groups bring political and social issues to the attention of the public and combat prejudicial and stereotypical attitudes about old age. Many Asian cultures by contrast revere the elderly for their experience and wisdom.

3. As older individuals enjoy healthier, longer lives, the retirement years may be the most pleasurable and rewarding of the life cycle if they are not complicated by poverty, illness, or loneliness.

VII. DEATH AND DYING

A. **Child's perspective**

1. A child's response to death is based on her level of awareness. An awareness of the meaning of death becomes more concrete as comprehension develops.
   a. **Children younger than 5 years of age** view death as **abandonment.** When they think about death, they do not understand its finality and irreversibility. They may say, "When Grandma comes back to life . . ." or "When Grandma comes to visit . . ." even when they are told explicitly about her death. For these reasons, they cannot fully mourn important individuals in their lives.
   b. By **middle childhood,** a **more realistic view** of death emerges, and children usually understand the finality of the event.
      (1) At this stage, anxiety about death concerns not only the loss of, or separation from, loved ones but also fears about mutilation (castration anxiety), suffering, and pain.
      (2) Because their thinking is **egocentric,** children often experience guilt and **view themselves as responsible** for their own or others' illness and death. They may view illness or death as punishment for bad behavior.
   c. **Adolescents** usually have an adult cognitive view of death and a **clear understanding** of its irreversibility. In addition, they usually have a capacity to mourn, especially by midadolescence.
      (1) Adolescents with chronic physical illness (e.g., cystic fibrosis) are regularly confronted with the death of their similarly affected peers. Therefore, they have a sense of the finiteness of life and often live their lives while waiting for the final stage of their own illness.
      (2) With a decrease in the egocentricity of their thinking and a diminished tendency to view illness or death as justified or deserved, adolescents experience both resentment and despair as they struggle to accept their own mortality.

2. **Parental response to a child's death.** A child's death is a devastating experience for the parents. If the death is not sudden, the parents often unconsciously undergo **anticipatory mourning,** during which they gradually relinquish strong emotional ties to the child. This process can be painful for both the child and the parents.
   a. The child senses the diminished emotional involvement by the parents. Thus, the child experiences abandonment, even though the parents may be physically present. The relationship often becomes superficial as the parents attempt to hide their distress. An emotional barrier is erected, conversation becomes trivial, and the subject that is most on the child's and parents' minds becomes taboo.

b. When the child dies, the parents feel guilty because they are not more upset by the child's death or because they are relieved that the ordeal is over. Unless properly counseled, they may consider themselves callous when in fact they have already grieved, although unconsciously and in advance.

B. **Adult's perspective**

1. Adults are anxious about their own death because of a dread of separation from their loved ones and concern about pain and suffering. They also fear that they will not leave an indelible mark on the world that will ensure their perpetual existence and thus avoid nothingness.

2. Elisabeth Kübler-Ross[7] states that dying patients experience **five stages** before death occurs. These stages, however, are not fixed or universal.
   a. **Denial** is the initial stage, in which the patient cannot believe that he is dying.
   b. **Anger** encompasses a range of reactions, including rage, bitterness, and confusion.
   c. **Bargaining** is characterized by a search for meaning in life, a return to religious institutions, and often a belief that some magical power will intervene.
   d. **Depression** involves two phases of grieving.
      (1) **Preparatory grief** often involves emotional detachment and a relinquishing of social and family bonds and responsibilities.
      (2) **Final grief** involves a patient's preoccupation with his own death and is often marked by reflections about existence and life.
   e. **Acceptance** is manifested as emotional detachment or neutrality or as a calm, even euphoric, state.

C. **Physician's response.** Several common responses occur in physicians who care for dying patients.

1. A sense of **failure** is common. Despite knowing otherwise, many physicians believe that if they had tried harder, the outcome might have been different.

2. Occasionally, a patient reminds the physician of a loved one, either a child, spouse, friend, parent, or colleague.

REFERENCES

1. Spitz RA: Anaclitic depression. *Psychoanal Study Child* 2:313–342, 1946.

2. Mahler MS, Pine F, Bergman A: *The Psychological Birth of the Human Infant.* New York, Basic Books, 1975.

3. Pasamaneck B, Knoblock H: Environmental factors affecting human development before and after birth. *Pediatrics* 26:210–218, 1960.

4. Piaget J: *The Origins of Intelligence in Children.* Madison, CT, International Universities Press, 1952.

5. Colarusso CA, Nemiroff RA: *Adult Development.* New York, Plenum, 1981.

6. Erikson E: *Childhood and Society.* New York, Norton, 1950.

7. Kübler-Ross E: *On Death and Dying.* New York, Macmillan, 1969.

STUDY QUESTIONS

DIRECTIONS: Each of the numbered items or incomplete statements in this section is followed by answers or by completions of the statement. Select the ONE lettered answer or completion that is BEST in each case.

1. Which one of the following statements describes parallel play?

(A) It is common in grade school children
(B) It describes group games such as hide and seek and team sports
(C) It describes healthy interaction between a mother and an infant
(D) It is seen in young children, who tend to play autonomously in the presence of other children
(E) It is primarily caused by separation anxiety

2. The mother of a 9-month-old infant visits the pediatrician with concerns about her child. Although the child used to be friendly with friends and neighbors and to do well with baby-sitters, he now refuses to be held by his aunt and he cries when the baby-sitter comes. The mother wonders what she can do to help her baby be more sociable. Which of the following would be the best advice from the pediatrician?

(A) The child should begin day care as soon as possible so he will be exposed to different people every day
(B) The crying is probably caused by too much sugar in the child's diet
(C) The child should be spanked each time he cries with his aunt, so he learns that his crying is wrong
(D) The child is exhibiting stranger anxiety, which is a normal phase and represents healthy cognitive development
(E) The child should have a psychiatric consultation to evaluate his irritability

3. Which of the following is the correct definition of egocentrism?

(A) The belief by a child that every moving object is alive and has feelings
(B) The inability of a child to put himself in the place of someone else
(C) The belief of a child that all things are made by humans and for humans
(D) The inability of a child to distinguish between physical and psychological causality
(E) The inability of a child to comprehend more than one property of an object at a time

4. A 12-month-old child is usually able to do all of the following EXCEPT

(A) walk when held by the hand
(B) say "mama" and "dada"
(C) have a vocabulary of about 50 words
(D) stand without support
(E) demonstrate full visual accommodation

5. Each of the following is true regarding the formal operational stage EXCEPT

(A) it is typical of adolescents
(B) it is a stage of cognitive development
(C) it features the capacity for abstract and propositional thinking
(D) an important feature of this stage is the Oedipus complex
(E) it follows the concrete operational stage

6. Normal features of early adulthood include all of the following EXCEPT

(A) development of the capacity for intimacy in a loving, sexually satisfying relationship
(B) the opportunity to resolve some lingering conflicts from childhood
(C) the need to face the prospect of dying
(D) the need to adjust to shifting demands of work and family
(E) the reemergence of issues of autonomy and dependency

Questions 7–11

For each definition, select the aspect of psychological development that it defines.

(A) Individuation
(B) Intimate differentiated attachment
(C) Object permanence
(D) Practicing phase
(E) Rapprochement crisis

7. A process of differentiation through which the child realizes that she is an entity distinct from the mother

8. The principal psychological task of the first year of life

9. Development of locomotion, which allows the child to explore the environment and return to the mother for emotional reinforcement

10. A period marked by shadowing and moving away

11. Development of a mental representation of objects and persons

ANSWERS AND EXPLANATIONS

1. The answer is D [III B 2 b]. Parallel play, which is characteristic of toddlers, describes the tendency of young children to play independently, even in the company of peers. For example, several three-year-olds with a set of blocks will likely each build alone, rather than building something together. Parallel play is unrelated to separation anxiety, which peaks at 18 months of age and involves clinging behavior toward the mother.

2. The answer is D [II B 3]. It is normal for a 9-month-old to become distressed in the presence of strangers, and even in the presence of family or baby-sitters who visit only occasionally. It is a mark of attachment to the mother and represents the beginning of the cognitive capacity to recall a mental image of her. No treatment, such as day care, is necessary. Diet is unrelated to separation anxiety. The baby should not be spanked for normal behavior and is not in need of psychiatric consultation. Educating the mother about this and other phases of development is the best course of action.

3. The answer is B [III A 4 a (2)]. A child who demonstrates egocentrism will be unable to put herself in the place of another person. Animism is the belief that all moving objects are alive. Artificialism is the belief that all things are made by and for humans. Each of these beliefs is characteristic of children 2 to 7 years of age, who are in the preoperational stage of cognitive development. Other features of this stage are the inability to distinguish between physical and psychological causality and the inability to comprehend more than one property of an object at a time.

4. The answer is C [Table 7-1]. A typical one-year-old is learning to walk and should be able to stand without support and walk if held by the hand or holding on to furniture. Speech should also be developing, and the child will use simple words such as "mama" and "dada" as well as a few other words. However, a 50-word vocabulary is more typical for an 18-month-old child. Visual accommodation should certainly be in place at age 1, because this usually occurs at about 4 months of age.

5. The answer is D [III A 4 b, B 1 a; IV A 2]. Formal operations describes the final stage of cognitive development; it follows concrete operations. This stage typically begins at approximately age 11 and is commonly seen in adolescents. The ability to think abstractly and to look at a problem from several points of view is characteristic of formal operations. The Oedipus complex is seen as part of the phallic stage of psychosexual development. It is not related directly to the stages of cognitive development.

6. The answer is C [V A 2]. Early adulthood, which includes the years between the ages of 20 and 40, typically presents a number of challenges. The development of a loving, committed relationship often occurs during this time. Beginning such a relationship, however, may rekindle old issues of autonomy and dependency, but may also provide an opportunity to resolve these and other lingering conflicts from childhood. When parenthood follows, it requires the ability to adjust to demanding changes and to deal with the conflicting priorities of work and family. Because many individuals in this phase are physically healthy and have not yet lost a friend or parent to death, facing the prospect of death is considered more typical of older adults.

7–11. The answers are: 7-A, 8-B, 9-D, 10-E, 11-C [II B 1, 3 a, 4 d, e (1)–(2)]. Individuation is the psychological separation of mother and child. It is the process by which personality is formed.

Intimate differentiated attachment is the foremost psychological task of the first year of life, in which the infant forms a bond to the mother or primary care giver. Formation of this attachment is essential to the development of future relationships.

The practicing phase is the period when the toddler practices his walking skills. Locomotion permits the toddler to explore the environment by moving away from the mother and returning to her for encouragement and emotional support.

During the rapprochement subphase, the child becomes aware of the separateness of the mother. The toddler may react intensely to this realization. By alternately following the mother carefully (shadowing) and running away from her (darting away), the toddler exhibits the wish for reunion and separation, respectively.

Object permanence is the infant's capacity to maintain a mental representation of the mother, even when she is not present. This ability allows the infant to recognize that a stranger is not the mother. Thus, the stranger represents the mother's absence, which creates stranger anxiety.

Part II
The Psychosocial Behavioral Sciences

Chapter 9

Human Sexuality

Robert L. Hendren
Barry Sarvet

I. **DEVELOPMENT OF SEXUALITY.** Sexuality is a basic function that is present throughout the life cycle. Its development is intertwined with physical maturation, growth, and psychological development.

A. **Infancy and Childhood**

1. Physical correlates of genital excitation, such as erection, can be observed beginning in newborns.

2. Loving human touch is necessary for the well-being of infants and young children. Aspects of adult sexual behavior are reminiscent of infant–mother interactions, such as breast suckling, hugging, rocking, kissing, and oral exploration.

3. **Awareness of gender** and concern about gender conformity are seen as early as the second half of the third year of life. This awareness usually follows a more generalized identification with the parent of the same sex.

4. Children engage in genital self-stimulation as infants and throughout childhood. Mutual sexual stimulation and exploration may be seen throughout middle childhood. When later associated with incorporated prohibitions against certain sexual behaviors, individuals may experience guilt that may be pathogenic. Organized fantasies and the goal of orgasm characterize masturbation beginning in early adolescence.

B. **Adolescence.** The adolescent period is characterized by relatively rapid **physical change** that leads to maturation of the sexual and reproductive anatomy (Table 9-1). In girls, the reproductive cycle is established.

1. During adolescence, long bone growth is accelerated and pubic and axillary hair appears in both boys and girls. Gender-specific maturation, such as breast development and menarche in girls and penis growth and onset of nocturnal emissions in boys, is noted. In girls, adolescent changes occur 1 to 2 years earlier than those in boys.

2. Adolescents may experience strong sexual urges that are released through masturbation or sexual experimentation. Masturbation allows the adolescent to "try out" sexual functioning with the aid of sexual fantasies. The content of the adolescent's sexual fantasy may become a source of considerable guilt or shame.

C. **Adulthood**

1. **Typical development of sexuality.** For many, adulthood involves a deepening of intimacy in marriage and the parenting of children. Expressions of sexuality change as each partner copes with these events and the aging of the body. Sexual problems may emerge as a result of poor communication between partners, with resultant sexual dysfunction, boredom, stereotypical behavior, and dissatisfaction. Monotony, feelings of being taken for granted, concerns with career, illness in either partner, and overindulgence in food and alcohol all interfere with sexual activity in both men and women.

TABLE 9-1. Tanner Stages of Sexual Maturity

Stage	Pubic Hair	Breasts (female)	Genitalia (male)
1	No pubic hair	Elevation of papilla only	Same as early childhood
2	Sparse, downy, straight hair at base of penis or along labia	Breast bud: enlargement of areola, elevation of papilla and breast as small mound	Enlargement of scrotum and testes, reddening and texture change of scrotum, minimal penile enlargement
3	Darker, coarser, beginning to curl, spread sparsely over pubes	Further enlargement of mound with separation in contour between areola and breast	Lengthening of penis, further enlargement of scrotum and testes
4	Hair resembles adult type (coarse, curly, abundant) but with smaller area of distribution	Projection of areola and papilla above the contour of the breast	Increased girth, length, and development of glans, darkening of scrotum and further enlargement of testes
5	Adult quantity and distribution, spread to medial thighs	Mature: areola recedes into contour of breast, projection of papilla only	Adult size

Adapted from Tanner JM: *Growth at Adolescence,* 2nd ed. Cambridge, MA, Blackwell Scientific Publications, 1962, pp 28–39.

2. **Changes with age. Sexual interest and activity persist but decline** throughout adulthood and older age (most noticeably between 46 and 55 years of age). The extent to which this decline occurs depends on earlier levels of sexual interest and activity. Men report greater interest and activity than do women.

    a. As **women** age, estrogen levels decrease and menopause occurs. Menopause generally occurs early in the sixth decade. It causes **changes in estrogen-dependent tissue,** such as that found in the breasts and vagina. Women may also have emotional symptoms such as mood lability and depression. Vaginal lubrication often decreases, and the vaginal vault expands less with sexual arousal. With age, changes are noted in the uterus, the labia majora and minora, and in the size of the clitoris. The orgasmic phase becomes shorter, uterine contractions may become spastic and painful, and there is a more rapid resolution phase.

    b. In **men,** sexual responsiveness is affected by biologic and emotional factors in middle age. Physiologic changes include delay in attaining an erection and decline in the fullness of the erection. The feeling of ejaculatory inevitability may vary, and the explosive force decreases, as does the volume of seminal fluid. Resolution is quickened, and the erection is lost more rapidly. The refractory period is longer. Ejaculatory control improves, but the desire for ejaculation may decrease.

D. **Older age.** Although the desire for genital sexual activity may wane and the capacity for genital sexual function decreases, sexuality, broadly defined, continues to be important. Touching, caressing, and hugging as well as emotional intimacy are very important to the well-being of the elderly.

1. Changes in estrogen- and androgen-dependent tissues and organs continue in older age.

2. The frequency of intercourse and masturbation decreases over the life cycle. Sexual activity is related to the quality of health and the availability of a partner. Cessation of intercourse is most often attributed to poor health in either partner or to sexual dysfunction in the man.

II. SEXUAL PHYSIOLOGY

A. **The sexual response cycle.** Masters and Johnson[1] described four phases of physiologic change that occur in the sexual response cycle (Table 9-2). These four phases are preceded by an **appetitive phase,** which refers to the onset of sexual desire before observable physiologic changes occur.

1. **Excitement phase**
   a. **Woman.** Pelvic congestion and myotonia cause the clitoris to enlarge and become more sensitive. The inner two thirds of the vagina "balloons" in length and width, and transudation (sweating) occurs, producing lubrication. The labia majora thicken and move away from the introitus. Nipples become erect and more sensitive; breast size increases. Voluntary and involuntary muscle tensing occurs in the lower abdominal and pubococcygeal regions. The heart rate and blood pressure increase as sexual excitement increases.
   b. **Man.** Penile tumescence and erection occur. The erection may be partially lost and regained during this phase. Tensing and thickening of the scrotal sac occur, with elevation of both testes as the spermatic cord shortens. Nipple erection may occur in addition to tensing of the abdominal and pelvic muscles. The heart rate and blood pressure increase.

2. **Plateau phase**
   a. **Woman.** The clitoris retracts against the anterior body of the symphysis pubis underneath the clitoral hood. Vasoconstriction of the outer third of the vagina and the labia minora causes this tissue to increase in size. This is referred to as the **orgasmic platform**. The uterus becomes fully elevated and the cervix elevates, producing a tenting effect of the vagina. The labia minora change in color from bright red to a deep wine, indicating impending orgasm. Bartholin's glands release a few drops of mucoid secretions. The **sex flush,** a maculopapular rash, may spread over the abdomen and chest at this time or during the excitement phase.
   b. **Man.** The penis increases in circumference at the coronal ridge. The testes increase in size and elevate further. These signs are indicative of impending ejaculation. Cowper's glands release a few drops of mucoid secretions. These secretions may contain a few active spermatozoa. The sex flush may appear during this phase.

3. **Orgasmic phase**
   a. **Woman.** Contractions in the orgasmic platform occur with increasing intervals and decreasing intensity. The musculature of the pelvic floor contracts, forcing blood out

TABLE 9-2. Male/Female Sexual Response

Phase	Woman	Man
Excitement phase	Clitoral enlargement Ballooning of vaginal vault Nipple erection	Penile tumescence Testes elevate Nipple erection
Plateau phase	Clitoris retracts Tenting of vagina Bartholin's secretion Sex flush	Increase in penile circumference Testes increase in size Cowper's secretion Sex flush

Orgasmic phase	Pelvic contractions
	Increase in pulse and blood
	   pressure
		Contractions
		Increase in pulse and blood
		   pressure

Resolution phase	Clitoral detumescence Loss of vasal congestion Descent of uterus and cervix	Penile detumescence Testes descend

of the area. This action may be one factor that is responsible for orgasm. Contractions of the uterus begin at the fundus and spread downward. The intensity of these contractions parallels the intensity of the orgasm. The rectal sphincter may contract, and the pulse rate and blood pressure may increase further. Orgasmic expulsions of lubricating secretions may be triggered by stimulation of the Gräfenberg spot on the anterior vaginal wall. Both vaginal and clitoral orgasms have been described.

    b. Man. Contractions of the prostate gland, vasa efferentia of the testes, epididymis, vas deferens and seminal vesicles, and urethra propel seminal and prostatic fluids to the exterior while the bladder sphincter closes. Involuntary contractions may occur as well as contractions of the anal sphincter. Heart and respiration rates increase. The increase in blood pressure is more pronounced in the man than in the woman.

4. Resolution phase

    a. Woman. The clitoris quickly returns to its normal position with more gradual detumescence. The vaginal walls and orgasmic platform lose their vasocongestion, as do the labia majora and minora. The uterus returns to its normal position, and the cervix descends to the seminal basin in the dorsal area of the vagina. Because the vasocongestion and myotonia subside less quickly in women than in men, the clitoral and perineal tissues are sensitive enough to respond almost immediately to continued stimulation.

    b. Man. The loss of vasoconstriction in the penis is rapid, with a resulting decrease in size and a slower involution to preexcitement levels. The testes descend, and the scrotum relaxes. The refractory time varies from less than 10 minutes to 45 minutes, and increases with age.

B. **Hormonal influences on sexual development and function**

1. Hormonal influence in utero

    a. The sex hormones are believed to influence the **sexual differentiation** of the human embryo. Androgens secreted by the testes in male fetuses during the first trimester are necessary for the differentiation of male external genitalia. Disorders of end-organ sensitivity to androgen, such as testicular feminization syndrome, and of excessive androgen production, such as andrenogenital syndrome, cause intersex disorders in which genital differentiation is incongruent with genotype and gonad type.

    b. Sex hormones influence **sex typing of the brain** during fetal development. Research with animal models suggests that either androgens or estrogens that are metabolically derived from androgens interact with receptors in the hypothalamus. In either case, the hormones derived from the testes or the lack thereof lead to a male or female pattern of gonadotropin release. Evidence suggests a similar hormonal neurodevelopmental basis for human sexual orientation (see IV C 2).

2. Hormonal and physiologic influence on the sexual response cycle. Testosterone is postulated to influence sexual desire in both men and women. In the absence of a deficiency state, however, administration of hormones is not useful in enhancing libido. Vaginal changes, such as lubrication associated with the excitement phase, are believed to be mediated by the local release of **vasoactive intestinal peptide (VIP),** a neuropeptide hormone that is secreted by nerves in the vaginal wall.

C. **Neurophysiologic influences on the sexual response cycle**

1. Aspects of the excitement phase are largely under **parasympathetic** control. Effects such as penile erection are the result of vasocongestion that is caused by dilation of local blood vessels in the penis.

2. The orgasmic phase is largely under **sympathetic** control.

3. Several areas of the **limbic system** are involved in sexual behavior, including the hippocampus and the amygdala. Connections between cortical areas, hypothalamic areas, and limbic nuclei may be responsible for various complex emotional, behavioral, and physiologic aspects of sexual functioning.

III. CULTURAL AND PSYCHOLOGICAL INFLUENCES ON SEXUAL EXPRESSION

A. **Sociocultural factors** that affect sexual expression include the customs, traditions, and attitudes of the family and the society in which an individual lives.

1. **Culture.** The culture in which an individual is raised or currently lives determines to a large extent how sexuality is expressed. Cultural influences can affect an individual's view of what is considered sexual and what is not; the purpose of sex (i.e., for procreation only or for enjoyment at other times); the role of the woman and the man; the appropriateness of nonmarital sex; choices regarding sexual positions, foreplay, and duration of the sexual act; and the ways in which sexual feelings are communicated.

2. **Family.** The sexual values of the family may reflect the cultural values or may be in conflict with them. Parents who have moved from one culture to another or who have differing cultural values may have conflicting feelings about sexual expression that may be shared by their children.

3. **Socioeconomic differences** also affect sexual behavior. A study of families of lower socioeconomic status, in which the marital relationship had a high degree of role segregation, showed less frequent and less satisfying sexual expression than occurred in families of middle socioeconomic status, in which the roles were more jointly organized.

4. **Religious teachings** vary from viewing sexuality as part of human relationships, to sex for procreation only, to sexual enjoyment as a sign of wickedness. Religious training early in life may continue to influence sexual behavior at a later age, even if the religious beliefs of the individual have changed.

B. **Psychological factors**

1. **Early experiences** with intimacy, sexuality, trust, and guilt exert continued influence on the individual through both conscious and unconscious attitudes.

2. **Early sexual traumas,** either within or outside the family, may provide a continuing source of anxiety and guilt later in life. Examples of trauma include incest, sexual abuse, sexual awkwardness due to lack of knowledge and experience, and impulsive "acting out."

IV. HOMOSEXUALITY. Homosexuality is an issue of sexual orientation. Homosexual individuals are attracted to others of the same sex. **Bisexual** persons are attracted to both men and women. Homosexuality must be distinguished from **transsexualism,** which is an issue of gender identity.

A. **Background**

1. Homosexuality is considered a normal variation of sexual behavior and not a mental disorder. Diagnostic classification systems proposed before the *Diagnostic and Statistical Manual of Mental Disorders,* 3rd edition (*DSM-III*) included homosexuality as a mental disorder.

2. Because of the persistence of sometimes severe forms of social stigma in the lives of many homosexuals, they often affiliate with a homosexual community, where they find acceptance. Homosexuals may feel alienated from the dominant culture, the culture of origin, and the family.

3. The development of homosexual relationships, commonly occurring in adolescence, may be associated with great emotional turmoil that is generated by psychological conflict. This turmoil may mimic a personality disorder, but may be distinguished by its transience.

4. Homosexual experimentation may occur during developmental periods, such as adolescence, and is not indicative of sexual orientation.

B. **Prevalence.** According to the Kinsey Institute study,[2] 4% of men and 1% to 3% of women in the United States are exclusively homosexual. Underreporting may flaw these data.

C. **Etiology.** The etiology of homosexuality remains controversial; however, several etiologic factors have emerged. Well-accepted data show that childhood gender nonconformity is associated with a higher incidence of homosexuality. This notion of early-onset predisposition is used to support both biologic and psychosocial theories of etiology. Currently, investigators favor an integrative model with a developmental perspective that draws on the following areas of research.

1. **Genetic.** Twin studies show a higher concordance rate of sexual orientation for monozygotic twins than for dizygotic twins. This finding suggests the presence of a genetic factor, although the concordance rate for monozygotic twins is far short of 100%, leaving room for nongenetic factors.

2. **Hormonal.** The study of a rodent model suggests that different patterns of prenatal interaction of androgens with fetal brain steroid receptors lead to gender-specific sexual behaviors that are associated with gender-specific patterns of hypothalamic function.

3. **Neuroanatomic.** The size of several human brain structures may vary with sexual orientation. Most notably, LeVay[3] found that the third interstitial nucleus of the anterior hypothalamus is smaller in both homosexual men and heterosexual women than it is in heterosexual men.

4. **Psychosocial.** The theory of the influence of a family constellation that consists of a dominant mother and a weak or rejecting father has been advanced as a cause of male homosexuality. This theory proposes that male homosexuals develop a sexual identification with the mother as a result of longing for male nurturance.

V. **SEXUAL DYSFUNCTION** is generally classified according to the phase of the sexual response cycle that is involved. Psychogenic and organic factors have been implicated. Most types of dysfunction have both male and female analogs.

A. **Disorders affecting the appetitive phase.** Two types are distinguished, but they may be related.

1. **Hypoactive sexual desire disorder** is defined as a relative or absolute lack of desire and fantasy regarding sexual activity. It may occur in the context of a specific committed relationship, or the deficiency of desire may be global. In the latter case, there is a greater likelihood of relevant organic factors, such as testosterone deficiency in men, side effects of medications (e.g., antihypertensives), and general physical illness. Depression may cause similar symptoms; however, in DSM-IV, these symptoms would be subsumed under the affective disorder diagnosis.

2. **Sexual aversion disorder** implies an extreme avoidance of sexual activity rather than a simple lack of desire. It is distinguished from simple lack of desire by its association with anxiety symptoms. It is believed to be related to phobia, and it may be associated with actual panic attacks. If panic disorder is present, specific treatment is essential in the overall clinical approach. The patient may have a history of sexual trauma, such as rape or incest.

B. **Disorders affecting the excitement phase**

1. **Male erectile disorder** is a persistent inability to maintain erection until completion of the sexual act. In some cultures, this disorder is extremely feared and may be self-reinforcing depending on the reaction of the partner and the resultant feelings of guilt and inadequacy. The incidence increases from approximately 4% in young adulthood to 80% in some elderly samples.

a. Common **biologic factors** include medical illness, most commonly diabetes (Table 9-3); medications, especially antihypertensives and antidepressants (Table 9-4); neurologic damage or illness; and endocrinopathies. Clues to the biologic or psychogenic etiology of this disorder are often discovered through careful history taking and the use of easily administered, noninvasive tests to measure nocturnal penile tumescence. The test is based on the expectation that normal erectile function would be demonstrated during rapid eye movement (REM) sleep, although results are occasionally misleading.

b. Common **psychological factors** include symptoms of anxiety and intimidation, fears of failure in sexual performance, and unconscious fears of sexual expression and excitement.

2. Female sexual arousal disorder is not as well understood as male erectile disorder. Affected women have impaired secretion of lubricant fluid and impaired swelling of vaginal tissues during sexual activity. Postmenopausal women may have similar symptoms because of a deficiency of estrogen. Intercourse is painful, although sexual desire is generally preserved. Because of related dyspareunia, however, affected women may avoid sex and experience more widespread sexual dysfunction. The cause of this disorder is unclear.

C. **Disorders affecting the orgasmic phase** include inability to attain orgasm despite sexual activity that is adequate in focus, intensity, and duration; or in men, inability to adequately control the timing of ejaculation. According to DSM-IV, these diagnoses only are made if the patient experiences marked distress or interpersonal difficulty.

TABLE 9-3. Diseases Implicated in Erectile Dysfunction

Cardiovascular diseases
Atherosclerotic disease
Aortic aneurysm
Cardiac failure

Pulmonary disorders
Respiratory failure

Neurologic disorders
Multiple sclerosis
Transverse myelitis
Parkinson's disease
Temporal lobe epilepsy
Traumatic or neoplastic spinal cord disease
Central nervous system (CNS) tumors
Amyotrophic lateral sclerosis
Peripheral neuropathies
General paresis
Tabes dorsalis

Endocrine disorders
Diabetes mellitus
Acromegaly
Addison's disease
Chromophobe adenoma
Adrenal neoplasias
Myxedema (hypothyroidism)
Hyperthyroidism

Surgical procedures
Perineal prostatectomy
Abdomino-perineal colon resection
Sympathectomy (frequently interferes with ejaculation)
Aortoiliac surgery
Radical cystectomy
Retroperitoneal lymphadenectomy

Hepatic disorders
Cirrhosis (usually associated with alcoholism)

Renal and urologic disorders
Chronic renal failure
Hydrocele or varicocele

Infectious and parasitic diseases
Elephantiasis
Mumps

Genetic disorders
Klinefelter's syndrome
Congenital penile vascular or structural abnormalities

Nutritional disorders
Malnutrition
Vitamin deficiencies

Poisoning
Lead (plumbism)
Herbicides

Miscellaneous
Radiation therapy
Pelvic fracture

Adapted from Sadock BJ: Normal human sexuality and sexual dysfunction. In *Comprehensive Textbook of Psychiatry*, 5th ed. Edited by Kaplan HI, Sadock BJ. Baltimore, Williams & Wilkins, 1989.

TABLE 9-4. Pharmacologic Agents Implicated in Male Sexual Dysfunction*

Drug	Impairs Erection	Impairs Ejaculation
Psychiatric drugs		
Tricyclic antidepressants[†]		
Imipramine (Tofranil)	+	+
Protriptyline (Vivactil)	+	+
Desipramine (Pertofrane)	+	+
Clomipramine (Anafranil)	+	+
Amitriptyline (Elavil)	+	+
Nortriptyline (Aventyl)	+	+
Selective serotonin reuptake inhibitors		
Fluoxetine (Prozac)	+	+
Sertraline (Zoloft)	−	+
Paroxetine (Paxil)	+	+
Monoamine oxidase inhibitors		
Tranylcypromine (Parnate)	+	−
Phenelzine (Nardil)	+	+
Pargyline (Eutonyl)	−	+
Isocarboxazid (Marplan)	−	+
Other mood-active drugs		
Lithium	+	−
Amphetamines	+	+
Major tranquilizers[‡]		
Fluphenazine (Prolixin)	+	−
Thioridazine (Mellaril)	+	+
Chlorprothixene (Taractan)	−	+
Mesoridazine (Serentil)	−	+
Perphenazine (Trilafon)	−	+
Trifluoperazine (Stelazine)	−	+
Reserpine (Serpasil)	+	+
Haloperidol (Haldol)	−	+
Minor tranquilizers[§]		
Chlordiazepoxide (Librium)	−	+
Antihypertensive drugs		
Clonidine (Catapres)	+	−
Methyldopa (Aldomet)	+	+
Spironolactone (Aldactone)	+	−
Hydralazine (Apresoline)	+	−
Guanethidine (Ismelin)	+	+
Commonly abused drugs		
Alcohol	+	+
Barbiturates	+	+
Cannabis	+	−
Cocaine	+	+
Heroin	+	+
Methadone	+	+
Morphine	+	+
Miscellaneous drugs		
Antiparkinsonian agents	+	+
Clofibrate (Atromid-S)	+	−
Digoxin (Lanoxin)	+	−
Glutethimide (Doriden)	+	+
Indomethacin (Indocin)	+	−
Phentolamine (Regitine)	−	+
Propranolol (Inderal)	+	−

Adapted from Sadock BJ: Normal human sexuality and sexual dysfunction. In *Comprehensive Textbook of Psychiatry*, 5th ed. Edited by Kaplan HI, Sadock BJ. Baltimore, Williams & Williams, 1989.
*Both increase and decrease in libido have been reported with psychoactive agents. It is difficult to separate those effects from the underlying condition or from improvement of the condition. Sexual dysfunction associated with the use of a drug disappears when the drug is discontinued.
[†]The incidence of erectile dysfunction associated with the use of tricyclic antidepressants is low.
[‡]Impairment of sexual function is not a common complication of the use of major tranquilizers. Priapism occasionally has occurred in association with the use of major tranquilizers.
[§]Benzodiazepines can decrease libido, but in some patients, the diminution of anxiety caused by those drugs enhances sexual function.

1. **Inhibited female orgasm** includes a potentially wide range of orgasmic responsivity to sexual stimulation. The most severe manifestation is the absolute inability to have an orgasm under any circumstance. The milder form involves dissatisfaction with a need for adjunctive clitoral stimulation during coitus to attain orgasm. This common disorder may arise from **psychological** factors, such as fear of losing control, internal conflicts related to sexuality, and conflict in the relationship. Alternatively, **biologic** factors, such as medication, diabetes, and endocrinopathies, may be responsible for this disorder.

2. **Inhibited male orgasm** is analogous to the female condition, but is less common. It has both mild and severe variants, and there are both conflict-derived and biologic explanations.

3. **Premature ejaculation** is a common disorder that may affect 30% of men. The control that is necessary for optimal timing of ejaculation may be comprised by anxiety, lack of experience, lack of familiarity with a partner, or sexual overstimulation.

D. | **Sexual pain disorders**

1. **Dyspareunia** refers to pain associated with sexual intercourse. It is much more common in women than in men. It is frequently caused by physical factors that affect the pelvic tissues, such as infection or surgical scarring. Pain with intercourse may be related to psychological issues as well. Men may have pain of vascular origin that is related to inhibited male orgasm. Dyspareunia also may be caused by spasm of the perineal musculature during ejaculation.

2. **Vaginismus** is recurrent involuntary spasm of the muscles that surround the outer portion of the vagina. Medical conditions, such as infection, may cause spasm, and must be excluded. Sexual aversion disorder may be associated, and the patient may have a history of sexual trauma. A possible psychodynamic factor is the association of sexual penetration with fears related to aggression. This association may be unconscious, and the patient may have normal sexual desire.

E. | **Clinical management of sexual dysfunction.** Before the work of Masters and Johnson[4] in the 1970s, sexual dysfunction was regarded primarily as a symptom of underlying individual psychopathology. Currently, a sexual problem, although understood as being frequently related to deep-rooted psychological conflicts, is considered an autonomous symptom that may respond well to intervention that addresses the problem directly.

1. **Evaluation**
   a. **Medical.** The physician should begin with a multisystem survey to explore potential organic causes. The following systems should be considered: **neurologic, endocrine, peripheral vascular, urologic, and gynecologic.** Medications, effects of angina, drug or alcohol abuse, and any general medical illness may be direct causative factors or part of a multifactorial formulation that also includes psychological or interpersonal problems (see Tables 9-3 and 9-4).
   b. **Psychiatric.** Affective disorder, panic disorder, severe personality disorder, and other mental illness require evaluation and specific treatment before treatment can be applied to the sexual problem. A general evaluation of each partner's psychiatric history and mental status is often undertaken at the outset of treatment. In addition, examination of the relationship of the couple may suggest the need for couples therapy before or during the treatment for sexual dysfunction.
   c. **Sexual history.** Treatment begins with gathering detailed information about both partners' sexual behavior; thoughts and feelings before, during, and after sexual activity; masturbation attitudes and behavior; sexual fantasies; and bodily responses. Assessment of communication patterns and the partners' awareness of their own and the other's sexual wishes and attitudes is also essential.

2. **Elements of sex therapy.** Currently, a flexible, short-term approach is favored.
   a. **Couples format.** Although one partner may be more easily identified as symptomatic, there is an assumption that both members are responsible for their sexual relationship. Problems are often maintained and exacerbated by poor communication and a resultant lack of awareness of a partner's needs and vulnerabilities. Emphasis

is placed on the development of communication skills and the enhancement of emotional sensitivity in relation to the sexual activity.

   (1) Education. To combat myths that may interfere with realistic understanding of the relevant problems, couples are given information about basic physiology and the psychology of sexual functioning.

   (2) Behavioral approach. Specific behavioral strategies are useful for specific types of sexual dysfunction.

   (a) Sensate focus exercises help couples become more aware of their sensory responsiveness. These exercises begin with nongenital stimulation and lead to genital stimulation. Couples are encouraged to heighten their awareness of basic sensations of touch, sight, smell, and hearing during exercises in which they imagine and practice sensual stimulation. Problems such as anxiety, guilt, and interpersonal conflict will arise, and can be discussed in therapy. This element is useful for most types of sexual dysfunction; however, it has an especially important role in disorders that affect the excitement phase of the sexual response cycle.

   (b) Anxiety management includes systematic desensitization and relaxation exercises. These exercises are useful when anxiety is a significant causal factor, especially with vaginismus and sexual arousal disorders.

   (c) Assertiveness training is useful in helping partners experience more control and confidence. Changes in these areas may help control anxiety-generated sexual dysfunction and improve overall communication between partners.

   (d) Specific techniques. Couples can learn methods of increasing or decreasing sexual stimulation for disorders that affect the excitement phase or premature ejaculation, respectively. For premature ejaculation, the **squeeze method** and the **stop–start technique** are used in conjunction with sensate focus techniques and efforts to improve communication. With this approach, partners can recognize in themselves and each other the stages of progression toward orgasm, and then use a behavioral technique to exercise control.

   (3) Psychodynamic methods. Inner psychological struggles, unconscious fantasies, and dynamic relationship issues are addressed through conventional psychotherapeutic intervention only as these issues are encountered in the form of resistance to the other elements of sex therapy. For example, when couples do not follow through with exercises or cannot otherwise participate in therapeutic work, this problem is progressively explored. These patients may benefit from a degree of insight into their behavioral patterns. If this limited psychodynamic approach is not effective, then more traditional forms of individual or couples therapy may be indicated as an adjunct or an alternative.

b. Other treatment approaches

   (1) Hypnosis may be useful for treating anxiety-generated sexual dysfunction; for altering psychosomatic response patterns, such as vaginismus; or for treating sexual excitement disorders. Hypnotic suggestion may be aimed at altering an unconscious thought process when it occurs during sexual activity. The induction of trance states may be combined with self-hypnosis to aid relaxation.

   (2) Group therapy. Sex therapy may be enhanced by the peer support and peer validation that are associated with group therapy.

   (3) Medical or surgical treatment. In addition to the management of specific organic factors that may arise in the general evaluation of sexual dysfunction, organic treatments may be used in conjunction with sex therapy or when other modalities are ineffective. When an organic therapy is used, its risks must be considered in relation to the suffering caused by the dysfunction and the availability of safer alternatives. These treatments include the use of a variety of medications that may increase or decrease sexual response in the context of sexual dysfunction, injectable vasoactive substances that produce erection, and surgical prosthetic devices that simulate erection. These interventions may be treatments of last resort for patients with uncorrectable organic dysfunction. Use of these treatments often necessitates adjunctive therapy to help partners adjust to the changes in sexual technique that are required.

VI. PARAPHILIAS AND GENDER IDENTITY DISORDERS

A. Paraphilias

1. Definition. Paraphilias encompass a variety of patterns of deviant sexual behavior or fantasies. These patterns of behavior are characterized by a preference for nonhuman objects, activities that involve suffering or humiliation, or sexual activity with nonconsenting partners. Examples of paraphilias include pedophilia, fetishism (use of inanimate objects), voyeurism, sexual sadism, sexual masochism, frotteurism (touching or rubbing against nonconsenting individuals), exhibitionism, and zoophilia.

2. Diagnosis and treatment

a. According to the *DSM-IV,* the **diagnosis** requires at least a 6-month duration of either repetitive behaviors or significant distress associated with deviant sexual fantasies. **Psychophysiologic testing,** such as measurements of penile tumescence during exposure to paraphilic stimuli, may be useful during assessment and treatment. A negative test result, however, is not a definitive finding.

b. Treatment of these patients involves a variety of psychotherapeutic approaches, with a strong emphasis on behavioral techniques. A major component of the treatment involves facing applicable legal consequences in addition to pairing other unpleasant associations with the sexual fantasies. These patients often have serious patterns of denial and disavowal of the problem that complicates treatment.

3. Prognosis. Factors that are suggestive of a **poor prognosis** include a poorly integrated or deficient sense of guilt associated with the paraphilic behavior, the early onset of paraphilic behavior, and a high frequency of paraphilic acts.

B. Gender identity disorders

1. Definition. Gender identity disorders are characterized by persistent distress about one's assigned gender associated with various degrees of preoccupation with or modeling of the stereotypical behaviors of the opposite sex. Biologic, familial, intrapsychic, and cultural factors may play a significant role in the cause of this disorder. It is important to distinguish gender identity disorders from transvestism. The latter is considered a paraphilia in which cross-dressing behavior is associated with strong sexual urges.

2. Treatment. Divergent treatment approaches are used. One approach emphasizes surgical or hormonal reassignment of gender in adults who have carefully weighed the risks and benefits of such treatment. Alternatively, patients undergo psychotherapy based on behavioral or insight-oriented principles, with the goal of helping the patients to cope with their orientation.

VII. SEXUALITY IN MEDICAL PRACTICE

A. Sexual history

1. General guidelines. Taking the sexual history of the patient should be a routine part of every patient evaluation. The manner in which the history is taken may vary according to the patient's age, social background, and culture as well as the reason for seeking medical help. Discussion of the patient's sexual history should not be avoided because of the practitioner's discomfort with sexuality. Studies have shown that only 10% of patients will initiate a discussion of sexual functioning, but 50% will discuss it if asked.

2. Approach. A method that uses the **chronology of sexuality** throughout the life cycle is often less threatening to the patient, provides a better understanding of sexual functioning, and implies that sexuality is a natural function. The clinician should proceed from the least to the most taboo topic. Open-ended questions prefaced by educational comments are often effective in encouraging the patient to share her concerns. For example, the physician could say, "Most well-adjusted people expect to have some experience with sexual dysfunction in their lives. Could you tell me some of your own experiences with this?"

3. **When the history suggests a problem.** If sexual dysfunction is present, more directed questions can be used to prompt a description of the problem. For example, if a patient reported a loss of interest in sexual activity, questions might be directed to life stress, marital satisfaction, and general health.

B. **Sexual counseling in primary care.** Unwanted pregnancy and sexually transmitted diseases are serious complications of sexual behavior.

1. **Family planning.** In assisting patients with choosing a **birth control method,** factors beyond safety and efficacy must be considered. These factors include the potential influences of the method on the patient's sexual functioning and body image. For example, the interruption entailed by the use of a condom must be considered as well as the psychological ramifications of more permanent interventions, such as implants or surgical procedures. A chosen method may interact unfavorably with underlying anxieties about nonprocreative sexual behavior, or other sexual dysfunction.

2. **Safe sexual practices**
   a. The primary care physician plays a vital role in the teaching of safe sexual practices and the clarification of unrealistic fears about the risks of contact with affected individuals. The emergence of acquired immune deficiency syndrome (AIDS) as a major public health problem has increased sensitivity to the problem of sexually transmitted diseases. However, anxieties about sexuality may lead to denial, distortion, or exaggeration of risks.
   b. The foundation of safe sexual practice involves reduction in the number of sexual partners and the use of condoms in both heterosexual and homosexual individuals to prevent unwanted pregnancy and sexually transmitted diseases, including AIDS. Condoms do not offer absolute protection from the transmission of AIDS. However, in combination with other prudent measures, such as disclosing sexual history and obtaining human immunodeficiency virus (HIV) testing when a high-risk history is present, patients often can find realistic reassurance.

C. **Sexuality during pregnancy and lactation**

1. **Sexual activity during pregnancy.** Bodily changes, societal expectations, personal feelings about pregnancy, and fear of harming the fetus are major factors that affect eroticism and the frequency of sexual intercourse for both men and women during pregnancy. Wide variation in frequency is reported.
   a. Both men and women, especially nulliparous women, experience a **decrease in sexual interest and frequency throughout pregnancy.** Some studies report greater sexual interest and performance in the second trimester than in the first and third trimesters.
   b. The frequency of sexual intercourse, masturbation, and orgasm during pregnancy is related to the relative frequency before pregnancy.
   c. Both men and women may experience conflict about the coexistence of motherhood and sexuality. This conflict can interfere with sexuality during pregnancy and afterward.
   d. A few conditions, such as premature labor and placenta previa, contraindicate sexual activity during pregnancy. If abstinence is necessary, the practitioner should provide a clear explanation of the reason.
   e. For the healthy pregnant woman, sexual activity during pregnancy is not harmful to either the mother or the fetus, with the exception of the forceful blowing of air into the vagina.

2. **Sexual activity during the postpartum period.** Most couples resume sexual relations within 6 weeks after delivery.

    a. Many women report increased sexual desire in the postpartum period, but the frequency of intercourse is often decreased because of pain and fatigue.

    b. Sexual activity usually returns to near prepregnancy levels by the end of the first year postpartum.

3. Sexual stimulation during **breast-feeding** is reported by many nursing mothers. The mother may experience conflicting feelings regarding sexuality and her child.

D. **Cardiovascular disease and sexuality**

1. Sexual activity after myocardial infarction. Myocardial infarction often results in decreased self-esteem of the patient, concerns about impotence, and a decrease in the frequency of sexual intercourse.

    a. Most commonly, the decrease in frequency is caused by psychological factors.

    b. Patients who have no medical complications may resume sexual activity 6 weeks after the infarction.

    c. Patients who participate in exercise training and education generally have a more satisfactory return to normal sexual activity. The educational program should include the patient's partner, who may have concerns that interfere with the resumption of sexual activity.

2. Cardiac symptoms during intercourse

    a. It is not unusual for patients with cardiovascular disease to experience symptoms (e.g., chest pain, shortness of breath) during intercourse.

    b. Myocardial infarction occasionally occurs during intercourse as a result of the physical and emotional stress of unusual circumstances.

E. **Sexuality and chronic illness**

1. General considerations. Chronic illness can decrease the patient's self-esteem and affect his sexual functioning and relationship with a partner. The health care provider's consideration of these effects is an important factor in the sexual adjustment of both the patient and her partner.

    a. The **sick role** (see Chapter 11 I A 2) places the patient in a dependent position that may lead to regressive behavior.

    b. Certain psychological symptoms associated with disease interfere with the physiologic functioning that is necessary for sexual response. These symptoms include **malaise, anxiety,** and **depression. Medications** that are necessary to treat the disease can also affect sexual response.

    c. Sexual roles often are altered as a result of illness; the healthier partner may assume a more nurturing role. The partners also may be physically separated as a result of the illness and hospitalization.

2. Chronic renal failure results in a high incidence of sexual dysfunction, especially in patients with untreated uremia, patients who are undergoing dialysis, and those who have undergone renal transplantation.

3. Diabetes mellitus results in a high incidence of sexual dysfunction that increases with the duration of the disease. The cause of the impotence is often organic, but psychological causes (e.g., impaired self-esteem, fear of impotence) should also be considered. Fifty to sixty percent of men with diabetes experience periods of organically based erectile dysfunction. Women with diabetes may experience problems with arousal and vaginal lubrication. These problems may be complicated by vaginitis.

4. Vascular disease related to hypertension, diabetes mellitus, or atherosclerosis may be the primary factor contributing to the sexual dysfunction that occurs with aging.

5. Other illnesses. The sexual functioning of patients with physical illnesses that interfere with sexual performance, such as arthritis, cancer, cerebrovascular accident, and spinal cord injury, should be determined. Developmentally disabled adolescents should also be evaluated for sexual dysfunction.

F. **Drugs that affect sexual functioning.** More than 6% of the general population abuse alcohol and other drugs.

1. **Alcohol.** Small amounts of alcohol may enhance sexual desire by decreasing inhibitions, but large amounts cause significant dysfunction in both men and women.
   a. **Extent of dysfunction.** Alcohol interferes with sexual functioning because of its depressant effect on the central nervous system (CNS). Diseases related to alcoholism (e.g., hypertension, cirrhosis, neuropathy) and psychological disorders exacerbated by alcohol abuse can cause sexual dysfunction, even after cessation of drinking. Chronic alcohol abuse causes irreversible sexual dysfunction in some individuals, whereas others recover sexual functioning completely after a period of abstinence.
   b. **Nature of dysfunction**
      (1) The most common types of sexual dysfunction in **alcoholic women** are inhibited desire, dyspareunia, and orgasmic dysfunction.
      (2) In **alcoholic men,** the most common types of sexual dysfunction are inhibited desire, erectile dysfunction, and delayed orgasm or ejaculation.

2. **Drugs of abuse**—often used initially to enhance sexuality—can cause sexual dysfunction.
   a. **Marijuana (cannabis).** The incidence of decreased libido and impaired potency is higher among cannabis users than among nonusers. Men who are chronic users have decreased plasma testosterone levels, sperm count, and sperm motility.
   b. **Chronic cocaine use** decreases sexual functioning and interest.
   c. **Narcotic addiction** causes nonemissive erections and impotence in men and amenorrhea, infertility, reduced libido, and spontaneous abortions in women.
   d. **Amphetamines** may help to increase physical performance initially, but larger doses cause loss of interest in sexual activity.
   e. **Barbiturates** may lower sexual inhibition; however, larger doses depress sexual performance.

3. **Prescription drugs** also may impair sexual functioning.
   a. **Antihypertensive drugs** that act by blocking the functioning of the sympathetic nervous system can cause sexual dysfunction. These drugs include methyldopa, reserpine, and trimethaphan. Other antihypertensive agents that interfere with sexual functioning are chlorothiazide, spironolactone, and clonidine.
   b. **Antidepressant drugs** may interfere with sexual functioning. Among the tricyclic antidepressants, the anticholinergic effects are primarily responsible for sexual dysfunction. Selective serotonin reuptake inhibitors (SSRIs) such as fluoxetine, sertraline, and paroxetine have been found to cause ejaculatory and erectile dysfunction as well as decreased libido. Monoamine oxidase (MAO) inhibitors interfere with sexual functioning because of their tendency to block peripheral ganglionic nerve transmission. Lithium carbonate also may interfere with sexual functioning.
   c. **Antihistamines,** with continuous use, may interfere with sexual activity because of their anticholinergic effects and blockade of parasympathetic nerve impulses.
   d. **Antispasmodic agents** may interfere with sexual functioning through ganglionic blockade.
   e. **Neuroleptic medication** can cause decreased sexual interest, erectile dysfunction, or retarded ejaculation in some individuals. Thioridazine can cause retrograde ejaculation.
   f. **Sedative-hypnotics,** in small doses, may improve sexual functioning in anxious individuals, but chronic use often causes impaired performance. Several benzodiazepines interfere with ejaculation.

REFERENCES

1. Masters WH, Johnson VE: *Human Sexual Response.* Boston, Little, Brown, 1966.

2. Kinsey AC, Pomeroy WB, Martin CE: *Sexual Behavior in the Human Male.* Philadelphia, WB Saunders, 1948.

3. LeVay S: A difference in hypothalamic structure between heterosexual and homosexual men. *Science* 253:1034–1037, 1991.

4. Masters WH, Johnson VE: *Human Sexual Inadequacy.* Boston, Little, Brown, 1970.

BIBLIOGRAPHY

American Psychiatric Association: *Diagnostic and Statistical Manual of Mental Disorders,* 4th ed. Washington, DC, American Psychiatric Association, 1994.

Byne W, Parsons B: Human sexual orientation: the biological theory reappraised. *Arch Gen Psychiatry* 50(3):228–239, 1989.

Gees J, Heiman J, Leitenberg H: *Human Sexuality.* Englewood Cliffs, NJ, Prentice-Hall, 1984.

Kaplan H: *The New Sex Therapy: Active Treatment of Sexual Dysfunctions.* New York, Brunner/Mazel, 1974.

Kolodny RC, Masters WH, Johnson VE: *Textbook of Sexual Medicine.* Boston, Little, Brown, 1979.

Masters WH, Johnson VE: *Human Sexual Inadequacy.* Boston, Little, Brown, 1970.

Masters WH, Johnson VE: *Human Sexual Response.* Boston, Little, Brown, 1966.

Sadock BJ: Normal human sexuality and sexual dysfunction. In *Comprehensive Textbook of Psychiatry,* 5th ed. Edited by Sadock BJ, Kaplan HI. Baltimore, Williams & Wilkins, 1989.

Woods NF (ed): *Human Sexuality in Health and Illness.* St Louis, CV Mosby, 1984.

▎ STUDY QUESTIONS

DIRECTIONS: Each of the numbered items or incomplete statements in this section is followed by answers or by completions of the statement. Select the ONE lettered answer or completion that is BEST in each case.

1. By which of the following ages are young children normally aware of their own gender and that of others?

(A) The first year of life
(B) Years 1 to 2
(C) Years 3 to 5
(D) Years 5 to 7
(E) Years 11 to 13

2. Which of the following sexual behaviors is cause for concern in an adolescent patient?

(A) Sexual "acting out"
(B) Nocturnal emissions in boys
(C) Masturbation
(D) Sexual fantasies
(E) Shyness related to late development of secondary sexual characteristics

3. During a routine physical examination, a healthy man in his early 60s mentions that he has been having increasing difficulty attaining and maintaining an erection over the last several years. He is worried that he is becoming impotent. His history and physical examination exclude medical and medication causes, including substance abuse. The best course of action is to

(A) initiate a medical workup for impotence
(B) counsel the patient that impotence is a normal part of aging
(C) ask to visit or speak with the patient's wife to learn more about his impotence
(D) explain that his symptoms are a normal part of aging, but are unlikely to result in impotence
(E) suggest that sexual intercourse is not a necessary part of older peoples' lives

4. During a routine physical examination, a 64-year-old woman hints that her sex life is not what it used to be. The most useful response during this initial visit is to

(A) ask direct questions about her sexual functioning
(B) gather a chronological sexual history
(C) reassure the patient that most elderly people lose interest in sex
(D) refer the patient to a specialist in sexual dysfunction
(E) suggest that the patient may need to use artificial lubrication because she is older

Questions 5–6

During the sexual history portion of the examination, a healthy 15-year-old boy states that he wonders whether he is homosexual because he participated in mutual masturbation with two different male friends in the last 2 years. He reports feeling embarrassed and uncomfortable and mentions that he has slept poorly for the last several nights.

5. Which of the following information is LEAST important to pursue in evaluating his question?

(A) History of sexual abuse
(B) Emotional turmoil regarding sexual preference
(C) Elements of a homosexual identity
(D) History of gender conformity
(E) Evidence of psychiatric disturbance

6. Additional information provided by the patient suggests that he has a pattern of heterosexual preference. Which of the following is the best response to the patient's question?

(A) "Fortunately, it does not seem that you are going to be homosexual."
(B) "Based on your experience so far, you will need to watch for latent homosexuality."
(C) "Sexual feelings can be confusing at your age. You are not necessarily homosexual; however, it may be helpful to talk with someone if you are very troubled about this situation."
(D) "If you don't stop this activity, you will become homosexual."
(E) "Your life will be much more difficult if you choose to be gay."

DIRECTIONS: Each of the numbered items or incomplete statements in this section is negatively phrased, as indicated by a capitalized word such as NOT, LEAST, or EXCEPT. Select the ONE lettered answer or completion that is BEST in each case.

7. All of the following are possible causes of homosexuality EXCEPT

(A) psychiatric disorder
(B) genetic predisposition
(C) influence of prenatal hormones
(D) gender nonconformity
(E) psychosocial influences

8. All of the following statements about the effect of cardiovascular disease on sexuality are true EXCEPT

(A) some patients have impaired sexual functioning after a myocardial infarction
(B) myocardial infarctions that occur during intercourse are often associated with unusual and stressful circumstances
(C) the most common reason for decreased frequency of intercourse after a myocardial infarction is anginal pain associated with intercourse
(D) there is a higher incidence of return to normal sexual activity by patients who receive exercise training and education than by those who are not involved in such programs
(E) the spouse of a patient who has had a myocardial infarction must be involved in educational programs because her fears can interfere with the resumption of sexual activity

DIRECTIONS: Each set of matching questions in this section consists of a list of three to twenty-six lettered options (some of which may be in figures) followed by several numbered items. For each numbered item, select the ONE lettered option that is most closely associated with it. To avoid spending too much time on matching sets with large numbers of options, it is generally advisable to begin each set by reading the list of options. Then, for each item in the set, try to generate the correct answer and locate it in the option list, rather than evaluating each option individually. Each lettered option may be selected once, more than once, or not at all.

Questions 9–11

For each sexual function presented below, select the hormone that influences it.

(A) Testosterone
(B) Vasoactive intestinal peptide (VIP)
(C) Androgen

9. Responsible for the development of male sexual genitalia

10. Responsible for sexual desire in men and women

11. Mediates vaginal lubrication

Questions 12–14

For each of the physiologic responses listed below, select the stage of the sexual response cycle during which it occurs.

(A) Excitement phase
(B) Plateau phase
(C) Orgasmic phase
(D) Resolution phase

12. Descent of the cervix in women and descent of the testes in men

13. Rhythmic contractions of the pelvic floor in women and of the anal sphincter in men and women

14. Sex flush over the abdomen and chest

ANSWERS AND EXPLANATIONS

1. The answer is C [I A 3]. By 2½ years of age, children can categorize people by sex and recognize their own sex. Gender identity disorders become evident in the preschool years.

2. The answer is A [I B 1–2]. Concerns about the timing of the onset of the development of sexual characteristics, nocturnal emissions, masturbation, and sexual fantasies are a normal part of adolescence. In general, early development is less stressful for boys, and average or late onset of sexual development is less stressful for girls. Sexual "acting out," or the expression of concealed sexual conflicts in poorly considered sexual activity, often carries significant risks for adolescents. The risks include pregnancy, sexually transmitted diseases, and unpleasant social and peer group consequences.

3. The answer is D [I C 2 b; I D 2; V B 1]. The first step is to reassure the patient that his difficulty is a normal part of aging rather than an indication of impotence. The physiologic changes associated with aging include delay in attaining an erection and decreased fullness of erection. Sexuality continues to be important for the well-being of older people. Because the history and physical examination do not reveal any medical or medication causes, a medical workup for impotence is not indicated at this time.

4. The answer is B [I D 1–2; VII A]. Education and counseling by the primary care physician can relieve many causes of sexual dysfunction. The belief that most elderly people lose interest in sex is inaccurate. Moving from open-ended to direct questions and reviewing the patient's sexual functioning are usually the most effective ways to gather a sexual history, especially with younger patients. With elderly patients, it is usually effective to ask general questions and establish a rapport before moving to direct questions about sexuality. Rapid referral to a specialist in sexual dysfunction is likely to make the patient uncomfortable. Gathering a history will help the primary care physician to determine whether referral is appropriate.

5. The answer is E [IV A 1–4]. Although a history of psychiatric disturbance is an important part of any routine history, it is probably the least important piece of information that is needed to respond to the patient's question. Sexual activity with a male partner may leave an adolescent boy feeling confused about homosexuality. Further discussion is needed to determine the patient's sexual preference.

6. The answer is C [IV A 1–4]. Sexual experimentation with friends of the same sex in early adolescence is not necessarily associated with homosexual orientation. It is important to gather a history of sexual preference and to support the adolescent in his evolving identity.

7. The answer is A [IV C 1–4]. Although psychiatric disorders may coexist with homosexuality, as with heterosexuality, they are not the cause of homosexuality. Genetic predisposition, hormonal influences, gender nonconformity, and psychosocial influences are all associated with the development of homosexuality although no one of them has been found to be responsible for the development of all homosexual orientation.

8. The answer is C [VII D 1–2]. The most common reasons for decreased frequency of sexual intercourse after a myocardial infarction are psychological. Patients who have had a myocardial infarction can have decreased self-esteem; men may have concerns about impotence. The stress associated with an unusual circumstance (e.g., an atypical sexual activity, inebriation, a new sexual partner) is often responsible for myocardial infarction during intercourse. Exercise and educational programs are effective in helping patients with cardiovascular disease to resume a normal life, but the involvement of the spouse in these programs is important.

9–11. The answers are: 9-C, 10-A, 11-B [II B 1–2]. Androgens secreted by the testes in male fetuses during the first trimester of pregnancy are necessary for the formation of male external genitalia. Testosterone is believed to influence sexual desire in both men and women. Vasoactive intestinal peptide (VIP) mediates vaginal changes that are associated with the excitement phase of sexual arousal.

12–14. The answers are: 12-D, 13-C, 14-B [II A 1–4]. During the plateau phase, a maculopapular rash known as the sex flush may spread over the chest and abdomen of both men and women. During the orgasmic phase, contraction of the orgasmic platform, including the pelvic floor, uterus, and anal sphincter, occurs in women. In men, there are contractions of the prostate gland, seminal vesicles, urethra, and anal sphincter. During the resolution phase, descent of the cervix into the dorsal area of the vagina occurs in women, and penile detumescence and descent of the testes occur in men.

Chapter 10

Social and Family Behavior

Frederick S. Wamboldt
Marianne Z. Wamboldt

I. **INTRODUCTION. General systems theory is a holistic model used by both physical and social scientists to explain how various systems function as complete entities.** The theory states that **phenomena are embedded in their environment,** not composed of separate, independent parts, as is stated in the **reductionistic model**. General systems theory is useful for the study of family and social behavior. It has particular relevance for important health-related issues.

A. **System. A system is a set of interrelated elements that function as a whole** (e.g., immune system, solar system, family system, international political system). Systems are characterized by their structure, organization, and environmental context. **The elements are dynamic entities; therefore, the system can disintegrate.**

1. **Structure.** The elements, or components, of a system and the relations among them define the structure of the system.
   a. **Recurrent structure.** Certain relations among elements of the system may occur with such regularity that the **structure of the system is predictable**. Recurrent structure is characteristic of a system at **equilibrium**.
      (1) **A boundary is a recurrent, interactive, relation between the elements and the environment** of the system. The recurrent relation between the dermis and the vascular components of the body in maintaining the epidermal boundary can be compared to the interactions within a family that determine what information should or should not be given to outsiders.
      (2) **A bond, or alliance, is a recurrent, interactive, relation among elements** of a system.
      (3) **Emergent properties.** Some interactions among elements in a system create new properties within the system. Depth perception is an emergent property that involves the interaction between the two retinal images in the visual system. In the same way, **personality attributes,** such as dependency or hatred, can be seen as emerging from and being maintained within certain relationships. If the relation changes, the emergent property may change or disappear. For example, American public opinion of the People's Republic of China shifted from untrustworthy enemies to industrious people after Richard Nixon's visits in the 1970s.
   b. **Novel structures** arise in a system that is attempting to adapt to stress. These novel structures may become recurrent structures if they permit the system to adapt and regain equilibrium. If they fail, the structures will disappear. For example, a family that values spontaneity over routine may suddenly become structured in response to a serious illness.

2. **Organization.** The organization of a system involves relations among components that are necessary for the system to retain its identity or membership within a specific class. The organization of a system usually allows a variety of potential structures. Therefore, systems usually have a significant ability to adapt. For example, to adapt to stress, water can assume three structures: ice, fluid, and vapor. Similarly, a family that values community involvement may be challenged when multiple sclerosis develops in a family member. This family can maintain its identity by shifting its involvement from other organizations to their local chapter of the Multiple Sclerosis Society. Conversely, a family that considers itself close-knit may have difficulty when a child decides to go away to college, especially if additional stress is present (e.g., a parent works two jobs because of financial hardship). By choosing not to go away to school, the child can be

seen as helping the family affirm its identity (i.e., we are close-knit and stay together). Some unexpected decisions by patients and family members may be attempts to preserve family identity.

3. **Environment. Living systems exist within an environment,** or context. They continually adjust their structure to preserve their organization in the face of stresses, demands, or changes in the environment. Successful systems adapt in ways that combine stability and change.
   a. **Morphostasis, or homeostasis (stability).** The system attempts to maintain the original structure as much as possible [e.g., the negative feedback effects of plasma cortisol on the hypothalamic–pituitary axis cause cellular activity to return to the steady state that existed before the release of corticotropin-releasing factor (CRF) and adrenocorticotropic hormone (ACTH)].
   b. **Morphogenesis (change).** The system undergoes maximal change or innovation in structure (e.g., the transition of water from liquid to gas in response to heat).

4. **Disintegration.** A system dissolves if it cannot adapt to environmental stress. For example, passage of sufficient electric current through an atmosphere of hydrogen and oxygen molecules disintegrates the system of separate hydrogen and oxygen molecules. They reorganize as water molecules. Similarly, some families cannot adapt to the demands of their environments. These families fragment, and their members enter new systems (e.g., foster homes, halfway houses, prisons).

B. **The biopsychosocial model** was proposed by Engel[1] as a model for medical science. It is based on general systems theory.

1. According to Engel, the **biomedical model** is the dominant conceptual model in contemporary medicine. It is **reductionistic** (i.e., it attempts to explain all complex phenomenon in the language of molecular biology), **dualistic** (i.e., it gives priority to somatic variables and ignores psychosocial variables), and **assumes causal linearity** (e.g., β-hemolytic streptococci cause pharyngitis). Although this model serves medical science as a heuristic guide, it neglects certain dimensions of human experience and does not answer many important medical questions (e.g., Why do many people have colonized β-hemolytic streptococcus in their throats and not have symptoms of pharyngitis? Why is increased stress associated with increased susceptibility to upper respiratory tract infection? Why would a woman wait until a breast lump reaches massive proportions, perhaps even eroding through her skin, before consulting her physician?).

2. Engel's **biopsychosocial model** proposes that, to understand human illness adequately, a physician must consider factors other than biomedical data. These factors include the following:
   a. **Intrapsychic factors** (e.g., an adolescent focused on his physical appearance may be noncompliant with his regimen of systemic steroids after he learns that they can cause a Cushingoid habitus)
   b. **Interpersonal behavior** (e.g., an individual who is accustomed to a leadership role may have difficulty assuming the role of patient)
   c. **Family dynamics** (e.g., family intervention can lower serum blood sugar levels in adolescents with diabetes mellitus and reduce psychotic recurrences in young adults with schizophrenia)
   d. **Social groups** to which the patient belongs (e.g., opinions differ as to whether individuals who abuse alcohol have a medical or moral problem; whether an individual whose drinking is out of control consults a physician for help is likely to be determined by the opinions of her peers)

II. INTERPERSONAL BEHAVIOR

A. **Interaction between people is inevitable.** One cannot choose not to interact or behave. Even silence is an interpersonal posture.

B. **Aspects of interpersonal relationships can be reliably quantified.** Historically, there are two major approaches to the quantification of relationships: **dimensional** and **categorical**.

C. The **structural analysis of social behavior model (SASB)** is a dimensional approach.[2,3] In this model, interpersonal behaviors are represented by dimensions that have a geometrically meaningful relation to each other (Figure 10-1). The geometric structure of such models facilitates clinical understanding.

1. **Units of interaction.** Within SASB, interpersonal behavior is defined as discrete units that occur between **two interacting partners,** or a **dyad.** A unit may be the entire speech of one speaker until someone else begins to speak, or a complete thought that conveys a single message to another person.

2. **Dimensions of interpersonal behavior.** Units of interpersonal behavior can be classified into dimensions of **interpersonal postures.** Assigning an SASB code to a specific interpersonal behavior involves three factors.
   a. **Focus** (see *other* and *self* surfaces in Figure 10-1). Is the individual **initiating an action** toward the other individual (focus on other) or **responding to an action** from the other (focus on self)?
   b. **Interdependence** (see *vertical axis* in Figure 10-1). Is the action an **attempt to control or influence** (focus on other) or an **offer for autonomy or independence** (focus on other)? Does the action show **submission** (focus on self) or an **assertion of independence** (focus on self)?
   c. **Affiliation** (see *horizontal axis* in Figure 10-1). Does the action show **hostility toward the other person** (focus on other), **friendliness** (focus on other), **withdrawal protesting a hostile act** (focus on self), or **approach enjoying a friendly act** (focus on self)?

3. **Patterns of dyadic interaction.** For any pair of people (e.g., doctor and patient, husband and wife, classmates) dyadic interaction tends to stabilize into characteristic patterns of interpersonal behavior. In the language of general systems theory, the behavior develops recurrent structure. Some of these patterns that have clinical importance are described with SASB.
   a. **Complementary postures** involve **similar degrees of affiliation and interdependence, but differing focus.** They are usually **stable** over time. For example, an **enmeshed dyad** typically includes one individual with prominent controlling behavior (high interdependence, focus on other) and one individual with prominent submissive behavior (high interdependence, focus on self).
   b. **Symmetric postures** involve **similar degrees of affiliation and interdependence as well as the same focus.** They are usually **unstable,** resulting in interaction of escalating intensity. Over time, they typically move toward complementary postures. For example, a **power struggle** involves two individuals with high controlling behavior (high interdependence, focus on other).
   c. **Antithetical postures** involve responding with a posture that **differs in focus and is directly opposite in degrees of affiliation and interdependence** from the partner's message. Antithetical postures can change the posture of a dyadic partner. For example, a parent who complains, "Come on doctor, you've been poking my daughter with needles for days and she looks sicker. When are you going to do something right?" may react better to the physician who responds with an antithetical statement (e.g., I'm disappointed too. I was hoping for more, but I want to keep trying to help you and your daughter.) than with a symmetric reply (e.g., Well, you know, you haven't done much of value either!) or a complementary response (e.g., You're right, I need to try harder.).

D. The **expressed emotion construct** is a categorical approach to quantifying behavior in which meaningful categories of behavior are clustered into discrete groups rather than arrayed as continuous dimensions. In the late 1950s, Brown and associates[4] interviewed parents of newly hospitalized patients with schizophrenia to study environmental influences on psychotic relapse. This work led to extensive study of the expressed emotion construct. The level of expressed emotion in a family is determined by the number of statements made

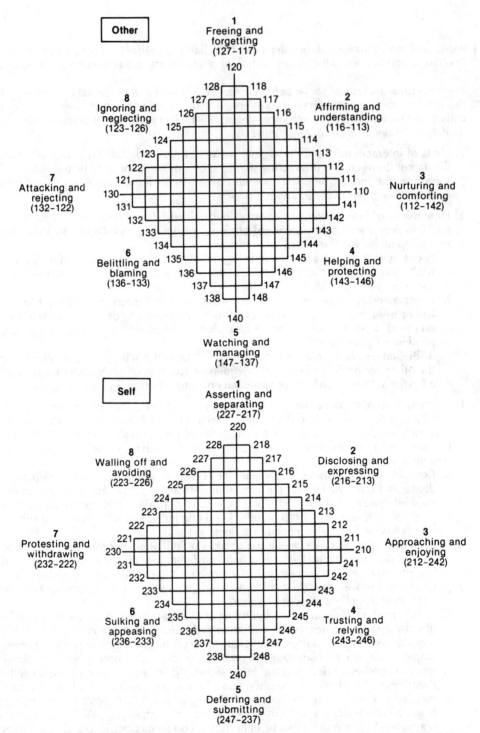

FIGURE 10-1. Cluster version of interpersonal surfaces of Benjamin's structural analysis of social behavior model (SASB). Benjamin's model allows classification of all behaviors in terms of three dimensions: **focus on other or self** (*surfaces*), degree of **friendliness** (*horizontal axis*), and degree of **interdependence** (*vertical axis*). The cluster version shows eight groups of behaviors per surface and is a condensation of the full SASB model, which describes thirty-six behaviors per surface. For example, cluster 5 from the *other surface* (watching and managing) contains 5 closely related behaviors from the full model (137: *intrude, block, restrict;* 138: *enforce conformity;* 140: *manage, control;* 147: *benevolently monitor, remind;* 148: *specify what is best*). (Adapted from Benjamin LS: Principles of prediction using structural analysis of social behavior (SASB). In *Personality and the Prediction of Behavior.* Edited by Zucker RA, Aronoff J, Rabin AJ. New York, 1984.)

by family members toward the patient that show **hostility, criticism,** or **emotional overinvolvement**. Families that score high in these areas have a high level of expressed emotion. Families that score low in these dimensions have a low level of expressed emotion.

1. Schizophrenic patients discharged to families with a high level of expressed emotion have a three- to sevenfold greater likelihood of relapse within 1 year than those who return to families with a low level of expressed emotion. In most studies, this effect is additive to the effect of antipsychotic medication.

2. **Interventions** aimed at reducing the level of expressed emotion through psychoeducational therapy to decrease the level of criticism, hostility, or emotional overinvolvement both lower the level of expressed emotion and extend the intervals between relapses in schizophrenic patients.

3. Family expressed emotion has been studied in patients with many other diagnoses including unipolar and bipolar depression, eating disorders, asthma, epilepsy, and inflammatory bowel disease. Expressed emotion may be a categorical construct that can identify chronically ill patients who are at higher risk for a more difficult clinical course because of familial interactional patterns.

4. Differences in **dimensional** interactional behavior occur between families with high versus low levels of expressed emotion. For example, families with a low level of expressed emotion show greater helping and protecting behaviors with SASB. Those with a high level of expressed emotion show greater belittling and blaming behaviors. Behavioral responses are considered more variable, and therefore probably less consistent, in families with a high level of expressed emotion.

5. Despite the promise of this research, caution is necessary.
   a. The tendency to equate a high level of expressed emotion with a "bad" family is both damaging and incorrect. It remains controversial whether a high level of expressed emotion causes poor outcome or if differences in patients (e.g., more negative symptoms of schizophrenia, poorer premorbid adjustment, unpredictable threatening behavior by the patient) cause families to increase their level of expressed emotion. Evidence favors the latter explanation. It is wise to consider expressed emotion a marker of families that are burdened by stress and not a causal variable. The level of expressed emotion decreases in some families after the patient's symptoms improve. A high level of expressed emotion in other care givers, physicians, nurses, social workers, foster parents, and even institutions may have as great an effect as a high level of expressed emotion in a patient's family. Treatment of any family is most effective when health care providers use a nonblaming approach and recognize the burden placed on families with ill members.
   b. A **vulnerability-stress-coping model** is used to explain the effect of environmental variables on conditions with clear genetic propensity. In the case of level of expressed emotion and schizophrenia, patients are assumed to have an underlying psychobiologic vulnerability that prevents them from coping with the stress of overstimulating social interaction. This vulnerability intensifies the effects of illness. Progress is being made in the search for the underlying biologic deficits in schizophrenia, but no underlying psychobiologic defect in social processing is known in any other illness in which level of expressed emotion correlates with clinical course.

E. Classification of **attachment style** is another categorical approach. Bowlby[5] wrote extensively about the need of infants to attach to their significant care givers. Attachment is a crucial developmental need in humans and many other mammalian species. Ainsworth[6] developed a structured behavioral observation procedure known as the **strange situation paradigm**. It classifies the quality of the attachment relationship between 12-month-old infants and their primary care givers (usually the mother) based on the infants' responses in a laboratory setting to reunion with the care givers after a separation of several minutes.

1. Three major categories of response are observed.
   a. **Secure attachment** is shown by the infant who seeks contact with or comfort from the care giver on her return. The mothers of these infants show consistent sensitivity to them during the first 12 months (as measured by home observations).

    b. Insecure/avoidant attachment is shown by the infant who avoids the care giver on her return. These infants have mothers who provide less physical contact during the first 3 months and show less sensitivity during the first 12 months.

    c. Insecure/resistant attachment is shown by the infant who shows angry and resistant behavior alternated with comfort-seeking behavior on the care giver's return. The mothers of these infants show inconsistent responses during the first 12 months.

2. The quality of infant attachment at 12 months is predictive of the child's subsequent progress in several areas, including cognitive development, persistence in problem solving, attention to tasks, and social functioning in preschool with teachers and peers.

3. The quality of **attachment relationships in older children and adults** also has been studied. These ratings show interesting correlates, including an association with how each partner perceives the current relationship and a correlation between the parent's attachment style and that of the children. Of particular clinical importance are reports that link specific patterns of adult insecure attachment to child abuse and neglect.

4. Healthy functioning is associated with secure attachment, in which the child is confident that the parent will be available, responsive, and helpful if he encounters adverse or frightening experiences. With this assurance, the child feels bold enough to explore the world and self-confident that he can handle challenges.

    a. A child with **insecure/avoidant attachment** expects that when she seeks help, she will not receive a helpful response, but will be rebuffed. Thus, she acts compulsively self-reliant or, in severe cases, delinquent.

    b. A child with **insecure/resistant attachment** is unsure whether the parent will be available or responsive. Thus, he is prone to separation anxiety, and tends to be clingy and anxious about exploring the world.

5. These attachment styles are not unchangeable, but without active intervention, they usually **remain stable over time.** Stressful family events (e.g., sudden illness, financial hardship) can change a secure attachment relationship to an insecure attachment style.

6. Recent studies extended the categories of attachment style to older children and adults. The results are promising, but the conceptualization of attachment is clearest for infants and their care givers. Many needs remain in later life, but the extreme, fixed dependence seen in the infant–care giver relationship does not. Therefore, it is not clear to what extent the construct of attachment style is valid in adult relationships. The most important factor seems to be the development of an **internal working model of how relationships function.** This model sets a pattern for other relationships.

F. **Interaction in larger groups.** As individuals are added to a group, the number of dyads increases geometrically. The social interaction becomes more complex and difficult to examine with either dimensional or categorical models.

1. Coreceivers, or a relevant audience, may exist for any seemingly dyadic interaction. For example, the attending physician on a surgery service asks particularly difficult questions of one medical student whose father is a prominent local physician and the attending physician's golf partner. In this case, superseding the dyadic message may be the message to the coreceivers (the other medical students): "Even though this student's father is my friend, I will not treat her preferentially."

2. Triads, or triangles, are inherently unstable during interaction. They usually evolve into a closely aligned dyad and a more distant third person. In **rigid triangles,** the alignment among the individuals does not vary over time. These triangles are often observed in dysfunctional interactions. Two types are described.

    a. In the **scapegoating triangle,** the individual in the distant position is blamed for the problems of the group.

    b. In the **inverted power hierarchy triangle,** one individual (of high rank) allies with another (of low rank). A third person (of high rank) is excluded. For example, families in which parent–child incest occurs often have a rigid cross-generation alliance between a child and one parent, with the other parent taking a childlike role.

III. **LARGE GROUP BEHAVIOR.** Individuals and families are embedded in a series of larger and more diverse groups (e.g., peers, neighborhoods, religious congregations). These groups have important effects on the behavior of the members. These effects involve the **framing and coordination of normative behavior** and the **provision of alternative social support**.

A. **Social coordination of behavior.** Social interaction requires procedures that make behavior predictable and adaptive to the environment.

1. **Cultural aspects of coordination.** Culture is the collective set of beliefs, values, and norms used by members of a large group to give understanding, meaning, and purpose to their lives. Culture involves the roles, rituals, and conventions that the members of a group use to organize their social interactions. The presence of a culturally bound rule is often inferred by the unexpected behavior exhibited by a member of another culture when such a rule is unwittingly broken. The **ease of communication** between two individuals is related to their degree of cultural similarity.

   a. **Explanatory models.** Individuals from different cultures may have varying ideas about how events, including medical illness, occur. When ill, they may have differing views about what constitutes a symptom or disease, the interpretation and presumed causes of disease, the classification of symptoms into syndromes, acceptable treatment, and the role of a physician in treatment. For example, in many Latin cultures, somatic complaints are acceptable symptoms to report to a physician, but psychological complaints are not. Therefore, depression or anxiety may be presented as a series of physical complaints. The physician must recognize the possibility of a psychiatric disorder, despite the patient's denial of emotional symptoms.

   b. **Cultural relativism** asserts that the cultural values and customs of any group are best examined in the context of that group and should be judged with regard to their utility within that group. **Ethnocentrism** is the common tendency to view an individual's own culture as superior and differing cultures as inferior.

   c. **Socialization** is the process through which cultural beliefs and practices are passed on to new members. This learning occurs primarily during childhood, but also at other times (e.g., medical school and residency). This information is conveyed in many ways, including modeling (i.e., learning by observing) and operant conditioning (i.e., learning based on reward and punishment).

2. **Consensual component of social reality.** Cultural beliefs and practices depend on continuing consensual validation by members of the culture. In most cases, consensual validation is so automatic that it goes unnoticed, but it is much more prominent in some situations. For example, when a physician examines a patient's genitals, the physician and patient must cooperate to maintain the idea that the examination is a medical procedure and is therefore acceptable.

3. **Structural component of social reality.** Although cultural beliefs and practices originate in consensual processes, over time they are established as social imperatives, regulations, and institutions. These social structures are not likely to change. For example, an increased incidence of perinatal complications is associated with lower socioeconomic status. This finding is affected by the structurally based limited availability of medical care to poor people. When good prenatal care is equally available, no difference in perinatal complications is found between socioeconomic groups.

B. **Social support systems.** Individuals form networks of attachments that promote adaptation to or mastery of difficult life events. An individual's social support system usually includes family members, but a viable network can be maintained with nonrelatives, especially those who share similar cultural beliefs and practices.

1. The **mediating and buffering role** of social support systems in medical care is drawing increasing attention. Effective social support systems can:

   a. Promote adherence to medical regimens

b. Enhance the effectiveness of medical treatment (e.g., effective social support systems reduce steroid doses required under stress in adults with asthma and reduce the complications of pregnancy in women who are at high risk)

c. Protect against depression and other psychological problems during adverse life events

d. Promote the return to normal growth and stability after severe medical illness (e.g., the effectiveness of a family's social support system predicts its development after a child dies of cystic fibrosis)

2. Conversely, the expectations of members of an individual's social support system may create additional **responsibility** for the individual.

IV. **FAMILY BEHAVIOR.** The family in which an individual grows up and the family created through marriage usually provide the individual's most influential and intense interpersonal relationships. Findings from many disciplines suggest the central role of family relationships in the health of family members.

A. **Definitions of family.** It is difficult to define family. Three major definitions are currently used.

1. Structural

a. Extended family. The United States Census Bureau defines a family as **any group of individuals related by blood, marriage, or adoption**. This definition emphasizes the **biologic and sociolegal legitimacy** of the connection between family members. This connection is often important to physicians (e.g., in genetic counseling).

b. In a **nuclear family,** the family members not only have legitimate connections but also **live together**.

c. The **family of orientation,** or family of origin, is the **nuclear family in which an individual has the status of child**.

d. The **family of procreation** is the **nuclear family in which an individual has the status of parent**.

2. Functional. A family is a **psychosocial system that consists of an adult and one or more other individuals** (children, adults, or both) **who have a commitment to mutual need fulfillment and nurturance**. This definition, by emphasizing **normative function** (i.e., need fulfillment), is identical to the concept of a social support system.

3. Transactional. The family is a **group of individuals who share affection and loyalty, a history and a future, and a sense of home**. This definition emphasizes **emotional and experiential bonds** that arise from recurrent face-to-face interactions.

B. **Demographics and current trends.** There is considerable controversy about whether the American family is in decline. The conclusions often depend on what period in history is used for comparison. Many conclusions are based on comparisons with the post-World War II 1940s and 1950s, which was a period of unusual family cohesion and stability. Certain changes are occurring, but most arguments concern whether these **changes** indicate **decline or diversity**.

1. Stable trends in family life

a. Most Americans (90%) live with relatives. Fewer than 5% of individuals live alone. Fifteen percent of nuclear family households contain members of three generations.

b. Marriage remains popular. Ninety-five percent of individuals marry. Ninety percent of those who divorce remarry. Married people are healthier than single people of similar age. The protective effect of marriage appears stronger for men than for women. **Marriage fosters better health** by:

(1) Providing a more stable, less risk-oriented lifestyle

(2) Increasing daily social contact and decreasing loneliness

(3) Allowing partners to develop a shared consensus of the world

(4) Providing a forum to discuss problems

c. Extended family. Despite increased geographic distance between extended family members, there is little evidence of reduced emotional and psychological support. In fact, patterns of telephone calls and holiday visits suggest that interaction among extended family members remains high. The extended family is the **primary source** of **support during major life transitions and crises**.

d. Family violence

(1) Incidence. The reported rate of physical and sexual abuse of children, spouses, and parents is increasing (5%–20% of families have an abused member, and 25% of murders occur among family members), but most of this increase is probably the result of improved case detection and reporting. Family violence is frequently associated with neglect, which is either the absence of care or excessive, poorly timed care. Mental or emotional abuse can be as harmful to a child as overt physical abuse. It is also more difficult to detect and treat within the existing social systems for the protection of children.

(2) Characteristics of abusers. Most abusers do not have a history of major psychiatric problems. The incidence of concurrent psychiatric problems is estimated at 5% to 15% of abusive parents, which is essentially the population norm. However, a history of violent acts is a relevant finding. Individuals who are likely to abuse family members often have a history of recurrent abuse or deprivation as a child. Most abusers (80%) were abused. However, only approximately one third of individuals who were abused are seriously abusive or neglectful parents. At least another one third escape the cycle of abuse parenting. The group that comprises the last third is vulnerable to poor parenting if exposed to significant environmental stress. A crucial factor for those who escape the cycle is the presence of a supportive person (e.g., parent, sibling, teacher) who helps them to realize that they did not deserve abuse. Many abusers offer bland, or idealized, portrayals of their parents, often with major discrepancies between their global appraisal and the details they report (e.g., She was the perfect mother. Well, there was the time I fell and broke my wrist, but didn't tell Mom or Dad for over a week because I knew they would get mad at me.). The tendency to abuse family is exacerbated by the following factors:

(a) Severe social and economic stress

(b) Poor social support systems

(c) Stressful interactions with the abused person (e.g., 25% of premature infants and 8% of full-term infants are abused; premature infants may be more difficult and demanding and, therefore, create more stress for their parents)

(d) Problems with drug and alcohol abuse (e.g., many violent acts are committed while the aggressor is intoxicated)

2. Changing trends in family life

a. The **number of children born to married couples is declining**. In 1992, the average American woman had 2.0 children. This figure was 3.6 in 1960. The number of couples who remain childless is increasing (as many as 25% of all couples). One half choose not to have children, and one half are infertile. Accordingly, the percentage of children in the United States population is now 25%, down from 35% in 1960.

b. The **divorce rate remains high,** but is not increasing. Approximately 40% of new marriages are predicted to end in divorce. Half of these divorces usually occur within the first 5 years of marriage. The increase in the divorce rate during this century is linked to the improvement in women's economic status as they entered the work force, although the economic status of most women declines after divorce and that of most men increases. Social attitudes toward divorce changed after this economic shift occurred. For example, the tax code favors single persons.

(1) Risk factors for divorce include:

(a) Short courtship

(b) Marriage at a young age

(c) Premarital pregnancy

(d) Persistent parental opposition to the marriage

(e) Limited social support system

(f) Extreme difference in background

(2) History of one divorce does not increase the likelihood of a second divorce. Many people find a better match the second time.

c. **The number of single-parent families is increasing rapidly.** Approximately 25% of American families are headed by a single parent. The figure is higher (55%) for black children. More than 90% of these single parents are women.

    (1) **Aggressive and delinquent behavior** is increased in children whose parents divorce. This effect is probably caused by decreased parental monitoring of the child's behavior and ongoing parental discord, not divorce itself. It is also seen in families with a high level of parental conflict and discord, regardless of whether divorce occurs. This pattern is not seen in children whose parents die.

    (2) Single-parent families typically have less social support, fewer financial resources, and decreased ability to adapt to parental illness. Families headed by single mothers are the fastest growing subgroup living below the poverty level, and single-parent families are a high-risk group for health problems.

    (3) When single-parent and other nontraditional families have access to necessary resources, they can meet the challenges of family life as well as two-parent families. There is no clear evidence of impaired child development in these nontraditional families.

    (4) An estimated 70% of American children born in 1980 will spend part of their childhood years in a single-parent home. Until the last several decades, this figure remained stable at 40% because the increase in the divorce rate was balanced by a corresponding decrease in the death rate. This statistic suggests a **growing acceptance of divorce** in the United States, especially in families with children.

d. **Working parents.** Nearly 60% of American children younger than 18 years of age live in families in which both parents work outside the home. For 15% of children, the father is the sole family wage earner. This figure was 42% in 1960.

C. **The family life cycle** is a normative model of family life that postulates that families face specific tasks at different stages of development. Healthy families differ, but the life cycle model can help the clinician determine areas of concern for his patients.

1. **Stage I: formation of a new family.** This stage begins when two individuals form a couple and ends when their first child is born. The major tasks of this stage include:
   a. Making the transition from two individuals to a dyad by creating a satisfactory balance between intimacy and autonomy
   b. Establishing working marital roles
   c. Restructuring relationships with both families of orientation

2. **Stage II: child rearing.** This stage of family development has several substages.
   a. **Stage IIa: preschool age.** The preschool stage extends from the birth of the first child until that child enters school. The major tasks of this stage include:
       (1) Dealing with the intense physiologic and psychological dependence of young children
       (2) Establishing a balance between intrafamily and extrafamily responsibilities (e.g., careers, child care arrangements)
       (3) Blending the roles of intimate partner and parent (e.g., many couples experience a decrease in marital satisfaction for at least 2 years after each child's birth)
       (4) Renegotiating relationships with the families of orientation (e.g., grandparents may expect a high level of involvement with grandchildren)
   b. **Stage IIb: primary school age.** The major tasks of this stage include:
       (1) Managing the tension that occurs when a child enters a larger social system; this process is more difficult when the family culture differs from the prevailing social system (e.g., minority and immigrant families may have difficulty during this stage).

(2) Maintaining a satisfying marital relationship during this demanding, child-centered period. Indeed, qualities of the marital relationship have been shown to predict aspects of the children's development such as self-esteem, academic achievement, and peer relationships.

c. Stage IIc: adolescence. The major task of this stage is fostering the development of identity and independence of the child while maintaining concern for her well-being.

3. Stage III: child launching. During this stage, the children leave home. The major tasks of this stage include:
   a. Transferring greater freedom and responsibility to the young adult
   b. Maintaining a supportive home base for the children
   c. Reestablishing individual parental interests and careers
   d. Reexamining the marital relationship
   e. Coping with the decline, increasing dependency, and eventual death of the grandparents

4. Stage IV: return of independence. This stage and the next stage usually account for more than half of a family's life. The major tasks of this stage include:
   a. Rebuilding the marital relationship
   b. Continuing involvement with individual interests and careers
   c. Maintaining ties with extended family in the older and younger generations

5. Stage V: dissolution of the family. The major tasks of this stage include:
   a. Maintaining integrity in the face of both partners' decline
   b. Planning for the dispersion of the family estate

D. **Crisis and the family life cycle.** A crisis is any event that requires an adaptive response from a family. Crises increase the level of stress within the family. If not mastered, they can lead to a decline in the family's health, or even disintegration of the family. **Adequate family functioning depends on the ability of the family to recognize and validate these sources of stress** and then to master them, either alone or with the assistance of a social support system.

1. Normative crises are the central developmental events in the family life cycle model (e.g., marriage, birth of children, children entering school). These events occur in all families, but they mark important transitions in family life and are considered crises because they require adaptive responses.

2. Paranormative crises are events that occur unexpectedly and distinguish each family's life cycle (e.g., miscarriage, divorce, disability).
   a. In more than 50% of families, at least one family member will have a diagnosable mental illness.
   b. More of these individuals are treated by primary care physicians than by psychiatrists or mental health professionals.

E. **Family therapy.** Many forms of family therapy are available to treat clinical problems. Outcome studies show that family therapy is effective. Family therapy is divided into three schools (Table 10-1).

1. Behavioral–psychoeducational approaches follow the principles of social learning theory. These principles assert that **interpersonal behavior is controlled, maintained, and shaped by current environmental events** and therefore is changed most effectively through the manipulation of these events.

2. Structural–strategic approaches. These independently developed methods borrow concepts from general systems theory. They view all problems as the result of dysfunctional attempts by the family to adapt to the current life context. Some approaches emphasize family **structure** (i.e., alliances, coalitions, hierarchies); others focus on the family's **organization and process** (i.e., rules for communication, circuits of interaction). These therapists typically use a variety of interventions, including behavioral techniques. They emphasize **cognitive reframing techniques and paradoxical interventions,** claiming that these techniques are powerful and are best used only by trained professionals.

TABLE 10-1. The Major Schools of Family Therapy

School	Attributes of a Healthy Family	Interventions
Behavioral–psychoeducational	Clear communication and expectations Predictable consequences Nonblaming posture	Identify dysfunctional behavior Apply social learning theory Provide communication training Provide problem-solving skill training Suggest contingency contracting
Structural–strategic	Clear generational boundaries Parental alliance Clear power hierarchy Clear, direct communication	Identify family structure Restructure faulty alliances Introduce cognitive reframing techniques Provide paradoxical interventions
Intergenerational–experiential	Positive effect Differentiation from family of origin Appropriate family development	Produce family genograms Clarify transgenerational patterns Facilitate communication Determine family identity Introduce model play and fantasy

   a. **Cognitive reframing** assumes that a family's view of a problem can interfere with the resolution of the problem. Typically, such views are critical of at least one family member. For example, "Our family would be perfectly all right if it wasn't for our daughter Mary, who has spent all her time recently moping and crying." By suggesting another explanation, the therapist opens other avenues for the family. For example, the therapist might say, "Maybe Mary is remembering Grandma Jean for all of you. After her death last year, you all got back to business as usual pretty quickly. Mary might be taking care of some important unfinished business for the family."
   b. **Paradoxical interventions** are counterintuitive suggestions that a therapist makes to a family to break a pattern of complex interpersonal reflexes that, once triggered, run their course. The therapist often prescribes the symptom in an attempt to change the context and inhibit the reflex. For example, a therapist urges a couple who has frequent arguments to have at least one argument before the next therapy session, even if one partner must provoke the other. With this approach, the therapist is attempting to inhibit the reflex to argue by raising the suspicion in each partner that the other is not really arguing, but simply following the therapist's orders.

3. **Intergenerational–experiential approaches** view dysfunctional behavior as the result of **family developmental fixation** (e.g., insufficient differentiation from or excessive obligation toward the families of orientation). Symptoms appear when a family cannot master a new developmentally related stress (e.g., first child goes to school, parent becomes ill) because of the family's developmental fixation. The success of this approach depends on the interpersonal skills of the therapist. Techniques are outlined in Table 10-1.

REFERENCES

1. Engel GL: The need for a new medical model: a challenge for biomedicine. *Science* 196:129–136, 1977.

2. Benjamin LS: *Interpersonal Diagnosis and Treatment of Personality Disorders*. New York, Guilford, 1993.

3. Benjamin LS: Principles of prediction using structural analysis of social behavior (SASB). In

Personality and the Prediction of Behavior. Edited by Zucker RA, Aronoff J, Rabin AJ. New York, Academic Press, 1984.

4. Brown GW, Monck EM, Carstairs GM, et al: Influence of family life on the course of schizophrenic illness. *Br J Prev Soc Med* 16:55–68, 1962.

5. Bowlby J: Developmental psychiatry comes of age. *Am J Psychiatry* 145:1–10, 1988.

6. Ainsworth MDS, Bell SM, Stayton DJ: Individual differences in strange situation behavior of one-year-olds. In *The Origins of Human Social Relations.* Edited by Schaffer HR. London, Academic Press, 1971, pp 17–57.

BIBLIOGRAPHY

Benjamin LS: Principles of prediction using structural analysis of social behavior (SASB). In *Personality and the Prediction of Behavior.* Edited by Zucker RA, Aronoff J, Rabin AJ. New York, Academic Press, 1984.

Benjamin LS: *Interpersonal Diagnosis and Treatment of Personality Disorders.* New York, Guilford, 1993.

Boss PG, Doherty WJ, LaRossa R, et al (eds): *Sourcebook of Family Theories and Methods: A Contextual Approach.* New York, Plenum Press, 1993.

Bowlby J: Developmental psychiatry comes of age. *Am J Psychiatry* 145:1–10, 1988.

Bretherton I, Waters E (eds): *Growing Points in Attachment Theory.* Chicago, University of Chicago Press, 1985.

Brown GW, Monck EM, Carstairs GM, et al: Influence of family life on the course of schizophrenic illness. *Br J Prev Soc Med* 16:55–68, 1962.

Coleman M, Popenoe D, Glenn ND, et al: An exchange on American family decline. *J Marriage Fam* 55:525–556, 1993.

Doherty WJ, Baird MA: *Fam Ther Fam Med.* New York, Guilford, 1983.

Engel GL: The need for a new medical model: a challenge for biomedicine. *Science* 196:129–136, 1977.

Engel GL: The clinical application of the biopsychosocial model. *Am J Psychiatry* 137:535–544, 1980.

Falloon IRH: Expressed emotion: current status. *Psychol Med* 18:269–274, 1988.

Gelles RJ, Maynard PE: A structural family systems approach to intervention in cases of family violence. *Fam Rel* 36:270–275, 1987.

Hahlweg K, Goldstein MJ (eds): *Understanding Major Mental Disorder: The Contributions of Family Process Research.* New York, Family Process Press, 1987.

Kavanaugh DJ: Recent developmental in expressed emotion and schizophrenia. *Br J Psychiatry* 160:601–620, 1992.

Oliver JE: Intergenerational transmission of child abuse: rates, research, and clinical implications. *Am J Psychiatry* 150:1315–1324, 1993.

Parke R (ed): *The Family: Review of Child Development Research,* vol 7. Chicago, University of Chicago Press, 1984.

von Bertalanffy L: *General Systems Theory.* New York, Braziller, 1968.

Wamboldt FS, Reiss D: Task performance and the social construction of meaning: juxtaposing normality with contemporary family research. In *The Diversity of Normal Behavior: Further Contributions to Normatology.* Edited by Offer D, Sabshin M. New York, Basic Books, 1991.

Wamboldt FS, Wamboldt MZ, Gurman AS: Marital and family therapy: the meaning for the clinician. In *Integrating Research and Clinical Practice: The Family Therapy Collections,* vol 15. Edited by Andreozzi LL, Levant RF. Rockville, MD, Aspen Systems Press, 1985.

STUDY QUESTIONS

DIRECTIONS: Each of the numbered items or incomplete statements in this section is followed by answers or by completions of the statement. Select the ONE lettered answer or completion that is BEST in each case.

Questions 1–5

A physician is asked to perform a psychiatric consultation on a 40-year-old black man, Mr. Sinclair, who is currently undergoing hemodialysis for end-stage renal disease secondary to severe hypertension. On the consultation request, his physician, Dr. Lewis, a 40-year-old white man, notes that Mr. Sinclair is entering a terminal stage of his illness. He requests an evaluation of Mr. Sinclair's "strange demeanor."

1. The biopsychosocial model would suggest that which one of the following influences should weigh most heavily in the evaluation?

(A) Mr. Sinclair's current blood pressure
(B) Cultural differences between the doctor and the patient
(C) An assessment of the patient's personality
(D) The patient's explanation of his situation
(E) All of the above

2. During the interview, Mr. Sinclair is cooperative, exhibits an appropriate sense of humor, and shows a philosophical view of his illness that is both simple and profound (e.g., I'm going to be a dead man soon, so why should I waste time worrying and fussing? I'm going to squeeze out all of the life I can get.). Examination and review of his medical record show no evidence of mental status impairment or personality problems. Rather, he seems to have realistically appraised his situation and reached a state of healthy acceptance. When this information is shared with Dr. Lewis, he glares and states, "Well, this is really a big help, all this shrink stuff." The consultant responds, "I'm telling you how I see things. If you know something about this case that I don't know, I'd like to hear it, because I am interested in giving you a consultation you find helpful." Dr. Lewis's response to the consultation is an example of

(A) a reductionistic statement
(B) a hostile, controlling statement
(C) an antithetical statement
(D) socialization

3. The reply to Dr. Lewis is an example of which type of interpersonal posture?

(A) An antithetical posture
(B) A power struggle
(C) A symmetric posture
(D) A complementary posture
(E) A stable posture

4. Dr. Lewis says that he "just can't talk to Mr. Sinclair." When the consultant questions him, Dr. Lewis states, "Maybe too much is happening in my own life." His younger brother recently died of acquired immune deficiency syndrome (AIDS), he and his wife are having marital problems, and his 11-year-old son is "hanging around with the wrong crowd." Dr. Lewis is spending more time at work because the other physician in his group practice just entered an impaired physician treatment program for alcoholism. Given this new information, which of the following influences is important in the assessment of the patient?

(A) The tension between the current family life cycle stages of Mr. Sinclair and Dr. Lewis
(B) The differing levels of environmental stress facing Mr. Sinclair and Dr. Lewis
(C) The cultural differences between Mr. Sinclair and Dr. Lewis
(D) All of the above

5. The consultant has a short, collegial talk with Dr. Lewis in an attempt to improve the relationship between Mr. Sinclair and Dr. Lewis. Still, Dr. Lewis is surprised that the other staff members are not having problems with Mr. Sinclair. Dr. Lewis suggests including the head nurse, Mrs. Dean, in the discussion. She states that to her knowledge, no one on the staff is having problems with Mr. Sinclair. A somewhat embarrassed Dr. Lewis then states his willingness to improve his relationship with Mr. Sinclair. Mrs. Dean's communication influenced Dr. Lewis through

(A) a systemic identity
(B) the consensual dimension of social reality
(C) morphostasis
(D) the structural aspect of social reality
(E) homeostasis

Questions 6–8

Jane, a 23-year-old white woman, maintained contact all her life with the physician who delivered her. The physician is aware that Jane grew up in a troubled home in which both of her parents had serious problems with alcohol abuse. During her adolescent years, Jane confided in her physician, who encouraged her to attend college. During her college years, she grew increasingly divorced from her parents. Because of their relationship, she asks her physician to attend her college graduation. After the ceremony, she introduces her physician to Rick, a classmate whom she plans to marry in 2 weeks. The physician asks Rick and Jane a number of questions about their plans.

6. Which of the following factors does NOT put the couple at increased risk for marital problems?

(A) Jane is 4 months pregnant
(B) Rick is a black man whose family lives in Trinidad
(C) Jane and Rick have known each other for slightly more than 4 months
(D) Rick's parents will provide financial and other assistance to the couple

7. According to the family life cycle model, during their first year of marriage, Rick and Jane are likely to need to do all of the following EXCEPT

(A) negotiate their relationship with both families of origin
(B) establish working marital and parental roles
(C) create an adequate mix of intimacy and individual autonomy
(D) reestablish individual interests and careers

The wedding and the birth of the baby, Bobby, go smoothly. Things seem to be going well. Two years after the marriage, Jane consults the physician about problems with Bobby. For a month and a half, Bobby has been waking frequently during the night. He is also aggressive, particularly toward Jane. Jane seems very unsure of her parenting abilities, and she mentions that she is giving a lot of thought to her own troubled childhood. The physician offers some advice, but learns several weeks later that the problem still exists. Jane, Rick, and Bobby are referred to a behavior-oriented psychologist for further assessment. A few weeks later, Jane reports that six therapy sessions proved helpful.

8. Which of the following interventions did Jane and Rick probably experience?

(A) Detailed exploration of their differing family histories
(B) Definition of their family identity
(C) A search for family developmental fixation
(D) Training in problem-solving techniques

DIRECTIONS: The incomplete statement in this section is negatively phrased, as indicated by a capitalized word such as NOT, LEAST, or EXCEPT. Select the ONE lettered answer or completion that is BEST.

9. Children learn the values and practices of their culture through all of the following processes EXCEPT

(A) ritual practices
(B) operant conditioning
(C) modeling
(D) ethnocentrism
(E) social interaction

DIRECTIONS: The set of matching questions in this section consists of a list of three to twenty-six lettered options (some of which may be in figures) followed by several numbered items. For each numbered item, select the ONE lettered option that is most closely associated with it. To avoid spending too much time on matching sets with large numbers of options, it is generally advisable to begin each set by reading the list of options. Then, for each item in the set, try to generate the correct answer and locate it in the option list, rather than evaluating each option individually. Each lettered option may be selected once, more than once, or not at all.

Questions 10–14

Match each treatment technique with the school of family therapy most associated with that technique.

(A) Behavioral–psychoeducational approaches
(B) Structural–strategic approaches
(C) Intergenerational–experiential approaches

10. Identification of transgenerational relationship patterns

11. Clarification of relationship patterns within the nuclear family

12. Training in social learning theory

13. Cognitive reframing

14. Definition of the family's identity

ANSWERS AND EXPLANATIONS

1. The answer is E [I B 2]. The biopsychosocial model postulates that to adequately understand illness, a physician must maintain a broad perspective to assess all relevant areas of human experience. Relevant sources of information include biomedical data, the patient's experience and behavior, and cultural factors.

2. The answer is B [I B; II C 2 a–c; III A 1 c]. The response shows focus on other, negative interdependence, and negative affiliation. Reductionism is a philosophy of science that holds that complex phenomena can be reduced to elementary principles. Antithetical statements are responses that differ from another person's statement by being opposite in focus and degrees of interdependence and affiliation. Socialization is a process of passing on cultural beliefs and practices.

3. The answer is A [II C 3 a–c]. An antithetical posture differs in focus and is directly opposite in degrees of affiliation and interdependence from the partner's previous message. A symmetric posture or a power struggle would require that the consultant respond in kind. A complementary posture would require the consultant to accept blame for the situation.

4. The answer is A [IV C 1–3]. Although the two men are the same age, they face different family life cycle tasks. Mr. Sinclair is preparing for his own death and the associated family changes. Dr. Lewis is dealing with the problems of a child-rearing family, balancing the demands of marriage, career, and children. Dr. Lewis is also experiencing family dissolution because of his brother's death. The similarities and differences between these men's life experiences, combined with the stress faced by Dr. Lewis, may explain their difficulty in communicating. Although Mr. Sinclair shows better adaptation to his life stress, it would be difficult to argue that Mr. Sinclair's anticipation of his own death is less stressful than Dr. Lewis's life circumstances.

5. The answer is B [I A 2, 3; III A 1–3]. An individual's beliefs about his social world are influenced by his interactions with significant others and by the structure of his society. Mrs. Dean's comment affected the former, the consensual aspect of social reality. Morphostasis and homeostasis are processes whereby a system responds to stress in a manner that maintains its original structure and its systemic identity.

6. The answer is D [IV B 2 b (1) (a)–(f)]. Greater risk of divorce is associated with short courtship, premarital pregnancy, and extreme difference in background. However, the support of Rick's parents provides an encouraging, buffering influence.

7. The answer is D [IV C 1, 2 a]. This couple is compressing into a short span of time the tasks of two stages of family development: formation of a new family and preschool age child rearing.

8. The answer is D [IV E 1–3]. The behavioral–psychoeducational approaches to family therapy are based on the principles of social learning theory. Problems are seen as related to current dysfunctional behavioral interactions that can be identified and changed. Problem-solving training, in this case related to the tasks of parenting, is frequently used. Exploration of family histories, definition of family identity, and search for family developmental fixation are usually associated with intergenerational–experiential approaches.

9. The answer is D [III A 1 a–c]. Children learn the values and practices of their culture through two major processes of socialization: modeling, or learning through observation, and operant conditioning, or learning through reward and punishment. Ritual practices are an important form of social interaction. Ethnocentrism, although typically one of the values learned, is the tendency of individuals to see their own culture as superior and differing cultures as inferior.

10–14. The answers are: 10-C, 11-B, 12-A, 13-B, 14-C [IV E 1–3]. Family therapy is roughly divided into three schools. The behavioral–psychoeducational approaches are grounded in social learning theory. Patients are frequently instructed in the principles of this theory during treatment. The structural–strategic approaches view family problems as misguided and dysfunctional attempts by the family to adapt to current circumstances. Clarification of current relationship patterns, such as alliances and coalitions, and cognitive reframing are techniques associated with these therapies. The intergenerational–experiential approaches view family problems as rooted in the family's fixation at a particular stage of development. Therapy attempts to discover the cause of this fixation by examining transgenerational patterns and defining the family's identity.

Chapter 11

The Physician–Patient Relationship

Thomas N. Wise

I. DEFINITION AND COMPONENTS OF THE PHYSICIAN–PATIENT RELATIONSHIP

A. **The physician–patient relationship** is the matrix within which medical care is maintained and delivered. It is a dyadic interaction wherein both physician and patient have roles and responsibilities. The most important factors for this dyadic structure are the psychological substrates that bond patient to healer.

1. **The physician's responsibilities** are to:
   a. Diagnose acute and chronic illness
   b. Cure disease whenever possible
   c. Maximize function and minimize pain in both acute and chronic conditions
   d. Provide solace and palliative treatment in terminal cases

2. **"The sick role"** is the name given to the patient's responsibility.
   a. **Elements of the sick role,** as defined by sociologist Talcott Parsons,[1] are as follows.
      (1) The sick person is considered exempt from normal social-role responsibilities and activities. Thus, the patient is not expected to go to work nor to care for the family if sick.
      (2) The sick person is not to be blamed for his illness and not to be expected to recover by himself. The illness and disease, therefore, require medical attention.
      (3) The sick person is obliged to want to get well and to cooperate with appropriate care givers.
      (4) The sick person is obliged to seek technically competent help.
   b. **Elements of illness.** The physician must measure the impact of the various aspects of illness to determine how to manage the patient. Failure to appreciate any of the following issues may distort the physician–patient relationship.
      (1) **Impersonal elements** of illness include physical limitations on activity; medications and their side effects; pain, immobilization, and malaise associated with the disorder or its treatment; dietary changes mandated by the disorder; financial burdens of the illness; and limitations on life span.
      (2) **Intrapersonal elements** of illness refer to the ways in which the patient reacts as a result of her personality to the stress of an illness.
      (3) **Interpersonal elements** of illness refer to the effects of illness on the patient's relationship with family, friends, employer, and environment.
         (a) Roles, boundaries, and communication patterns within a patient's family may change. Tasks normally delegated to certain family members may be renegotiated or relinquished.
         (b) Friends may withdraw in the face of serious illness, or the patient may isolate herself from support systems.
         (c) Illness may limit occupational ability and force a new relationship with the patient's employer.
         (d) Illness can affect the patient's relationship with the environment. For example, strangers may shun a person infected with human immunodeficiency virus (HIV) or recoil from a person who has undergone a disfiguring surgical procedure.
   c. **Impediments to sick-role behavior** include:
      (1) Financial limitations that prevent the sick person from seeking medical care
      (2) Responsibilities that cannot be abandoned, such as single parenthood or being a family's sole wage earner

(3) Inability to recognize an illness because of lack of knowledge, lack of symptoms, or psychological inability to face illness

(4) A different view of disease causation because of cultural differences. For example, many cultures explain anxiety and somatization as humoral imbalances.

B. **Components of the physician–patient relationship**

1. **Trust and confidence.** The physician must attempt to practice medicine in the best interest of the patient.

2. **Instillation of hope and minimization of fear and doubt.** The physician must reassure the patient that the best possible treatment will be provided and that pain and suffering will be minimized, without misleading the patient when an ominous symptom or a terminal diagnosis exists.

3. **Empathy,** wherein the physician places himself in the patient's position, helps the physician understand how the patient feels.

4. **A personal relationship based on concern** should be afforded every patient. The patient should be seen as a total human being, rather than a vector of altered physiology, and should receive treatment for both illness and disease.
   a. **Disease** is a pathologic alteration in normal anatomy or physiology that produces signs and symptoms, affects quality of life, and is apprehended by the objective diagnostic skill of the physician.
   b. **Illness** is experienced by the patient and is perceived as subjectively unique in terms of feeling unwell and creating suffering for both the patient and her family.
   c. **Treatment** of disease requires knowledge and technical skill, whereas treatment of illness requires knowledge and empathy. Both activities require communication between the patient and the physician.

5. **Communication**—an important aspect of the physician–patient relationship—is a difficult task that requires training, experience, and skill. By allowing a patient to relate his story and voice his concerns, a physician helps to strengthen the important relationship they share.

6. **Bridging cultural gaps.** Cultures differ in how they view disease causation and treatment. Treatments that may be labeled "folk remedies" by Western medicine should be understood by the physicians. Failure of the physician to acknowledge the patient's cultural beliefs will result in poor communication with the patient and limited compliance by the patient of Western medical treatments.

C. **Historical and current issues.** The physician–patient relationship is based on the historical evolution of medicine. A learned profession, a priestly caste, and a technical craft form the heritage of the contemporary physician.

1. The **Hippocratic oath,** which has been recited by generations of graduating medical students, contains elements of a profession as well as a technical body of skills to be learned:
   a. A code of ethical behavior to be regulated by the profession
   b. An obligation to transmit medical knowledge and venerate one's teachers, which denotes the need to stay informed of modern developments in one's specialty

2. The rise of **managed health care** has introduced a third element—the **"payor"**—into the previously dyadic relationship between physician and patient. This change threatens to disrupt a harmony that has existed for many generations.
   a. The basic covenant and contract remain in the physician–patient relationship, despite the rise of managed care and the growth of consumerism.
   b. The fiduciary relationship between healer and patient differs from a typical business relationship.[2] The first mandate of such a trust is **primum non nocere** (first do no harm). The physician must be knowledgeable and educated and must behave in an ethical manner.
   c. This role of the physician has been labeled the **apostolic function,**[3] but goals remain the same and obligations to the patient persist.

II. **MODELS OF THE PHYSICIAN–PATIENT RELATIONSHIP.** Emanuel and Emanuel[4] described the four basic models of the physician–patient relationship. All four of these models may be used in different situations (Table 11-1).

A. **Paternalistic model.** In this model, the physician decides what is best based solely on medical information and the physician's judgment. The physician acts as a guardian and determines from his perspective what is best for the patient. This style is exemplified by the physician who demands that his patient with carcinoma of the breast without nodal extension undergo a modified radical mastectomy despite the patient's wishes to preserve her breast. The problem with this model is that the patient and the physician may have different values. This model is best reserved for emergency care.

B. **Informative model.** In this model, the physician gives the patient all of the relevant information about his disease and possible treatments without attention to the patient's values. The physician is a purveyor of technical expertise. For example, a physician could offer a patient with metastatic colon carcinoma statistics on the success of chemotherapy without considering the patient's life situation, personality, or views on pain, suffering, and death. Such an approach would very often cause the patient anxiety and distress. This approach lacks the compassion that is necessary in a physician and unrealistically views the patient as totally autonomous. This model may be appropriate when a patient is seen for a minor illness, on a one-time basis, such as in a walk-in clinic. Many patients cannot decide independently what is the best treatment and must work with the physician to develop a mutually acceptable plan.

C. **Interpretive model.** This model combines the informative model with a consideration of the patient's life history, values, and personality. This model is most appropriate for patients with conflicting values so that they can best understand the nature of the conflicts and come to an informed decision based on both medical information and personal values. This approach demands that the physician understand the patient's needs and desires. Concurrent with this understanding, the physician provides technical information about the specific disease and treatments available. The physician is an advisor or counselor. For example, the physician treating a patient with metastatic colon cancer who has a controlling, orderly personality style would outline the risks and benefits of chemotherapy in a factual manner but also emphasize the ability to provide palliative care and minimize suffering in whatever course of treatment is chosen by the patient. This style demands that the physician develop skills in fully elucidating the patient's value system in the context of her life history. Such data are not always available for the consultant specialist who sees the patient on a limited basis. Nevertheless, it is imperative that every physician, no matter how limited the relationship, ascertain the patient's personality style and understanding of and reaction to the disease.

D. **Deliberative model.** In this model, the physician acts as a teacher or friend who articulates and persuades the patient to pursue the "best course" based on mutual understanding of the patient's values and medical information. The limitation of this model is that it is not the physician's task to judge values. However, a physician may involve herself in

TABLE 11-1. Use of Physician–Patient Relationship Models

Model	Clinical Setting
Paternalistic	Emergency situations
Informative	Walk-in clinic
	One-visit situation with minor illness
Interpretive	Ongoing clinical care
Deliberative	Public health setting

health-related issues in the context of clinical care. Thus, it is appropriate for a physician to strongly advise a homosexual man to practice safe sex as a health precaution against HIV infection, but not to castigate the patient for his sexual orientation. This model may be preferred in public health settings. It is used de facto when screening for organ transplantation, such as when a patient with end-stage liver disease who is still actively alcoholic is denied transplantation.

III. **TRANSFERENCE AND COUNTERTRANSFERENCE.** It is common for patients to react to physicians based on attitudes formed toward important persons in their past. In turn, physicians may exhibit emotionally motivated behavior toward patients.

A. **Transference** refers to the displacement of feelings and attitudes from important relationships in the patient's past to the physician. Through transference, the patient may regard the physician as a paternal or maternal figure, a teacher, or a rescuer. Such attitudes can be positive, or they can be negative, as shown in the following examples.

1. A patient who views her physician as an all-powerful or ever-caring parental figure will be disappointed by any deviation from total availability.

2. A patient who views her physician as a harsh, punitive parent or an authority figure who gives orders but does not fundamentally care about her well-being may react with counterproductive action (e.g., noncompliance).

3. A patient who reacts with anger or suspicion may have had an earlier experience wherein parental figures were untrustworthy. This type of patient may also seek many consultations in an effort to have a stable, trusting relationship. Negative transference reactions (e.g., hostility, suspicion, competitiveness) may elicit inappropriately angry (rather than curious or understanding) responses from physicians.

B. **Countertransference** refers to the complementary, unconscious attitude of a physician toward her patients. Overly critical attitudes and erotic fantasies are examples of countertransference phenomena.

IV. **PERSONALITY TYPES FOUND IN MEDICAL PRACTICE.** The theoretical and practical implications of transference and countertransference reactions are important. Having a working idea of various character types helps the physician understand how certain personality patterns commonly have specific transferences.

A. **Personality styles.** Personality refers to an enduring pattern of distinctive traits and tendencies that characterize an individual's reaction to specific circumstances. It is essential to have a general impression of each patient's personality. Personality disorders describe the chronic and maladaptive traits that promote difficulties in patients as well as in their interactions with others. Personality can be conceptualized as either an underlying dimensional or categorical nosology. Traits such as emotionality, neatness, sociability, and agreeableness reside along a dimension similar to quantitative levels of height, weight, and blood pressure. Understanding either categorical or dimensional approaches to personality is essential because the physician must recognize how a patient reacts to the threat of illness and the challenge of treatment, whether it is taking medication, undergoing a procedure, or modifying behavior, such as committing to a diet or exercise program.

B. **Categories of personality disorder** (Table 11-2). The *Diagnostic and Statistical Manual of Mental Disorders,* 4th edition (DSM-IV), uses a categorical designation wherein an individual may have more than one disorder. The disorders are grouped into three clusters.

TABLE 11-2. Categories of Personality Disorder

Cluster A: odd, eccentric
   Paranoid
   Schizoid
   Schizotypal
Cluster B: dramatic, unstable
   Antisocial
   Borderline
   Histrionic
   Narcissistic
Cluster C: anxious
   Avoidant
   Dependent
   Obsessive-compulsive

1. **Cluster A** includes odd and eccentric personality disorders.
   a. Individuals with **paranoid personality disorder** exhibit pervasive distrust and suspicion, and often perceive motives as malevolent. A paranoid individual may be distrustful of a physician who inquires about his personal life and may fear that treatments are harmful.
   b. Individuals with **schizoid personality disorder** neither desire nor enjoy close relationships. They live a solitary life with little interest in developing friendships. They exhibit emotional coldness, detachment, or a constricted affect. Because patients with schizoid personality disorder may feel threatened if the physician attempts to become close, these patients should be treated in a formal manner.
   c. Individuals with **schizotypal personality disorder** exhibit odd behaviors based on a belief in magic or superstition, and may report unusual perceptual experiences. They may be suspicious and demonstrate inappropriate affect. Schizotypal individuals may confront their physicians with odd ideas about symptoms. Like paranoid personalities, schizotypal personalities become suspicious and feel threatened if they experience side effects as a result of treatment.

2. **Cluster B** involves individuals with dramatic and unstable characteristics that often result in behavioral difficulties.
   a. Individuals with **antisocial personality disorder** have a lifelong history of inability to conform to social norms. They are irritable and aggressive, and may have repeated physical fights. These individuals also have a high prevalence of comorbid substance abuse disorders.
   b. Individuals with **borderline personality disorder** are acutely sensitive to real or imagined abandonment and have a pattern of repeated unstable but intense interpersonal relationships that alternate between extremes of idealization and devaluation. Such individuals may abuse substances or food, or be sexually promiscuous. They may have recurrent suicidal behavior and have marked mood swings from intense euphoria to depression and anxiety. These individuals have chronic feelings of emptiness and inappropriate intense rage reactions that include gestures and threats. The physician must recognize the tendency of these patients to use the splitting defense mechanism dramatically: The physician may be idealized as the omnipotent healer one day, and then devalued and feared the next. These patients may be sexually seductive, and the physician must set clear boundaries.
   c. Individuals with **histrionic personality disorder** attempt to be the center of attention through the use of theatrical and self-dramatizing behavior. The physician should treat these patients in a professional manner because they tend to eroticize any relationship.
   d. Individuals with **narcissistic personality disorder** have a pervasive sense of self-importance. They are preoccupied with fantasies of unlimited success, power, and

brilliance. They view themselves as special, and they often demand excessive admiration and attention. Concurrently, they lack empathy and are unwilling to recognize or identify with the needs of others. They appear arrogant and haughty. These patients may threaten the physician and devalue her competence. It is useful for physicians to recognize this style and not become threatened or angry.

3. **Cluster C** involves disorders in which subjective anxiety plays a central role.
   a. Individuals with **avoidant personality disorder** are fearful of becoming involved with people because of excessive fears of criticism or rejection. Although these individuals wish to be in social situations, they become intensely anxious in such settings and believe that they are socially inept or inferior to others. Extreme avoidant behaviors lead to social phobias. These patients may use health complaints as a way of socializing, especially if the physician is empathic and understanding. Identification of avoidant personality patterns is important because psychiatric treatment with psychotherapy and pharmacotherapy can modify such behaviors.
   b. Individuals with **dependent personality disorder** cannot make even daily decisions without excessive advice and reassurance. These patients need others to assume responsibility for them. Dependent patients can make inordinate demands by means of repeated telephone calls, and they may be unwilling to comply with treatment. These patients also have trouble relinquishing the sick role and leaving the hospital setting when appropriate.
   c. Individuals with **obsessive-compulsive personality disorder** are preoccupied with details, rules, lists, and schedules to the point that tasks often cannot be completed. They devote an excessive amount of energy to work to the exclusion of leisure and social life. They may be unable to discard worn out or worthless objects and often are rigidly stubborn. These patients often describe excessively detailed histories that may seem circumstantial. They require a careful and detailed explanation of any treatments offered.

C. **Dimensions of personality** (Table 11-3). The previous discussion designates categorical personality styles. A **dimensional approach** places the various traits of personality along a continuum. The following dimensions are included.

1. **Neuroticism** denotes a tendency toward anxiety, depression, a sense of self-consciousness, and vulnerability. Neurotic individuals tend to be worriers, and they often magnify and augment normal somatic sensations. The physician should understand that the patient with a tendency toward neuroticism may be particularly frightened by normal side effects of treatments.

2. **Extroversion** denotes an outgoing, sociable personality. **Introverted** persons are more solitary and aloof, by contrast. Introverted patients have a tendency toward dysthymia.

3. **Agreeableness** refers to the personality trait of readiness or willingness to consent. Overly agreeable patients may agree to all treatments suggested, but not comply. Individuals with a tendency toward disagreeableness have an antagonistic and hostile style.

4. **Openness** refers to a willingness to hear and consider or to accept and deal with. The overly open patient may be attracted to a variety of alternative therapies that have no basis for efficacy. The rigidly conservative patient, closed in his thinking, may have trouble with modern approaches to medical care.

TABLE 11-3. Dimensions of Personality

Neuroticism
Extroversion
Agreeableness
Openness
Conscientiousness

5. Conscientiousness refers to a dimension of organized, goal-directed behavior in completing tasks. Individuals who are not conscientious may have few goals in life, and have tendencies toward disorganization, procrastination, and inability to complete tasks. Patients who are not conscientious often will not comply with taking medications. Therefore, a patient with diabetes who is not conscientious may do better with a broad-based dietary regimen rather than one that involves strict caloric control.

V. **THE PHYSICIAN–PATIENT RELATIONSHIP UNDER STRESS.** Understanding the transferential elements and the personality style of each patient can help the physician manage the stress that can arise in the physician–patient dyad.

A. **The somatizing hypochondriacal patient**

1. The physician needs to recognize that these patients are subjectively suffering. These patients tend to **amplify their somatic sensations,** and they react anxiously with a fear of serious illness.

2. Mood disorders (e.g., major depression, chronic dysthymias) often coexist in these patients.

3. The complaints of these patients must be seriously considered, but extended evaluations and complicated laboratory studies can be avoided if the physician recognizes the psychogenic basis for the complaint.

4. Regular appointments may modify the tendencies of these patients to doctor shop and therefore may prevent unnecessary treatment.

B. **The patient who refuses medical advice.** This patient presents a challenge to the physician's authority. The physician should not react to this behavior as an affront, but instead should attempt to determine the factors that led to the patient's refusal.

1. **Denial** of the illness that necessitated hospitalization or treatment can be fostered by the fear and anxiety of the consequences of disease. An example of denial is ignoring a breast mass, chest pain, or increasing fatigue.
   a. To **manage denial,** the physician must assess the patient's understanding of her illness and its treatment. **Correction of misinterpretations and unfounded fears** may alleviate the patient's anxiety and foster acceptance of information offered by the physician.
   b. If the patient continues to deny serious illness, the physician should appeal to family members to urge the patient to comply with necessary treatment. If such appeals fail, determination of patient competence and consideration of **involuntary treatment** may be necessary. Involuntary treatment, however, is not a routine clinical option, and it requires legal proceedings, which vary by locality. In an emergent situation, however, the physician can institute life-saving measures.

2. **Cognitive impairment** as a result of dementia or delirium can cause a patient to be confused and not to fully understand the reason for hospitalization. These patients need treatment for the organic brain syndrome that causes the confusion. Table 11-4 delineates the acute and chronic syndromes of organic brain disease that can coexist. Treatment for these syndromes involves identification of the drugs or disease states that are compromising cognitive function (see Chapter 15 III A–B).

3. **Personality disorders.** Patients with personality disorders characterized by problems with authority or fear of confinement may find hospitalization and treatment threatening. Drug addicts may not tolerate hospitalization, and may leave to continue their addictive behaviors. Patients who display an extreme aversion to authority cannot easily tolerate the structured hierarchy of hospital life.
   a. The reason for this behavior must be ascertained (e.g., leaving to search for drugs, anger at having to wait a long time for a surgical procedure, anger toward authority).

TABLE 11-4. Features of Delirium and Dementia

Delirium	Dementia
Secondary to a medical or neurologic disorder	Results from a primary disease or host of conditions
Acute presentation	Chronic course
Fluctuating states of consciousness	Clear consciousness
Presence of hallucinations	Rare hallucinations or delusions
Shifting psychomotor activity	Intellectual deterioration
Coexisting systemic illness	. . .
Drug toxicity	. . .
Global slowing on electroencephalogram	. . .

    b. A frank discussion of the problem can alleviate some of the patient's concerns. By acknowledging that hospital life often is uncomfortable, inconvenient, and stressful, the physician validates the patient's distress.

  4. Noncompliance with treatment is a frustrating aspect of the physician–patient relationship. To manage noncompliance, the physician can:
    a. Simplify the regimen and make financial burdens more realistic
    b. Simplify a complex drug schedule
    c. Use a visiting nurse to augment compliance
    d. Use a unit diet rather than strict calorie count for some patients with diabetes
    e. Discuss the treatments and provide sufficient information to encourage patient cooperation
    f. Discuss potential side effects and, when indicated, change medication that causes unpleasant side effects

C. **The patient with chronic pain.** This patient may frustrate the physician so that inadequate treatment is provided, both patient and physician become angry, and the patient stops seeing the physician. Appropriate management demands that the patient's pain and suffering be considered genuine: The cause of the discomfort may be exaggerated as a result of anxiety, but the subjective experience is authentic. The **goal of chronic pain management** is to minimize narcotic medication and maximize function.

  1. Narcotics with dosages that must be increased because of the development of tolerance should be avoided. Aspirin or acetaminophen should be used as adjunctive medication, with amitriptyline given to potentiate analgesic medications if needed.

  2. Liberal use of **physical therapy** is important. The patient should be told that pain will be involved, but that tolerance as well as pain relief is the goal.

  3. Analgesic medication should be given on a scheduled basis, not "as needed." The dosages, then, can be adjusted according to a given schedule and not erratically.

  4. If pain persists despite these measures, and if the patient continues to use excessive narcotics, referral to a **pain clinic** should be considered. Such settings focus on reducing discomfort and addictive behaviors and helping the patient to maximal function.

  5. If there is litigation or financial compensation pending, maximal recovery can be delayed until a legal settlement is reached. This should be explained to patients whose injury and pain complaints are seen in the context of such litigation.

D. **The patient with cancer.** This patient presents a considerable challenge to the physician–patient relationship. Although it may be terrifying, cancer is not necessarily a terminal illness. The physician must recognize the following psychosocial stages of cancer.

  1. Diagnosis. Patients may ignore warning signs or may not heed a physician's warning to stop smoking or to get annual mammograms. When the diagnosis is made, patients may fear that the physician will be angry with them, blame them, or abandon them.

2. **Treatment** of neoplastic disease often involves referral to a specialist or surgeon. The involvement of other physicians may cause a sense of loss for both the primary care physician and the patient. The primary care provider should continue to play a part in the patient's care, even if it is limited to visits, telephone calls, or availability for questions. The side effects from chemotherapy and radiation therapy can include nausea, malaise, confusion, and depression. These reactions must be acknowledged by the physician and treated as effectively as possible.

3. **Remission** necessitates ongoing follow-up and vigilance. Patients may experience anxiety and fear that the neoplasm has recurred. The physician must support and reassure the patient, but must not provide a false sense of security that limits ongoing follow-up.

4. **Recurrence** may lead to terror and despair, but the physician must continue to instill hope that there are treatments available. Words such as "control the tumor" and "stop the spread of the disease" are welcomed by the patient although cure or total removal of a lesion may not be possible.

5. The **terminal phase** demands ongoing physician interaction to provide emotional support and palliation of pain and fear. Abandonment and lack of candor only increase suffering.

E. **Other issues affecting the physician–patient relationship**

1. Patients entering hospitals are now offered the option of completing a **living will,** which is an advance directive that no heroic measures will be taken to prolong a terminal state. It is essential that each patient understand that palliative care will be performed and that such directions can be rescinded at any time. Further, the physician must determine whether the patient is competent to sign such a directive. It is best for the patient's physician to discuss the concept of an advance directive before the patient is offered such an option. The living will does not permit physician-assisted euthanasia, but prevents actively implemented measures to sustain life.

2. The patient who requests **physician-assisted suicide** presents an extraordinary challenge.
   a. Physician-assisted suicide is defined as a physician intentionally and willfully helping a patient to end his life by overtly providing information on the lethality of drugs or by actually providing materials for termination of life. Koenig[5] reviewed the topic and noted that the following issues must be considered.
      (1) What constitutes intolerable suffering and intractable pain?
      (2) How terminal must an illness be?
      (3) How can we define the request as rational?
   b. A patient's depression or delirium may modify her understanding and ability to make rational decisions. Further, neurotic interactions with family members can lead to irrational choices to end life. Management of pain and suffering should be the first focus of the physician. Currently, there is a legal barrier to physician-assisted suicide. It is important for the physician to focus on pain management and to elucidate the patient's concerns, such as financial stress. Rather than aiding suicide, the appropriate role for the physician is taking the necessary steps to reduce suffering.

REFERENCES

1. Parsons T: *The Social System.* New York, Free Press, 1951.

2. Slavney PR, McHugh PR: *Psychiatric Polarities: Methodology and Practice.* Baltimore, Johns Hopkins University Press, 1987.

3. Balint M: *The Doctor, His Patient and the Illness.* London, Pitman, 1973.

4. Emanuel EJ, Emanuel LL: Four models of the physician–patient relationship. *JAMA* 267:2221–2226, 1992.

5. Koenig HG: Legalizing physician assisted suicide: Some thoughts and concerns. *J Fam Pract* 37:171–179, 1993.

BIBLIOGRAPHY

American Psychiatric Association: *Diagnostic and Statistical Manual of Mental Disorders,* 4th ed. Washington, DC, American Psychiatric Association, 1994.

Appelbaum PS, Grisso T: Assessing patients' capacities to consent to treatment. *N Engl J Med* 319:1635–1638, 1988.

Appelbaum PS: Legal liability and managed care. *Am Psychol* 48:251–257, 1993.

Balint M: *The Doctor, His Patient and the Illness.* London, Pitman, 1973.

Deblanco TL: Enriching the doctor–patient relationship by inviting the patient's perspective. *Ann Intern Med* 116:414–418, 1992.

Emanuel EJ, Emanuel LL: Four models of the physician–patient relationship. *JAMA* 267:2221–2226, 1992.

Ford CV: *The Somatizing Disorders: Illness as a Way of Life.* New York, Elsevier North Holland, 1983, pp 223–248.

Goldberg RJ, Novack DH: The psychosocial review of systems. *Soc Sci Med* 35:261–269, 1992.

Joos SK, Revler JB, Powell JL, et al: Outpatients' attitudes and understanding regarding living wills. *J Gen Intern Med* 8:259–263, 1993.

Kahana RL, Bibring GL: Personality types in medical management. In *Psychiatry and Medical Practice in a General Hospital.* Madison, CT, International Universities Press, 1964, pp 108–123.

Kleinman A, Sung LH: Why do indigenous practitioners successfully heal? *Soc Sci Med* 13B:7–26, 1979.

Koenig HG: Legalizing physician assisted suicide: Some thoughts and concerns. *J Fam Pract* 37:171–179, 1993.

Lipowski ZJ: Delirium (acute confusional states). *JAMA* 258:1789–1792, 1987.

Matthews DA, Suchman AL, Branch WT: Making "connexons": Enhancing the therapeutic potential of patient–clinician relationships. *Ann Intern Med* 118:973–977, 1993.

Parsons T: *The Social System.* New York, Free Press, 1951.

Schwenk TL, Romano SE: Managing the difficult physician–patient relationship. *Am Fam Physician* 46:1503–1509, 1992.

Slavney PR, McHugh PR: *Psychiatric Polarities: Methodology and Practice.* Baltimore, Johns Hopkins University Press, 1987.

Smith RC, Hoppe RB: The patient's story: Integrating the patient- and physician-centered approaches to interviewing. *Ann Intern Med* 115:470–477, 1991.

Starr P: *Social Transformation of American Medicine.* New York, Basic Books, 1983.

Szasz TS, Hollender MH: A contribution to the philosophy of medicine. *Arch Intern Med* 97:585–592, 1956.

Weisman AD: A model for psychosocial phasing in cancer. *Gen Hosp Psychiatry* 1:187–195, 1976.

Wise TN: Psychiatric management of patients who threaten to sign out against medical advice. *Int J Psychiatry Med* 5:153–160, 1974.

Wise TN: The emotional reactions of chronic illness. *Prim Care* 1:373–382, 1974.

Zinn W: The empathic physician. *Arch Intern Med* 153:306–312, 1993.

STUDY QUESTIONS

DIRECTIONS: Each of the numbered items or incomplete statements in this section is followed by answers or by completions of the statement. Select the ONE lettered answer or completion that is BEST in each case.

1. Which one of the following scenarios is an example of countertransference?

(A) A physician feels irritated when he is called in the middle of the night for a minor complaint, but he does not express his feelings
(B) A physician is very sad when a long-time patient is diagnosed with an inoperable brain tumor
(C) A physician is aware of his frustration when a diabetic patient does not comply with a diet and is readmitted to the hospital with ketoacidosis
(D) A physician angrily scolds his elderly female patient for complaining of chronic indigestion and fatigue

2. For physicians who understand their task to be the diagnosis and treatment of significant physical disease, which of the following patients would be perceived as being the most difficult?

(A) A somatizing patient
(B) An emphysematous person who continues to smoke
(C) A patient with senile dementia
(D) A patient who requests a second opinion
(E) Another physician

DIRECTIONS: Each of the numbered items or incomplete statements in this section is negatively phrased, as indicated by a capitalized word such as NOT, LEAST, or EXCEPT. Select the ONE lettered answer or completion that is BEST in each case.

3. All of the following foster ideal adherence to the sick role EXCEPT

(A) recognition that one is ill and in need of care
(B) a chronic, lingering illness with protracted malaise
(C) a supportive family, willing to take up the patient's responsibilities
(D) adequate financial resources to cope with an illness
(E) good physician–patient communication

4. All of the following are examples of transference responses EXCEPT

(A) a patient who fears that her physician will become too intimate
(B) a patient who sees another physician for a second opinion
(C) a patient who fears loss of control
(D) a patient who fears he will not be appreciated as a person who is suffering
(E) a patient who is excessively dependent on her physician

5. A 78-year-old man is hospitalized for nausea, vomiting, and anorexia. He is found to be jaundiced and to have an elevated serum ammonia level, and his electroencephalogram shows diffuse slowing. On the third hospital day, the patient says he wishes to leave the hospital and does not need any more treatment. All of the following would explain this patient's behavior EXCEPT

(A) he has a metabolic encephalopathy and is confused
(B) he is frightened about his surroundings
(C) he feels that the hospital he is in is not a good enough facility
(D) he wishes to die outside of a hospital setting
(E) he feels his situation is hopeless

6. All of the following are societal expectations of the sick role EXCEPT

(A) the obligation to get well
(B) functioning as usual until symptoms become severe
(C) exemption from usual social-role responsibilities
(D) the obligation to seek technically competent help
(E) exemption from blame for the illness

DIRECTIONS: The set of matching questions in this section consists of a list of four to twenty-six lettered options (some of which may be in figures) followed by several numbered items. For each numbered item, select the ONE lettered option that is most closely associated with it. To avoid spending too much time on matching sets with large numbers of options, it is generally advisable to begin each set by reading the list of options. Then, for each item in the set, try to generate the correct answer and locate it in the option list, rather than evaluating each option individually. Each lettered option may be selected once, more than once, or not at all.

Questions 7–10

Match each description with the psychosocial stage of cancer it best characterizes.

(A) Diagnosis
(B) Treatment
(C) Remission
(D) Recurrence
(E) Terminal phase

7. Period of short-term focus, when palliation of pain and patient support are paramount

8. Period during which denial may prevent proper management

9. Anxious waiting may cause emotional pain during this phase

10. Malaise, nausea, and vomiting may foster noncompliance

ANSWERS AND EXPLANATIONS

1. The answer is D [III B]. Countertransference is unconscious reaction of the physician to attributes in the patient that revivify feelings about early important figures in the physician's life. In this example, the physician may have been reacting to behaviors in the patient that reminded him of his own mother.

2. The answer is A [V A]. By definition, somatizing patients do not have a physiologic abnormality underlying their chronic complaints. Such patients are typically perceived as being especially difficult (i.e., frustrating and infuriating) by those physicians who have come to believe that their efforts, attention, and respect are merited only when significant physical disease is present or is likely to be so. In this narrow biomedical model of practice, the psychosocial aspects of the illness (e.g., the patient's personality) are ignored.

3. The answer is B [I A 2]. The sick role is best exemplified by a patient with an acute, time-limited illness. Chronic medical conditions that limit patient function, have ongoing debilitating symptoms, and require various treatments often stress not only the patient, but also her family and health care providers. Such chronic illness can foster depression and demoralization if return to premorbid functioning is not possible.

4. The answer is B [III A]. The transferential attitude of a patient can engender a variety of responses, depending on the patient's experience with important persons in her life or in previous medical experiences. It is the physician's duty to recognize indications of transference or countertransference and to maintain a reasonable balance in the context of a physician–patient relationship.

5. The answer is C [V B 2]. This patient is suffering from a hepatic encephalopathy, characterized by fluctuating levels of consciousness and documented by a diffusely abnormal electroencephalogram. His sense of hopelessness and confusion are part of the sensorial clouding and cognitive defects that characterize such a brain syndrome. Feeling that one is in an inferior hospital is not characteristic of someone in his mental state.

6. The answer is B [I A 2]. Sociologist Talcott Parsons has described four societal expectations that are basic to the sick role. These include the obligation to get well, the obligation to seek technically competent help, exemption from blame for the illness, and exemption from usual social-role responsibilities. The sick person is not expected to function as usual until his symptoms become severe.

7–10. The answers are: 7-E, 8-A, 9-C, 10-B [V D]. It is important for the physician to recognize the psychosocial stages that patients with neoplastic disease may experience, as the goals and difficulties of each phase differ. The diagnostic phase requires the physician's attention to possible patient denial of the disease and to ultimate acceptance of the need for treatment. The actual treatments of neoplastic disease often involve serious side effects (malaise, nausea, vomiting) that may promote noncompliance. The period of remission may involve anxious waiting for signs of the disease, which can lead to hypochondriacal complaints and lack of return to full functioning. Patients in the terminal phase of cancer need to be in a supportive setting without abandonment and should be provided with adequate palliation of pain and discomfort.

Chapter 12

Communication and Interviewing

Robert L. Hendren
James R. Phelps

I. INTRODUCTION

A. **Communication.** Research shows that the ways in which a physician communicates with a patient significantly affect:

1. The patient's **medical outcome** (e.g., diabetic control)

2. The patient's **adherence** to the treatment plan (e.g., continuing to take medication with unpleasant side effects)

3. The patient's **satisfaction** (e.g., the likelihood of a lawsuit in the event of poor clinical outcome)

4. The **quality of the data** gathered (e.g., accurate information about risk behavior)

5. The detection of **emotional disturbance** (e.g., recognizing underlying depression)

B. **Interviewing.** The interview is the most common procedure performed by physicians. It is a "rate-limiting step" toward a good patient outcome. Cohen-Cole and Bird propose that the interview has three functions: building rapport, gathering information, and patient education and treatment planning (See reference 1 for a complete explication of the "three-function" model).

II. RAPPORT-BUILDING SKILLS

A. **Responding to patients' emotions** is a crucial step in building rapport. Physicians sometimes concentrate on obtaining the information that they need and overlook the emotional aspects of patients' experience of their illness and of the interview itself.

1. **Learning more** about the emotion from the patient increases the physician's **understanding** of the issue. The **disclosure** process is often therapeutic for the patient as well. Some patients have difficult personality styles that interfere with this process (see IV B). Three methods for learning about the patient's emotions are:

   a. **Exploring** the emotion. The physician asks the patient to provide additional detail (e.g., "Could you stay with that thought for a moment and tell me more about it?")

   b. **Reflecting** what the patient says. The interviewer invites further comment nonverbally (e.g., "Your husband has not been very helpful around the house?").

   c. **Empressing empathy.** The physician offers the patient a label for his or her emotion. Disclosure can be helpful in itself, but accurately labeling feelings shows the patient that the physician truly understands what is disclosed. This understanding is also powerfully therapeutic. Empathy is a three-step process.

      (1) The first step is to **recognize the emotion** (e.g., anger, unhappiness, fear).

      (2) The second step is to choose a **label** that the patient can accept (e.g., confused, blue, frightened)

      (3) The third step is to offer the label as a **hypothesis**. Phrases such as "sounds like," "I wonder if," and "seems like you might be feeling" can be helpful. For example, the interviewer may say, "sounds like your husband's behavior sometimes makes you angry." Phrasing this message as a question (using an upward

inflection of voice) invites the patient to correct inaccurate guesses and conveys the physician's desire to understand the patient's concerns.

2. **Acknowledging the emotion** without asking the patient for further clarification may be necessary when time does not permit in-depth discussion. Because the following methods can interfere with the physician's ability to fully understand the patient's emotions, they should be used **only when time is limited**.
   a. **Support or partnership** is expressed through verbal and nonverbal indications of interest, concern, and willingness to help (e.g., "Arthritis can be difficult to handle, but we will work together on it and do all we can to get it under control").
   b. **Legitimization** indicates that the patient's experience is normal (e.g., "Most people worry about their ability to teach their children discipline").
   c. **Reassurance** tells the patient that her worries are not likely to be realized. However, this approach can be interpreted as dismissing the patient's concerns. This approach is common among physicians (e.g., "Don't worry; this won't hurt much").

B. **Positive regard** from care givers is an essential element in therapeutic relationships. The physician can demonstrate positive regard in a number of ways.

1. **Respect.** A physician shows respect for a patient by using the patient's last name (in some cases, this practice can be viewed as condescending, such as with adolescents); using easily understood language; avoiding medical jargon; arriving promptly for appointments; and apologizing when patients have to wait for long periods.

2. **Openness.** The physician should **avoid judging** the patient's behavior as good or bad, wise or foolish. The physician should find a way to approach the patient with the conviction that he is a good person worthy of the physician's full efforts. Some patients present a challenge in this regard.

C. **Active listening** shows the patient that she is being attended to closely.

1. **Nonverbal behavior.** The physician's posture should be attentive, yet relaxed. Research indicates that leaning forward slightly conveys interest. Because patterns of eye contact are culturally variable, the physician should follow the patient's pattern.

2. **Facilitating techniques** encourage the patient to provide greater detail.
   a. The physician may **repeat** the patient's last word, look **questioningly** at the patient, or ask a **direct question**.
   b. Research shows that an **encouraging utterance** (e.g., "mm-hmm") or a **nod** often leads the patient to provide more information.
   c. The physician can clarify a patient's concerns by **paraphrasing** the patient's words (e.g., "So, you're saying that your job is your biggest source of stress?").
   d. The physician can **summarize** the patient's words to verify that he is understood (e.g., "So, your sore throat started on Saturday, the fever started last night, and this morning you are having difficulty swallowing?").
   e. The physician can **request correction** with a slight inflection at the end of a statement or a direct question. In addition to ensuring accurate information, this practice shows that the physician recognizes the importance of understanding the patient correctly.

D. **The process of interviewing**

1. Beginning interviewers usually focus their attention on **content** (i.e., what to say next, what to ask next, what they need to know). With experience, this focus on what is said broadens to include how it is said, or the **process** of the interview.

2. **Process communication** is a form of emotional expression in which **unacknowledged or unspoken feelings** guide behavior.
   a. **Momentary anger** at a minor irritation may indicate underlying **fear or apprehension**. For example, a patient who becomes angry when her physician is late for an appointment may fear that the physician will not be available when she needs him.

b. Current concerns may be expressed by **recalling the past**. For instance, a patient who states, "I didn't like my last doctor; she never told me anything about my illness," may be requesting that his current physician share information with him.

c. Important messages may be contained in trivial remarks, asides, and casual jokes. The comments that a patient makes before or after the history is gathered are often revealing. For example, a patient who is leaving the office and comments, "Oh, by the way, doctor, could you speak to my husband? He is very concerned about me," may need additional explanation and reassurance about her illness.

d. Shifts in conversation away from or toward certain topics may occur. For example, during the interview, a middle-aged man with a recent myocardial infarction frequently mentions his athletic activities. His focus on this topic indicates his concern about his ability to be active in the future.

e. Body language often offers clues to a patient's concerns. A patient who repeatedly clenches and unclenches his fists while calmly discussing his reaction to an illness may have underlying concerns that he is reluctant to express.

f. Repetition of a topic indicates the importance of the topic to the patient.

g. Repeated requests for information may signal concern. For example, a patient who repeatedly asks for information about a recommended surgical procedure may fear that he will do poorly during surgery or the recovery period.

3. **Responding to the emotions expressed** in process communication is as important as responding to more overtly expressed feelings.

III. INFORMATION-GATHERING SKILLS

A. Agenda

1. The principle reason for the patient's visit should be determined. For **acute problems,** this reason is known as the **chief complaint**.

2. For **outpatients with complex medical histories,** it is often helpful to establish an agenda before addressing the first issue. An agenda can be established as follows:
   a. All of the issues that the patient would like addressed in this visit are identified.
   b. The patient's record is reviewed to identify medical problems that require follow-up.
   c. Health risk factors to address in this visit are selected based on the patient's age, sex, and ethnicity. Disease prevention issues such as smoking cessation should always be included unless raising such issues would conflict with addressing an acute symptom.
   d. The order in which these items are addressed is determined. Some issues may be addressed at a later visit.

B. History

1. **Open-ended questions** (i.e., questions that cannot be answered yes or no, such as "What brings you in today?") elicit the most information from patients.
   a. The first moments of information gathering determine whether the process will be led primarily by the doctor or the patient. In outpatient settings, a **patient-led process is associated with greater patient satisfaction**. In a patient-led process, the patient is allowed to "tell the story" of his or her chief complaint (e.g., chest pain). The physician gathers necessary information by encouraging the patient to provide further detail in critical areas (e.g., duration of pain, quality of pain).
   b. A patient-led process adds approximately 1 minute to office visits compared with physician-led interviews. In a **physician-led process,** the patient answers questions posed by the physician (e.g., Where do you feel the pain? How severe is the pain? How long have you felt it? Does it radiate anywhere? Do you have shortness of breath?)

2. **Interrupting the patient interferes with information gathering.** In one outpatient study, patients had an average of 18 seconds to respond to the physician's opening question before being interrupted. Moreover, after the interruption, the patients did not return to the concern that they were describing.

3. **Closed questions** (e.g., "Have you had a fever also?") may be used to fill in missing information.

4. The following **specific dimensions of a problem** provide helpful information:
   a. Location (e.g., midthoracic area)
   b. Duration and course (e.g., 1 week; steadily increasing)
   c. Quality (e.g., sharp pain)
   d. Quantity (e.g., 4 on a 1–10 relative scale)
   e. Radiation (e.g., spreads to shoulders)
   f. Aggravating factors (e.g., worse with coughing)
   g. Ameliorating factors (e.g., better with shallow respirations)
   h. Associated symptoms (e.g., muscle aches)

C. Structure

1. **Facilitating techniques** can be used to elicit additional information (see II C 2 a–e).

2. The inquiry can be **narrowed** by progressing from open questions to closed questions.
   a. Before a new area of inquiry is begun with an open-ended question (e.g., "What other ongoing medical problems do you have?"), the interviewer should **summarize** the previous point (e.g., "So, your throat has been bothering you for 3 days, with a fever beginning yesterday and difficulty swallowing since this morning").
   b. A clear nonverbal invitation for correction, or a verbal request, (e.g., "Have I got that right?") can be used to **verify** the accuracy of the summary.

D. It is important to determine the **patient's perspective** on this visit.

1. For acute care, the interviewer should determine why the patient came in today rather than yesterday or a month ago. The interviewer should also identify the **patient's hypotheses** about possible causes or diagnoses.

2. For ongoing care, the interviewer should identify the patient's **primary health concerns**.
   a. These concerns should be reflected in the agenda, but patients do not always volunteer their greatest fears during the agenda-setting process.
   b. If the patient has no specific concerns, the interviewer should review the patient's awareness of health risk factors.

IV. PATIENT EDUCATION AND TREATMENT PLANNING SKILLS

A. Collaboration. A collaborative approach involves the patient as an active participant. A weakness of current medical care is physicians' inattention to patients' low adherence rates. Treatment efficacy is dramatically increased when physicians take the following steps.

1. The **patient's perspective** on treatment should be determined (e.g., What is her understanding of the diagnosis? What information does she need to understand the diagnosis and its implications? What ideas, requests, or concerns does she have about treatment?).

2. **Treatment options.** Offering a single treatment approach increases the risk of low adherence. The physician should enlist the patient's help in identifying possible approaches (e.g., a diabetic patient can be asked to identify strategies for reducing her consumption of refined carbohydrates).

3. **Selecting a treatment option.** The physician should help the patient to choose among the options by helping him to identify the advantages and disadvantages of each approach, and how to weigh them; offering her own opinion only cautiously; and conveying the idea that the patient is the best person to select the treatment because he must carry it out.

4. **Barriers to adherence**
   a. One of the most useful steps that a physician can take to increase adherence is to ask "What could get in the way of carrying out this plan?".
   b. Barriers to adherence are varied and are often overlooked by the physician. They include finances, lack of time, and motivational issues.

5. **The best approach to patient education and treatment planning is asking, not telling, the patient how to proceed.**

B. **Motivation.** Increasing or maintaining patient motivation for treatment is a physician's responsibility. Most common major illnesses (e.g., diabetes, heart disease, cancer) are associated with health-related behaviors. Physician interventions can motivate patients to change potentially harmful behaviors (e.g., smoking, remaining sedentary, engaging in unprotected sex).

1. **Change in health-related behavior proceeds in stages** (See reference 2 for more on the "stages of change" model).
   a. Patients in the **later stages** of change (i.e., determination, action, maintenance) may be helped by **instruction in techniques** for behavior change. For example, a smoker who is determined to quit may be helped by learning strategies to control the weight gain that often accompanies smoking cessation.
   b. Patients in the **early stages** of change (i.e., precontemplation, contemplation) need **motivation,** not instruction in technique.

2. Research data indicate that **physician style influences** the **willingness of patients to consider change**.
   a. An aggressive, authoritarian, confrontational style is associated with **resistance to change**.
   b. A nonjudgmental, empathic approach is associated with **openness to change**.

3. **Avoiding arguments and expressing empathy are central elements in effective motivational interviewing** (See reference 3 for more information on motivational techniques).

V. COMPONENTS OF THE MEDICAL HISTORY

A. **Different settings require different approaches** to history taking. Table 12-1 outlines the elements of a traditional inpatient history, a risk-oriented history, and a practical outpatient history.

B. **Choosing an appropriate format.** The formats shown in Table 12-1 and additional variations are helpful in different circumstances. The model is chosen according to the context, including supervisor requirements. The style of presentation (e.g., detailed description versus outline) varies similarly.

C. **Components of each category**

1. **Patient identification** includes the patient's name, age, sex, ethnicity, marital status, and occupation.

2. **Chief complaint.** The patient's reason for seeking care is stated briefly, in the patient's own words.

TABLE 12-1. Three Versions of a Medical History

Traditional Approach	Risk-oriented Approach[4]	Practical Outpatient Approach
Identifying data	Identifying data	Identifying data
Chief complaint	Chief complaint	Past problem list
History of current illness	History of illness	Today's agenda
Medical history	Risk factor assessment*	History: agenda item 1
Family history	Fixed risks*	History: agenda item 2
Social history	Demographic risks: age, sex, ethnicity*	Brief medical history
Review of systems	Genetic risks*	Social history
Physical examination findings	Acquired risks*	Living situation
Laboratory tests	Environmental risks: exposure, travel*	Primary relationships
Problem list	Lifestyle/behavioral risks: substance use, sedentary lifestyle, sexual practices*	Work situation
Assessment and plan	Health maintenance habits: immunizations, disease detection*	Pertinent physical examination findings
	Disease-associated risks: illnesses*	Assessment by agenda item
	Treatment-associated risks: surgery, medications, allergies*	Plan
	Medications: prescribed, over-the-counter*	
	Social history	
	Review of systems	
	Physical examination findings	
	Laboratory tests	
	Problem list	
	Assessment and plan	

*Difference from traditional approach.

3. **History of current illness** is the most important part of the clinical history. The following information is obtained.
   a. The **last symptom-free period** (e.g., "patient was well until 3 weeks ago, when . . .")
   b. The **initial symptoms and course**
   c. **Review of symptoms for the relevant organ systems,** with pertinent negative findings noted. For example, for a patient with abdominal pain, gastrointestinal symptoms, changes in bowel function, urinary tract symptoms and function, and genitourinary symptoms and findings are reviewed. Findings that confirm or exclude likely diagnoses are noted.
   d. **Risk factors** that might predispose the patient to specific diagnoses

4. Requirements for a past medical history vary considerably according to the context.
   a. A **basic outpatient past medical history** includes the following elements:
      (1) Ongoing health problems
      (2) Medications
      (3) Risk factor evaluation (e.g., Do you smoke? How much alcohol do you consume? Do you know your cholesterol level?)
   b. A **more detailed outpatient history** includes additional risk factors (e.g., noting any depression or anxiety, noting the amount of physical activity, noting preventive health practices). **Other elements** of the past history are gathered as needed (e.g., childhood illnesses, surgery, mental health care).

   c. For **inpatients,** an inventory of hospitalizations, surgeries, and medical problems is usually included in this section of the history.

   d. **A risk-oriented format** for the past medical history helps to organize the information in a way that is useful for diagnosis and preventive care (see Table 12-1).

5. Family history is shown efficiently with a genogram (Figure 12-1).

   a. The **structure of the patient's family** (e.g., number of siblings, number of children, members of the patient's immediate family unit) is shown easily. Patients often enjoy helping to construct this diagram.

   b. The **immediate family unit** (i.e., those who live together) is circled.

   c. If time permits, the **cause of death and age at death** for each immediate relative are listed.

   d. **Family risk history** is shown by noting illnesses with known genetic risk (e.g., heart disease, cancer, substance abuse). The physician should inquire about the illnesses that the patient's problems suggest are pertinent. It is not necessary to inventory all common diseases.

6. Social history often provides the key to understanding an episode of illness. Studies indicate that more than 50% of outpatient visits are caused by or complicated by emotional disturbance.

   a. The **three variables that are most commonly involved** in emotional disturbance should be examined routinely for inpatients. For outpatients, these variables should be examined when time permits or when emotional factors affect the illness (more than 50% of cases). These variables include:

    (1) Home situation, especially relationships with those in the home

    (2) Family constellation, especially first-degree relatives, whether nearby or distant

    (3) Work situation, including unemployment, job-related stress, relationships with superiors, and personal or family finances

   b. **Other variables** to consider, depending on the patient's symptoms and on time constraints, include:

    (1) Social network (e.g., friends, religious affiliation or involvement, social activities)

    (2) Typical activities (e.g., hobbies)

    (3) Recent losses (e.g., illness or death in the family)

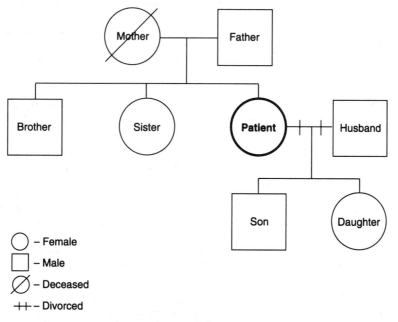

FIGURE 12-1. Sample genogram. This genogram depicts a female patient and her first-degree relatives: deceased mother, living father, living brother, living sister, living son and daughter; and ex-husband.

7. The **review of systems** can be used to obtain a **complete inventory** of the patient's symptoms. Most clinicians use this inventory to assist with complex diagnostic problems in the inpatient context. For outpatients, it is used selectively (see V C 3).

VI. VARIATIONS IN TECHNIQUE

A. **Age and developmental level.** Communication with children, adolescents, and older people may be improved with modifications in interviewing style.

1. **Children.** The interview with a child requires modifications based on the child's **use and understanding of language**.
   a. **Children usually respond to a patient, nurturing physician** who understands their methods of communication.
   b. **Play and fantasy** may help to establish rapport so that the child can speak comfortably.
   c. **Illness and hospitalization are often frightening to children** and cause concern about separation from family members.

2. **Adolescents usually respond best to clearly stated questions that are asked directly and simply** after initial rapport is established.
   a. The physician should approach the adolescent in a **warm, respectful manner** that is not condescending or overly familiar. The use of teen slang or age-inappropriate comments is not usually effective in building rapport.
   b. Many adolescents become less responsive when asked a number of indirect and open-ended questions. Direct questions usually yield the most information on sensitive topics, such as sexual issues or substance abuse.
   c. Many **adolescents fear that illness and hospitalization will limit their ability to engage in normal adolescent relationships and activities**.

3. **Elderly people** usually respond best to an interviewer who conveys a **sincere interest**. It is important for the interviewer to be **patient and gentle** as the older person describes his life and his concerns about bodily functions.
   a. Direct questions about sensitive issues are best asked later in the interview, after rapport and trust are established.
   b. **Illness and hospitalization cause concerns about separation from and loss of significant others.**

B. **Personality type.** Physicians encounter patients with different personality styles and characteristic defense mechanisms. The following suggestions can help physicians who encounter some of these personality styles.

1. **Dependent.** The physician who cares for dependent, demanding patients should:
   a. **Convey enthusiasm about caring for the patient.** Failure to do so may aggravate dependent or demanding behavior.
   b. **Set limits when necessary,** but not as an expression of impatience or anger. For example, refusing to increase pain medication following the patient's repeated demands is accepted more readily if the physician is not abrupt or critical of the patient's demands.
   c. **Interact directly and openly** to avoid passive-aggressive power struggles.
   d. **Avoid direct confrontation** by turning the responsibility for the patient's behavior back to him.

2. **Controlling.** The physician who cares for orderly, controlling patients should:
   a. **Inform the patient** methodically and in sufficient detail about her illness and treatment. Providing adequate detail helps the patient to establish intellectual control over her anxiety.

    b. Include the patient as much as possible **in decision making and** in **management** of her medical care.

    c. Acknowledge and encourage the patient's stengths to help build feelings of greater control.

3. **Dramatizing.** The physician who cares for dramatizing, emotional patients should:

    a. Compliment appropriately without misleading the patient; these individuals need reassurance that they are attractive and desirable.

    b. Discourage the patient's emotional involvement, and proceed calmly and firmly.

    c. Offer reassuring explanations about the illness and medical procedures to help the patient to distinguish reality from alarming fantasies.

    d. Allow the patient to discuss fears freely so that pent-up emotions can be discharged.

4. **Self-sacrificing.** The physician who cares for long-suffering, self-sacrificing patients should:

    a. Overcome the tendency to avoid these patients and thus intensify their behavior.

    b. Remain nonjudgmental, but do not reinforce the **sick role**.

    c. Offer support and guidance to family members. These relatives can often provide accurate information.

    d. Establish gentle, firm limits of interaction because the patient may become reliant on the physician.

5. **Suspicious.** The physician who cares for guarded, suspicious patients should:

    a. Inform these patients as fully as possible of diagnostic procedures and treatment to reduce suspicion.

    b. Adopt a formal, courteous attitude that precludes becoming too closely involved.

    c. Acknowledge the patient's suspicions without reinforcing them.

6. **Superior.** The physician who cares for **patients who perceive themselves as superior,** or special, should:

    a. Help the patient to feel comfortable by implicitly **acknowledging her as a person of worth**.

    b. Affirm his own expertise, especially when challenged by the patient. The patient needs assurance that she is receiving competent care.

7. **Reclusive.** The physician who cares for aloof, reclusive patients should:

    a. Respect the patient's need for privacy and distance, but not allow him to withdraw excessively.

    b. Approach the patient with **considerate interest and quiet reassurance,** without expecting a reciprocal response.

8. **Impulsive.** The physician who cares for impulsive patients should:

    a. Set firm limits before beginning treatment in an attempt to control impulsive behavior.

    b. Avoid open confrontations that are likely to lead to angry words and actions.

    c. Hold the patient responsible for his impulsive actions.

C. Assessing cultural factors within a health history[5]

1. The physician should **demonstrate respect** for individual cultural differences and stengths by listening to the patient carefully, asking questions, and modifying the management plan when appropriate.

2. The physician should **accommodate cultural differences** in communication (e.g., etiquette, emotional expression, taboo topics).

3. **Assessment** should include:

    a. Ethnic origin and identification

    b. Language preference

    c. Family structure and dynamics

    d. Cultural health beliefs and practices

    e. Socioeconomic influences

REFERENCES

1. Cohen-Cole S, Bird J: *The Medical Interview: The Three-Function Approach.* St Louis, Mosby-Year Book, 1991.

2. Lipkin M, Putnam S, Lazare A (eds): *The Medical Interview: A Textbook on Medical Interviewing.* New York, Springer-Verlag. In press, 1994.

3. Miller W, Rollnick S: *Motivational Interviewing.* New York, Guilford, 1991.

4. Sheagren JN, Sweifler AJ, Woolliscroft JO: The present medical database needs reorganization: it's time for a change. *Arch Intern Med* 1990; 150(10): 2014–2015.

5. Davis BJ, Voegtle KH: Culturally Competent Health Care for Adolescents. Chicago, American Medical Association, 1994.

▮ STUDY QUESTIONS

DIRECTIONS: Each of the numbered items or incomplete statements in this section is followed by answers or by completions of the statement. Select the ONE lettered answer or completion that is BEST in each case.

1. Certain techniques for gathering information from and communicating with patients are used frequently, whereas others are used infrequently. Which one of the following techniques should be used only when time is limited?

(A) Open-ended questions
(B) Summation
(C) Early reassurance
(D) Reflection
(E) Learning more about an emotion

2. An apprehensive patient expresses concern to her physician about the pain that may be involved in a bone marrow biopsy that he recommends for diagnostic evaluation. The physician interrupts the patient and quickly reassures her that there will be little pain. He then carefully explains the procedure to her. The patient asks no more questions, but before the procedure, the physician is surprised to find the patient tearful and shaky. What is the most likely reason that the physician's reassurance was not sufficient?

(A) The physician did not explain the procedure adequately
(B) The patient cannot tolerate anxiety
(C) The patient is overly demanding
(D) The physician did not allow the patient to fully express her concerns about the procedure
(E) The physician is unconcerned about the patient

3. Which technique of communication is likely to be the most effective in gathering a thorough history from an adolescent patient?

(A) Exclusive use of open-ended questions
(B) Direct questions about the adolescent
(C) Silence until the adolescent feels like talking
(D) Early expression of sympathy
(E) Confrontation of inconsistencies and contradictions in the history as they appear

4. A 78-year-old man is admitted to the hospital for a transurethral resection of his prostate gland. Initially, the staff finds him engaging and solicitous, but after his surgery, he becomes increasingly demanding and complains that the nurses and the attending physician are ignoring him. How can this problem be addressed?

(A) Point out the fallacy of the accusations
(B) Confront the patient's excessive demands
(C) Inform the patient of times that the physician will visit and times that the nurses will respond to reasonable requests
(D) Respect the patient's need for privacy and decrease the frequency of visits
(E) Suggest to the nursing staff that they avoid the patient to decrease the patient's dependency needs and thus decrease his unreasonable demands

Questions 5–6

A fourth-year medical student is assigned to obtain a history from and to examine a 55-year-old accountant who has a recent history of substernal chest pain on exertion because of myocardial ischemia. During the interview, the patient is controlling and provides excessive detail, making it difficult for the student to gather a complete history in the 45 minutes he has available before a required lecture by the attending physician. The frustrated student interrupts the patient and tells him that he must stop the interview. The patient becomes angry and begins to shout at the student.

5. Which approach is most likely to be successful?

(A) Leaving the room because rapport is unlikely to be reestablished
(B) Explaining respectfully to the patient that he has an unavoidable conflict and state when he will return to complete the history
(C) Spending the next hour completing the history, even though he will miss the lecture
(D) Confronting the patient's unreasonable demands
(E) Explaining the tribulations of being a medical student

6. When the student attempts to complete the interview, he finds the patient withdrawn and tense. How can the student reengage the patient in the interview?

(A) Confront the patient's withdrawn behavior as a sign of hurt feelings
(B) Encourage the patient to discuss his feelings about the seriousness of his heart disease
(C) Interpret the patient's anger as a sign of his controlling personality
(D) Encourage the patient to speak about his feelings regarding the abrupt termination of the interview
(E) Inform the patient that he will return later when the patient feels more like talking

7. A 36-year-old married woman enters the hospital for diagnostic tests. She is excessively friendly and complains that her physician does not pay enough attention to her. What is the physician's most effective response?

(A) Withdraw to keep the boundaries of the professional relationship clear
(B) Confront her excessive dependency
(C) Allow her to express her fears
(D) Transfer her to another member of the house staff to avoid excessive involvement
(E) Spend extra time with her to assure her that she is receiving appropriate care

8. A 42-year-old homeless man comes to a university hospital emergency room with sores on his legs and feet that do not heal. The physician assigned to interview the patient finds him reserved and suspicious of the emergency room staff. Which approach is likely to be helpful?

(A) Greeting the patient in an outgoing manner and reassuring him with a friendly pat on the shoulder
(B) Informing the patient as fully as possible of the purpose of the interview and the procedures that will take place
(C) Informing the patient that he can obtain better care at the outpatient clinic and that he should schedule an appointment there because he is not in need of emergency service
(D) Inform the patient that unless he cooperates he will not be able to get help and must leave
(E) Help the patient to label his feelings by pointing out that he is suspicious and paranoid

9. A 54-year-old night watchman is admitted to the hospital for evaluation of a chronic cough and a lung mass that is suspected to be cancerous. The patient is a loner who has no friends or family. How can the physician help this aloof, reclusive patient to feel comfortable in the hospital?

(A) Allow him to seclude himself in his room with few outside interruptions
(B) Not be offended if he does not respond to expressions of interest
(C) Encourage him to discuss his loneliness
(D) Occasionally stop by his room
(E) Consistently encourage him to identify and express his feelings

DIRECTIONS: Each of the numbered items or incomplete statements in this section is negatively phrased, as indicated by a capitalized word such as NOT, LEAST, or EXCEPT. Select the ONE lettered answer or completion that is BEST in each case.

10. What is the LEAST important component of empathy?

(A) Recognition of another's emotion
(B) Rapid reassurance of another's concern
(C) Acknowledging another's emotion
(D) Labeling another's emotion
(E) Checking one's perception of another's feelings

11. Active listening is described by all of the following techniques EXCEPT

(A) paying attention to nonverbal signals
(B) repeating the last word or phrase
(C) offering summaries
(D) controlling the interview with active guidance
(E) requesting correction and clarification

ANSWERS AND EXPLANATIONS

1. The answer is C [II A 2]. Open-ended questions, summation, reflection, and clarification are nonintrusive methods of gathering information from a patient. They do not imply undue familiarity and are not likely to cause a defensive or guarded response from the patient. Reassurance, when offered before exploration, empathy, and reflection, may not allow the patient to express his emotion, which is usually beneficial.

2. The answer is D [II A; III B 2]. The physician did not allow the patient to express her concerns about the procedure. Thus, his careful explanation of the procedure occurred before her anxiety decreased enough for her to listen fully. Her response is not unusual, and there is no clear indication that she cannot tolerate anxiety or is overly demanding. It is not clear that the physician is unconcerned about the patient, but his response did not address the patient's concerns.

3. The answer is B [VI A 2 a–b]. Adolescents usually respond best to clearly stated questions that are asked directly and simply. Indirect and open-ended questions and the use of silence often do not engage an adolescent. Early expressions of sympathy can appear insincere and condescending, and confrontation often leads to power struggles.

4. The answer is C [VI B 1]. Dependent, demanding patients fear that others will reject them and frequently test the limits of this fear. Challenging or confronting this patient or decreasing the frequency of visits will likely be regarded as a rejection, and may result in regression and further demands. Setting reasonable limits on his behavior and providing consistent, predictable contacts are likely to be effective in controlling his demanding behavior and improving his relationship with the staff.

5. The answer is B [II A 2; VI B 2]. The patient fears losing control and needs to feel respected. He also needs to feel that his physician knows how to be in control of himself. Leaving the room abruptly does not reflect respect for the patient, and staying in the room does not indicate that the student is in control of what he is doing. An apology that acknowledges the lack of respect for the patient's feelings and a brief explanation of the circumstances are most likely to leave the patient feeling that he is respected.

6. The answer is D [II A 2; VI B 2]. Confrontation, empathy that misses the point, interpretation, and avoidance probably represent the student's uncomfortable feelings and will further alienate the patient. Acknowledging the awkwardness of the situation and encouraging and accepting open expression of the patient's feelings are the responses that are most likely to reestablish rapport.

7. The answer is C [VI B 3]. Dramatizing, emotional patients often require reassurance to help them to distinguish reality from alarming fantasies. They also need to express their fears to discharge pent-up emotions. However, they may become overly involved emotionally and are best approached calmly and firmly. Withdrawing from the patient or transferring her to another staff member will probably leave her feeling rejected and unattractive, and may aggravate her behavior.

8. The answer is B [VI B 5]. Suspicious and reclusive patients have difficulty trusting others and are best approached with considerate interest and quiet reassurance. They should be informed as fully as possible of diagnostic procedures to reduce suspicion. An overly friendly manner is likely to cause the patient to withdraw. Referral to another facility may be perceived as rejection, especially if it is done quickly, and would decrease the likelihood that the patient would seek help. Threats and confrontation are not likely to be effective.

9. The answer is B [VI B 7]. The aloof, reclusive individual does not want intrusions. This wish should be respected, but the patient should not be allowed to withdraw completely. The physician should approach the patient with considerate interest and quiet reassurance, but should not expect the patient to reciprocate. Trying to obtain an emotional reaction from these patients often upsets their deep-seated defensive structure and may result in a worsening of the physician–patient relationship. Scheduled visits are less disruptive to solitude than are unscheduled visits.

10. The answer is B [II A 1 c]. Accurately recognizing the emotions of another is an important component of empathy. It also involves letting the patient know of the physician's understanding and helping her to recognize the emotion in herself. Reassurance, especially if it is given too quickly, may not be accurate and may not allow the patient to recognize her own emotions and to feel that the physician is genuinely interested.

11. The answer is D [II C 1–2]. Active listening demonstrates close attention to the patient by observing nonverbal behavior, repeating the patient's last comment in a questioning manner, summarizing what the patient says, and seeking correction and clarification. Active listening does not mean active direction of the interview, although active guidance may become necessary later in the interview.

Chapter 13

The Mental Status Examination

Joan K. Barber

I. **INTRODUCTION.** The mental status examination is a systematic method for evaluating a patient's behavioral, emotional, and cognitive processes. It involves observation (e.g., of behavior and facial expression), questioning (e.g., of thought content), and testing (e.g., of memory). The mental status examination should be used, as appropriate, **in conjunction with a complete medical and psychiatric history** (including medication and drug use), a complete physical examination (including details of autonomic activity), a neurologic examination, and laboratory tests and x-rays. The *Diagnostic and Statistical Manual of Mental Disorders,* 4th edition (DSM-IV), attributes many psychiatric syndromes to general medical conditions. A bedside or office mental status examination can help to prevent misdiagnosis. Many psychological testing situations require standardized and replicable conditions (see Chapter 14). In contrast, the mental status examination is often administered under difficult conditions (e.g., a noisy emergency room, a crowded room with a television set blaring). When this problem occurs, important sections of the examination can be readministered in a more favorable setting. A standard form is used to score the examination (Figure 13-1).

II. **APPLICATIONS.** Although some information regarding a patient's mental status is gathered during every clinical contact (e.g., facial expression, level of consciousness, ability to answer questions), at times a complete and systematic evaluation is indicated, as in the following situations.

A. It establishes a **baseline level of performance** and permits the clinician to follow the progress of a patient with acute or fluctuating changes in mental state.

B. It aids in **assessment of psychiatric patients with acute onset of symptoms.**

C. It helps to **distinguish among psychotic syndromes** that have many symptoms in common.

D. It also **provides information that is helpful for monitoring the course of high-risk patients,** such as:

1. The elderly
2. Patients taking drugs with central nervous system (CNS) effects
3. Patients with metabolic and endocrine disorders
4. Those in the intensive care unit (ICU) and those who are postsurgery
5. Patients with head trauma
6. Anoxic patients
7. Malnourished patients
8. Patients with structural brain disease

Mental Status Examination Score Sheet

Check or circle appropriate answer
0 = normal   1 = mild to moderate impairment   2 = severe impairment

I. Level of consciousness

Alert	yes ___	no ___			
Lethargic (somnolent)	yes ___	no ___			
Stuporous	yes ___	no ___			
Comatose	yes ___	no ___			
Fluctuating	yes ___	no ___			

Inappropriate to

verbal content	0	1	2
Fearful	0	1	2
Anxious	0	1	2

E. Interview behavior

Cooperative	yes ___	no ___		
Angry outbursts	0	1	2	
Impulsive	0	1	2	
Irritable	0	1	2	
Passive	0	1	2	
Demanding	0	1	2	
Negativistic	0	1	2	
Evasive	0	1	2	
Apathetic	0	1	2	
Withdrawn	0	1	2	
Silly	0	1	2	
Helpless	0	1	2	
Unconcerned	0	1	2	
Euphoric	0	1	2	

II. Attention, vigilance

A. Clinical assessment

Attention	0	1	2
Concentration	0	1	2

B. Formal testing
  Digits forward ___
  Digits backward ___
  Continuous
    performance test   0   1   2

III. Behavioral observations

A. Appearance

Clothing	0	1	2
Grooming	0	1	2

B. Motor activity

Increased	0	1	2
Decreased	0	1	2
Tics	0	1	2
Repetitive acts	0	1	2
Other (specify)	0	1	2

C. Facial expression

Angry	0	1	2
Happy	0	1	2
Sad	0	1	2
Anxious	0	1	2
Inappropriate to verbal content	0	1	2

D. Mood/affect

Angry	0	1	2
Sad	0	1	2
Apathetic	0	1	2
Fluctuating	0	1	2
Happy	0	1	2

IV. Speech, language, thought, memory

A. Handedness   L ___   R ___   mixed ___

B. Language comprehension

Oral	0	1	2
Reading	0	1	2

C. Spontaneous speech

Rate increased	0	1	2
Rate decreased	0	1	2
Muteness	0	1	2
Dysarthria	0	1	2
Dysprosody	0	1	2
Aphasia	0	1	2

D. Writing

Dictation	0	1	2
Self-originated	0	1	2
Dyspraxia	0	1	2

E. Thought
  1. Form

Reduced content	0	1	2
Incomplete sentences	0	1	2

FIGURE 13-1. Standard form for scoring the mental status examination.

Mental Status Examination Score Sheet (continued)

Circumstantiality	0	1	2
Derailment	0	1	2
Tangentiality	0	1	2
Flight of ideas	0	1	2
Clang associations	0	1	2
Confabulation	0	1	2
Neologisms	0	1	2
Echolalia	0	1	2
Perseveration	0	1	2
Word salad	0	1	2

2. Content

Illusions	0	1	2
Delusions	0	1	2
Hallucinations			
Auditory	0	1	2
Visual	0	1	2
Olfactory	0	1	2
Tactile	0	1	2
Assaultive thoughts	0	1	2
Homicidal ideas	0	1	2
Homicidal plans	0	1	2
Feelings of			
hopelessness	0	1	2
Feelings of			
worthlessness	0	1	2
Feelings of guilt	0	1	2
Suicidal thoughts	0	1	2
Suicidal plans	0	1	2
Obsessions	0	1	2
Phobias	0	1	2
Sexual themes	0	1	2
Somatic			
preoccupations	0	1	2
Religiosity	0	1	2

F. Memory

Sensorium—orientation to:

Time	yes ___	no ___
Place	yes ___	no ___
Situation	yes ___	no ___
Person	yes ___	no ___

Short-term memory

Recall of last few days	0	1	2
Four words	0	1	2
Retelling story	0	1	2

Remote memory

Details of medical history	0	1	2
Significant anniversaries/birthdays	0	1	2
Naming of presidents in patient's lifetime	0	1	2

V. Problem solving, learned material

Constructional ability	0	1	2
Calculations	0	1	2
Fund of information	0	1	2

VI. Abstract thinking, conceptual ability

Judgment and insight

Similarities	0	1	2
Proverbs	0	1	2
Abstract thinking	0	1	2
Conceptual ability	0	1	2
Insight	0	1	2
Understand need for hospitalization	0	1	2
Understand degree of illness	0	1	2
Understand need for help	0	1	2
Judgment	0	1	2

VII. Summary of positive findings

1. History

    Mental status examination

    Physical examination

    Neurologic examination

    Laboratory

2. Formulation

VIII. Differential diagnosis

Axis I   _____

Axis II   _____

Axis III _____

Axis IV _____

Axis V   _____

III. STRUCTURE OF THE EXAMINATION

A. **Neuropsychological hierarchy.** While the components of the mental status examination are fairly standardized, the way in which they are presented is not. The mental status examination organization used in this chapter is based on a neuropsychological hierarchy. It follows a **staircase, or ladder, model,** which proceeds from **lowest (consciousness) to highest (abstractions, insight, and judgment) function**. The areas of the brain that are involved with specific functions are shown in Figure 13-2.

B. **Hierarchical approach and diagnosis.** This hierarchical approach can help the clinician narrow the differential diagnosis, since, for many mental disorders, the symptoms tend to cluster a particular "level." **Dysfunction at lower levels of brain function interferes with functions at higher levels.**

    1. For example, a patient with delirium with a fluctuating level of consciousness and poor attentional ability (levels I and II; see Figure 13-1) also may show deficits in higher areas (e.g., short-term memory loss, delusions, hallucinations, and poor judgment).

    2. Similarly, a patient with language and communication problems (level IV; see Figure 13-1) may also show reduced reasoning capacity and judgment (level VI; see Figure 13-1).

IV. COMPONENTS OF THE EXAMINATION. All of the DSM-IV diagnoses discussed in this chapter are described more fully in Chapter 15.

A. **Level I: consciousness**

    1. **The brain site affected** is the pontine and midbrain **reticular activating system (RAS;** see Chapter 2 C 3 a–b).

    2. **Reduced consciousness has a metabolic cause** in 70% of cases and is caused by subtentorial lesions in 12% of cases. Rarely, widespread cortical damage occurs (e.g., as a result of carbon monoxide poisoning). A reduced level of consciousness is **rarely** seen in mental disorders other than delirium, intoxication, and withdrawal.

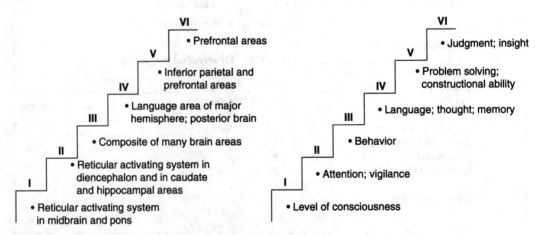

FIGURE 13-2. The mental status examination schema is ranked upward from the lowest (arousal) to the highest (executive) level of mental functioning. *Roman numerals* refer to numbered sections on the score sheet. Behavior (*level III*) is a composite of many brain areas, including the limbic system, striatum, and frontal areas.

3. **Assessment** involves clinical evaluation only. The patient's mental state is evaluated according to the following criteria.
   a. **Alert.** The patient is awake, aware, interacting, and responsive to stimuli. This state is **not** the same as being attentive.
   b. **Lethargic.** The patient can be roused but does not maintain arousal.
   c. **Stuporous.** The patient can be roused slightly with intense stimulation.
   d. **Comatose.** The patient cannot be roused, even with painful stimuli.
   e. **Fluctuating.** The patient's mental state varies during the course of the day.

B. **Level II: attention and vigilance** (Figure 13-3). **Attention is the capacity to focus on a single stimulus** and to screen our irrelevant stimuli. **Vigilance (concentration) is the ability to focus attention over an extended period.**

1. **Brain sites** that are affected include the RAS, the RAS–thalamic projection system, the reticulocortical and corticoreticular connections, and the RAS hippocampal and caudate areas. The development of these areas is complete at puberty.

2. **Causes of reduced concentration** include metabolic disorders, intoxication, withdrawal syndromes, infections, hypoxia, postoperative states, electrolyte imbalance, attention deficit disorders, severe depression, preoccupation with hallucinatory experiences, and severe anxiety.

3. **Assessment.** Clinical assessment consists of observing the patient's ability to be task oriented while the history is obtained and the examination is conducted. The patient is considered distracted if his attention shifts from one stimulus to another.
   a. **Digit span (forward and reversed) measures attention of less than a 10-second duration.**
      (1) The examiner should intone the numbers, without inflection, at a rate of approximately one per second. Numbers should be read from a prepared list to ensure smooth delivery of difficult sequences. Figure 13-4 shows a typical list of numbers.
      (2) The same numbers may be used for digits reversed. For this test, the patient is asked to reverse the sequence of the numbers that are read aloud. The ability to reverse digits requires more concentration than forward repetition. Patients who perform poorly on this test usually also do poorly on vigilance or continuous performance testing (CPT; see IV B 3 b).
      (3) If this test is repeated to evaluate a patient's clinical progress, the numbers should be changed daily.
   b. **Auditory vigilance** is measured by CPT. This test **measures concentration of approximately 1-minute duration**.
      (1) The patient is asked to tap with a finger or a pencil whenever an A is read aloud from a list of letters. The examiner should read the letters aloud, with an

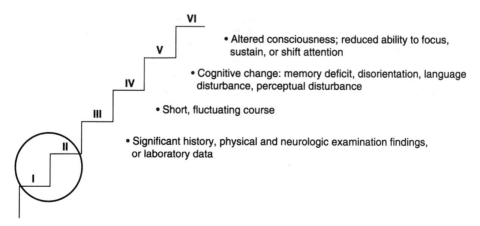

FIGURE 13-3. Delirium. The *circle* shows the primary area of dysfunction.

37
416
5318
26593
614783
9362514

FIGURE 13-4. A typical list of numbers for the digit span test appears left. A normal score for adults is six digits forward and five digits reversed. A normal score for elderly patients is five digits forward and three to four digits reversed.

uninflected and monotonous delivery, at a rate of approximately one letter per second. Figure 13-5 shows a typical list of letters.

   (2) Scoring. A normal adult usually makes no errors on this test.

C. **Level III: behavior** (Figures 13-6, 13-7, 13-8)

1. **Brain sites.** Behavior has roots in many cortical and subcortical areas (e.g., limbic system, prefrontal area, caudate area).

2. **Clinical assessment.** Observations of a patient's mood, facial expression, clothing, and ability to relate to the examiner are usually helpful in establishing a diagnosis. Observations are clustered into **appearance, motor activity, facial expression, mood and affect,** and **interview behavior**.

   a. **Appearance.** Observations about appearance and grooming are helpful in the diagnosis of almost all clinical syndromes. Notable features include the sometimes bizarre dress of patients with schizophrenia and mania, the seductive dress of patients with histrionic personality disorder, and the soiled and stained clothing of demented and intoxicated patients.

   b. **Motor activity**
      (1) Increased motor activity is seen in patients with agitated depression, mania, some attention deficit disorders, and delirium.
      (2) Reduced motor activity is seen in patients with depression, catatonia, some frontal lobe syndromes, parkinsonian states, and delirium.
      (3) Tics are simple motor actions that involve a few muscle groups. Examples are blinking and grimacing.
      (4) Repetitive acts are complex movements that involve entire limbs or a limb and the head (e.g., a movement resembling haircombing).

   c. **Facial expression.** Patients with little or no facial expression may have depression, a neurologic syndrome (e.g., Parkinson's disease, minor hemisphere stroke), or a drug-induced parkinsonian syndrome.

   d. **Mood and affect.** Affect is the immediate overt expression of an emotional state. Mood is the sustained or underlying emotion.

   $$Affect = Moment$$
   $$Mood = Hour$$

   Significant mood or affect abnormality suggests an affective disorder (i.e., depression, mania, hypomania, anxiety). The absence of facial expression may complicate diagnosis, but a patient's mood can usually be determined from other clues. Knowledge of a patient's thought form and content (see IV D 2 a–b) is essential in establishing a diagnosis of elevated or depressed mood.

   e. **Interview behavior.** Some patients show significant behavioral changes, even during a short interview. A manic or delirious patient may exhibit irritability, demanding behavior, anger, and euphoria. Helplessness and demanding behavior are common signs of an underlying personality disorder.

LPTEAAICT
DALAANIAB
FSAMRCOAD
PAKLAYJYO
EABAAEFMU
SAHEVARAT

FIGURE 13-5. A list of letters for the auditory vigilance test.

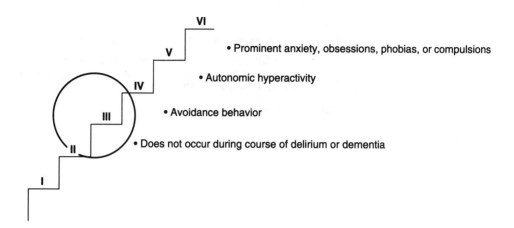

FIGURE 13-6. Anxiety disorder. The *circle* shows the primary area of dysfunction.

D. **Level IV: language, thought, and memory** (Figures 13-9, 13-10)

1. Language

    a. Brain sites. The mental status examination assesses the language areas of the major (usually the left) hemisphere. These areas include the sensory cortices, secondary and tertiary association areas of the inferior parietal lobe, subcortical pathways to the frontal and prefrontal areas, and pathways from the prefrontal area to the motor cortex involved with speech (Broca's area).

    b. Causes of impairment

        (1) Structural brain disease in one or more areas causes language disorder (e.g., a vascular lesion in Broca's area that produces impaired motor output of speech).

        (2) Delirium, which may be caused by intoxication or substance withdrawal, causes serious deficits in attention, with subsequent abnormalities in rate of speech, thought form (e.g., derailment, flight of ideas), and memory (e.g., failure of short-term memory secondary to loss of concentration).

        (3) Abnormalities in neurotransmission, which may occur in affective disorders and schizophrenia, cause language deficits.

        (4) Metabolic disorders cause abnormalities in thought form and content (e.g., myxedema madness, manic-like syndromes seen in hypercortisolism).

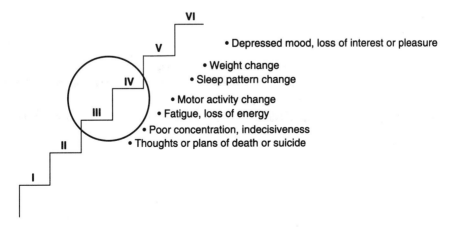

FIGURE 13-7. Mood disorder, depressed. The *circle* shows the primary area of dysfunction.

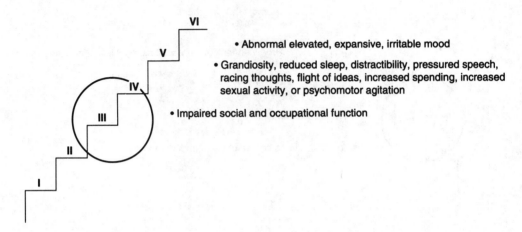

FIGURE 13-8. Mood disorder, manic. The *circle* shows the primary area of dysfunction.

c. **Assessment**
   (1) **Handedness**
       (a) Knowledge of handedness is important in the evaluation of any patient who has difficulty speaking or understanding spoken or written language. The examiner asks the patient or the patient's family which hand the patient uses to write, eat, and throw a ball.
       (b) Hemispheric dominance is associated with contralateral hand preference. In most individuals, even the left-handed, critical language function is located in the left hemisphere of the brain. Patients with mixed dominance are assumed to have more bilateral language representation. These patients have better recovery after strokes that involve the language areas.
   (2) **Language comprehension**
       (a) **Brain sites.** Lesions in the left temporal perisylvian region cause loss of ability to understand spoken or written language. Occasionally, the ability to read is preserved.
       (b) **Causes.** Vascular lesions of the middle cerebral artery and its branches are the most common causes of these aphasias.
       (c) **Testing.** If the examiner finds that an English-speaking patient does not understand what is asked or said, a full aphasia screening is required. In patients with fluent aphasia, the speech production mechanisms are intact, but the utterances are mixtures of words or phrases that have little meaning. This condition may be mistaken for a psychotic process with severe degrees

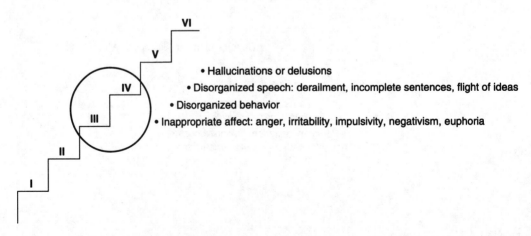

FIGURE 13-9. Psychotic disorder. The *circle* shows the primary area of dysfunction.

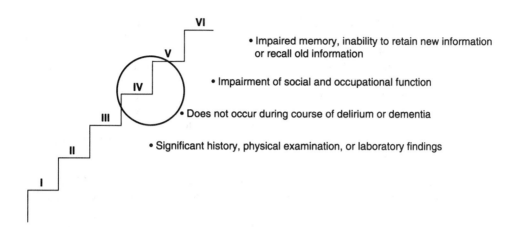

FIGURE 13-10. Amnestic disorder. The *circle* shows the primary area of dysfunction.

of derailment, tangentiality, or flight of ideas. To test for understanding, the patient is asked to follow a series of commands.

(i) The patient is given a series of increasingly difficult commands (e.g., show me your nose, hand, ankle, shoulder blade, brow). To exclude apraxia, in which a patient cannot act on a command despite intact receptive and motor capacity, the patient is asked a series of simple to complex questions that require only a head movement to indicate a positive or negative response. Possible questions include: Is this a hotel? Did you eat breakfast? Do you have dinner before breakfast?

(ii) The patient should be asked to read a passage aloud and then answer questions at approximately a fifth-grade level. Literacy is defined as the ability to read and understand at this level. Figure 13-11 shows a passage that can be used for this section of the test.

(3) Spontaneous speech. The patient is evaluated on the basis of observation alone; no special testing is required.

(a) Changes in rate of speech are common in many psychiatric disorders (e.g., depression, mania, schizophrenia, attention-deficit disorders). These changes are not attributed to specific structural lesions.

(b) Complete muteness is seen in some psychiatric syndromes (e.g., catatonia, elective mutism) but not in aphasia. Even patients with severe motor aphasia can phonate some sounds.

(c) Dysarthria is a nonspecific term for difficulty in articulation, intonation, and phonation.

(d) Dysprosody is the loss of melodic aspects of speech. Utterances are uninflected and monotonous. Patients with minor (right) hemisphere lesions, in an area that corresponds to Broca's area in the left hemisphere of the brain, may lose their ability to **encode** emotion into speech.

(4) Writing deficits are usually associated with frontal lesions. Evaluation of writing ability may be omitted if the patient does not appear to have aphasia.

> *The helicopter is a most unusual aircraft. It can rise straight up, descend straight down, fly forward, or fly backward. It can also fly very slowly and even remain in one place while in midair. These special flying features of the helicopter make it valuable in search and rescue missions because it has the ability to take off and land in a small amount of space.*

FIGURE 13-11. A sample passage for the language comprehension test.

      (a) Agraphia is the inability to write dictated material (with no paresis of the arm or hand). It is caused by posterior perisylvian lesions, and it rarely occurs alone. The inability to write is usually associated with other types of aphasia. Writing samples of aphasic patients often contain spelling and grammatical errors.

      (b) Dysgraphia is the faulty production of letters and words. It occurs in many situations, such as in children who are learning to write, children with learning disorders, and patients with delirium and dementia.

      (c) Testing. The patient is asked to write a dictated sentence and to write an original sentence.

2. Thought disorders may affect **content** (**what** is said) or **form** (**how** it is said). **When disorders of both form and content are present, the patient is usually considered psychotic.**

  a. Thought form disorders occur in many severely disturbed psychiatric patients.

    (1) Reduced content is a poverty of ideas that is often associated with vague, repetitive, abstract speech that contains little information. The patient's speech is usually adequate in amount and contains no syntactic or vocabulary errors. This disorder is sometimes called "empty philosophizing."

    (2) Circumstantiality is a condition in which a patient has trouble reaching the point because he includes unnecessary detail and parenthetical information.

    (3) Derailment is a shift in thinking in which the patient's ideas move from one unrelated topic to another. The patient is not aware of the incongruity of the juxtaposed ideas. This condition is also known as **loosening of associations**. It must be distinguished from circumstantiality.

    (4) Tangentiality is shifts in topic that at first may be related but progressively move further from the initial topic.

    (5) Blocking is a sudden cessation of speech that the patient attributes to losing her thought or having her mind become blank. Many patients who are distracted by inner perceptual disturbances (hallucinations) experience blocking.

    (6) Flight of ideas is a speech pattern that includes accelerated speech and rapid shifts in topic. Speech may become disorganized and incoherent, but syntax and vocabulary are usually intact.

    (7) Clang associations are a form of derailment in which the patient changes topic because of the sound rather than the meaning of words (e.g., we went up the hill, pill that he is).

    (8) Confabulation is the apparent fabrication of facts or events to fill gaps in memory. This disorder is common in patients with organic amnestic syndromes (e.g., Korsakoff's syndrome), but it rarely occurs in patients with amnesia associated with dementia.

    (9) Neologisms are word inventions or distortions of standard words (e.g., the grass is grumps).

   (10) Echolalia is the echoing of the words or phrases of others. It is often associated with meaningless repetition of the same words. This condition occurs in children with developmental language disorder, in individuals with transcortical aphasia, and rarely in patients with schizophrenia.

   (11) Perseveration is the persistent repetition of words and phrases. It occurs in patients with developmental language disorder, organic syndromes, and, rarely, schizophrenia.

   (12) Word salad is a form of disorganized speech in which syntax is lost and vocabulary use is idiosyncratic. It is usually caused by fluent aphasia.

  b. Thought content disorders occur in many medical, neurologic, and psychiatric syndromes.

    (1) An **illusion** is a misperception of a real external stimulus (e.g., a moving shadow of a tree on a bedroom wall appears to be a figure outside the window). Illusions are common in delirium and dementia.

(2) A **delusion** is a **fixed false belief** that is based on an incorrect interpretation of reality (e.g., a telephone ringing only once is absolute documentation of a government plot against the patient). Delusions are common in many clinical situations. Schizophrenic patients have organized and fixed delusions (e.g., the patient's thoughts are being controlled, her thoughts are being broadcast on television). Delirious patients have delusions that are more fleeting and are often based on illusions or hallucinations.

(3) **Hallucinations** occur in patients with psychosis caused by **intoxications, delirium, dementia, schizophrenia, and mood disorders**. The nature of the misperception suggests the underlying disorder (e.g., auditory hallucinations in schizophrenia, tactile hallucinations in withdrawal delirium), but exceptions are very common. Several types of hallucinations occur.

    (a) **Auditory** hallucinations are usually experienced as a human voice or voices. Other sounds are less common. Patients with complex partial seizures (e.g., temporal lobe epilepsy) report a variety of simple or complex sounds or music.

    (b) **Visual** hallucinations usually consist of focused images, such as a human form, an object, or, less commonly, lights. These hallucinations occur in all psychotic states.

    (c) **Olfactory** hallucinations usually occur as an unpleasant odor (e.g., burning rubber). These are frequently reported by patients with complex partial seizures (e.g., temporal lobe epilepsy), and they may be accompanied by gustatory hallucinations.

    (d) **Gustatory** hallucinations are usually perceptions of an unpleasant taste.

    (e) **Tactile (haptic)** hallucinations involve the sense of touch. **Formication** is a sense of something crawling or creeping. It usually occurs in patients who are experiencing alcohol withdrawal delirium or who are recovering from cocaine intoxication.

(4) **Assaultive thoughts** are wishes or intentions to harm an individual, a group, or, rarely, an institution or organization.

(5) **Homicidal thoughts** are wishes or intentions to kill another person. These thoughts may be specific, poorly formulated, or impulsive and momentary.

(6) **Homicidal plans** suggest that an intention or wish to kill is a real threat. In several states, mental health professionals are required by law to report to potential victims the possibility of an assaultive or murderous attack. The homicidal patient is involuntarily hospitalized if he will not accept voluntary hospitalization.

(7) **Feelings of hopelessness** occur in a variety of situations. They usually accompany depression or grief.

(8) **Feelings of worthlessness** are common. Sometimes they are simply a bid for reassurance, but they also accompany severe depression.

(9) **Anhedonia** is the inability to derive pleasure from ordinarily pleasurable activities.

(10) **Feelings of guilt** vary from regret over mild social solecisms to a sense of overwhelming culpability that often occurs in patients with serious depression.

(11) **Suicidal thoughts** can be expressed variously by the statement, ''I wish I were dead,'' by a student who is momentarily overwhelmed with work to an expression by a patient who is voicing death as the only way to end psychic pain or reunite with a dead, longed-for loved one. It is important to distinguish between a desperate wish to end pain and the manipulative and angry suicidal thoughts of a jilted lover or of a teenager who feels that her parents are insufficiently understanding.

    (a) Any depressed patient or patient who expresses a wish to die should be carefully evaluated. It is important to determine the probability that a suicidal plan will succeed (e.g., if the patient says that he might shoot himself, are there guns at home?).

    (b) In the United States, a patient who is a danger to himself can be involuntarily hospitalized. An examiner who believes that a patient is imminently suicidal should take the necessary legal steps for hospitalization.

(12) Obsessions are recurrent, persistent ideas, images, or impulses that the patient experiences as being intrusive and unwelcome (i.e., they are **ego-dystonic**). Obsessions occur in both psychotic and nonpsychotic states, including obsessive–compulsive disorder, eating disorders, and depression.

(13) Phobias are irrational and persistent fears of an object, activity, or situation. Patients attempt to avoid the fear-producing stimulus because it causes increased anxiety and overactivity of the autonomic nervous system.

(14) Sexual concerns are experienced by many patients. Some concerns are real, and others occur as obsessions (e.g., the patient thinks that his penis is too small), delusions (e.g., the patient has the most powerful penis in the world), or phobias (e.g., the patient has an exaggerated fear of venereal disease).

(15) Somatic preoccupations are seen in patients in all branches of medicine. These preoccupations are often unrelated to any underlying pathologic processes. They may occur with other disorders, such as anxiety disorders, mood disorders, somatoform disorders, factitious disorders, and psychoses.

(16) Religiosity is a preoccupation with religion. The preoccupation may be a delusion (e.g., the patient believes that she is God) or an obsession. Some patients experience guilt and worthlessness. Religiosity occurs in many psychiatric illnesses.

3. Memory

   a. Brain sites. Some neuroanatomic structures are associated with memory, but further study is needed. Tests of attention (e.g., the digit span test; see IV B 3 a) measure immediate recall, which some authorities classify as a function of memory. However, the RAS and the primary auditory cortex play a major role in memory, and the digit span test can be considered a test of attention only. The hippocampus, mammillary bodies, striatum, and dorsal medial nuclei of the thalamus are essential subcortical links in the storage and retrieval of verbal and nonverbal memory. Memory traces are presumed to occur in the neocortex, although many subcortical structures participate in the memory process.

   b. Assessment

   (1) Sensorium

   (a) Orientation. Many mental status examinations start with orientation questions. These questions about time, place, situation, and person are essentially tests of awareness and memory. Inability to answer some or all of these questions suggests an organic syndrome, such as delirium, a combination of delirium and dementia, or amnesia. It is important to determine whether a disoriented patient has delirium or dementia. In most cases, the patient's performance on the digit span test and CPT clarifies this differential diagnosis. Many demented patients perform well in tests of attention until late in the course of the disease.

   (b) Memory testing. A patient who is undergoing evaluation of memory must be attentive and be capable of cooperating with the examiner and of understanding the task requirements.

   (i) Orientation for time is evaluated by asking the patient to identify the day, month, year, time of day, and season.

   (ii) Orientation for place is assessed by asking the patient where he is. When the patient is uncertain, the examiner may provide alternatives (e.g., hotel, school, or hospital).

   (iii) Orientation for situation is determined by asking the patient to describe what is happening.

   (iv) Orientation for person is rarely lost. In a patient who has no relevant medical history or whose findings suggest a serious CNS disorder, loss of orientation for person suggests psychogenic amnesia or fugue.

   (2) Short-term memory testing requires the patient to retain new information for at least 5 minutes. The patient must be able to concentrate, then recognize, register, retain, and retrieve the information when asked.

    (a) Accurate recall of the last 24 hours may require a relative or friend for corroboration. This test assesses the patient's ability to process new information.

    (b) Formal testing can be performed by asking the patient to learn new material. In some testing formats, the patient is given four words that are diverse semantically and phonetically (e.g., shovel, yellow, anger, sofa). To evaluate attention and registration, the patient is asked to repeat these words three times. The patient is asked to repeat the words after 1 minute and after 5 minutes to determine whether any deficit occurs at either interval.

    (c) Scoring. A normal adult recalls all four words. Recall of three words is normal in elderly patients. Recall of only two words suggests a problem with short-term memory.

  (3) Remote memory testing. Problems with remote memory are usually detected while the medical history is taken. The degree of loss can be determined by asking the patient to recall important people and events in his lifetime (e.g., presidents, wars) and by asking him to identify important family dates and anniversaries if the family is available to verify the accuracy of this information. Patients rarely forget their own, their parents', or their siblings' birthdays. Women usually remember wedding anniversaries and their children's birthdays.

E. **Level V: constructional ability, calculations, and learned material** (Figure 13-12)

1. Brain sites. Many brain areas (i.e., parietal lobe, language area, frontal and prefrontal lobes) are evaluated at this level. Inability to perform specific tasks does not have specific localizing significance. The ability to perform well on all of the tasks suggests the integrity of many neural structures and their connecting pathways.

2. Assessment

  a. Constructional (graphomotor) ability is the ability to copy or draw two- or three-dimensional shapes or designs. This task is complex and involves visual, perceptual, and analytic functions of the occipital and parietal lobes and motor planning and action functions of the prefrontal and frontal lobes. Although both hemispheres are involved in the task, damage to the right (minor) parietal lobe causes severer impairment in performance.

    (1) The patient is asked to copy simple two- and three-dimensional objects and shapes, such as a cube and a flower in a pot.

    (2) Scoring is 0 for perfect or near-perfect reproduction; 1 for minimal distortion or rotation; 2 for moderate distortion or rotation and loss of the third dimension.

    (3) This screening test is excellent because a good performance suggests the integrity of many neural structures. Patients with an early stage of dementia (e.g., Alzheimer's disease) usually perform poorly.

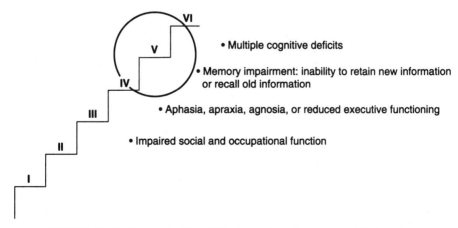

FIGURE 13-12. Dementia. The *circle* shows the primary area of dysfunction.

b. **Calculations** measure the ability of a patient to perform mental arithmetic. In normal individuals, performance is highly correlated with concentration, intelligence, and education. These factors must be considered when a patient performs poorly.

   (1) **Impaired performance** is caused by lesions in one or both hemispheres. Lesions of the major hemisphere usually cause greater impairment than similar lesions of the minor hemisphere. Patients with diminished attention and concentration and significant anxiety show impaired performance. Results are not reliable in these patients.

   (2) **Testing**

      (a) **Simple mental arithmetic**

         (i) The test begins with single-digit addition and proceeds to multiple-number addition and subtraction.

         (ii) **Scoring** is dependent on the patient's intellectual and academic level.

      (b) **Serial subtraction**

         (i) The patient is asked to subtract 7 from 100 and to continue subtracting 7 from the remainder, giving only the answer. Serial 3 subtraction may be used if the patient does not succeed with this task.

         (ii) **Scoring.** A normal adult with a high-school education should be able to complete this task.

c. **Learned material.** The patient is asked questions that assess her **store of knowledge or general information**. Responses are affected by the patient's intelligence and education, so the examiner should consider the patient's background when interpreting answers. Possible questions include: How many minutes are in an hour? What is the function of the kidneys? How many miles lie between San Francisco and New York?

F. **Level VI: abstract thinking, conceptual ability, judgment, and insight.** This level of the mental status examination measures the highest cortical functions, known as **executive ability**.

1. **Brain sites.** These abilities are dependent on the integration of all cortical areas, but the prefrontal and language cortices are critical to these functions.

2. **Abstract thinking**

   a. **Similarities.** The patient is asked to identify the essential relation between word pairs consisting of objects and ideas. Inability to provide appropriate abstract responses suggests a deficit in higher cortical function. This deficit may be caused by progressive brain disease (e.g., dementia).

      (1) **Assessment.** The patient is asked how word pairs are alike (e.g., turnip and cauliflower, chair and table, painting and symphony).

      (2) **Scoring** is 0 for the best abstract answer; 1 for an answer that identifies properties similar or shared, and 2 for a response that describes properties of only one of the pair or a generalization that does not apply.

   b. **Proverb interpretation** is dependent on the patient's cultural, intellectual, and educational background. Many well-educated young adults are unfamiliar with proverbs, so responses must be interpreted with care. The ability to provide an abstract response requires an intact fund of general information and the ability to apply generalities to new information.

      (1) **Brain sites.** The prefrontal and frontal cortices are involved in this skill. Language processing skills must be intact as well [see IV D 1 c (2)].

      (2) **Assessment.** The examiner should ask the patient to explain the following proverbs: "Rome was not built in a day"; "A bird in the hand is worth two in the bush"; "Birds of a feather flock together"; "A rolling stone gathers no moss"; and "An apple falls near its tree."

      (3) **Scoring** is 0 for the most abstract response (e.g., it takes time to do things well); 1 for a partial abstract response (e.g., don't do things too fast), and 2 for a concrete response (e.g., it took a long time to build Rome).

3. **Conceptual ability**

   a. **Brain sites.** Conceptual ability is dependent on many intact cortical areas. Prefrontal damage may destroy this capacity but leave many language and other cognitive functions intact.

```
(a) A  C   E  G _____  (l)
(b) 1  4  7  10 _____  (13)
(c) AZ  BY  CX  D _____  (W)
(d) Hydrangea      763047168
    Jewel          49823
    Hat            _____  (any three-digit numeral)
```

FIGURE 13-13. Sample letter and numeral sequences for the conceptual ability test.

- **b. Assessment**
  - **(1)** Overall conceptual ability is difficult to evaluate. One method of testing is to ask the patient to solve unfamiliar and complex verbal problems. A more formal assessment is done by asking the patient to complete a series of numbers, letters, or words that are presented in written form.
  - **(2)** The patient is asked to complete a series of letter and number sequences that are printed on a card (Figure 13-13).
- **c. Scoring.** Most patients can complete half of these examples. Completion of fewer suggests some impaired function in verbal reasoning ability.

4. Judgment and insight
- **a. Judgment** is the patient's understanding of what he has done or will do in various situations. The patient should be asked specific questions about his ability to cope with difficult or emergency situations. Possible questions include: What would you do if you smelled smoke in your apartment? What would you do if you had severe chest pain while you were alone at home? What would you do if you saw a 2-year-old child playing at the end of a pier?
- **b. Insight** is the patient's awareness of the significance of her symptoms and illness. It may range from partial to complete understanding of the origin, nature, and prognosis of the condition.

BIBLIOGRAPHY

American Psychiatric Association: *Diagnostic and Statistical Manual of Mental Disorders,* 4th ed. Washington, DC, American Psychiatric Association, 1994.

Leigh H, Reisen M: *The Patient.* New York, Plenum Press, 1980.

Lishman W: *Organic Psychiatry,* 2nd ed. Oxford, Blackwell Scientific Publications, 1987.

Luria A: *Higher Cortical Functions in Man.* New York, Basic Books, 1966.

Strub R, Black F: *The Mental Status Examination in Neurology.* Philadelphia, FA Davis, 1985.

STUDY QUESTIONS

DIRECTIONS: Each of the numbered items or incomplete statements in this section is followed by answers or by completions of the statement. Select the ONE lettered answer or completion that is BEST in each case.

1. Short-term memory dysfunction often accompanies intoxication, mania, and withdrawal syndrome because of

(A) excitement
(B) diminished brain stem reticular activating system (RAS) activity
(C) severe anxiety
(D) hallucinations
(E) hippocampal–diencephalic damage

2. During the course of an emergency room interview, a 27-year-old man shows behavior that varies from cooperative to erratic and demanding and from unconcerned to irritable. He shows poor attention and needs constant prompting and reminding about questions. He brags about his wealth and importance. Which of the following findings would help to confirm a diagnosis of mania?

(A) Delusions
(B) Negative toxicology blood screen
(C) Normal electrocardiogram (ECG) reading
(D) Intact long-term memory
(E) Intact design copying ability

Questions 3–4

A 72-year-old senior partner in a law firm comes to a physician's office with his son. The patient believes that his wife of 45 years is having affairs with tradesmen who visit the house. He is angry and is verbally and physically abusive to his wife. On mental status examination, the patient is belligerent and annoyed by the questions and the questioner. Because of the patient's limited cooperation, the examiner is certain of only the following findings: intact serial seven subtraction, repetition of three digits reversed, orientation, and good performance on similarity testing.

3. Which of the following diagnoses best fit the findings at this point?

(A) Delirium
(B) Mania
(C) Psychotic disorder not otherwise specified
(D) Borderline personality disorder
(E) Anoxic heart failure

4. Further questioning of the patient and his family shows that for 3 days the patient has been taking an over-the-counter preparation four to five times daily. Which of the following drugs might cause the signs demonstrated by the patient?

(A) Anti-inflammatory drugs
(B) Antacids
(C) Long-acting cold capsules
(D) Nasal spray (with decongestants)
(E) Hemorrhoidal preparations

5. A 76-year-old morbidly obese woman is admitted to a medical unit after complaining that gases in her apartment caused her to experience shortness of breath. Staff working with the patient hear her say that the gas is part of a deliberate attempt on her life by neighbors (whom she cannot name). She also believes that inspectors from the city government are involved in the plot because they said that they could not detect any evidence of toxic fumes. The patient denies any psychiatric problems. Positive findings on mental status examination are limited to the paranoid delusion. Attention and concentration, short- and long-term memory, general information, calculation, and similarity testing are all normal for her age. Medical, neurologic, and laboratory test results are essentially normal. Which of the following diagnoses best fits this brief clinical description?

(A) Residual schizophrenia
(B) Dementia
(C) Delirium
(D) Psychotic disorder not otherwise specified
(E) Anxiety disorder

6. A 55-year-old man is admitted to the psychiatric inpatient service because of depression and suicidal ideation. Which one of the following mental status examination findings is unusual in a major depressive disorder?

(A) Somatic delusion
(B) Poor performance on continuous performance testing (CPT)
(C) Disorientation for time, place, and situation
(D) Lack of insight
(E) Poor serial seven subtraction

7. A 63-year-old retired editor is seen by her physician because her family is concerned about her recent difficulties in performing usual household tasks. For example, her standard of meal preparation declined far below her usual standards. Physical, neurologic, and routine laboratory findings are normal. Mental status examination shows an alert, cooperative woman with excellent attention and concentration. Her affect is uniformly pleasant, and she denies anxiety, worry, and mood changes. She provides many details of her life and medical history. Which of the following mental status examination components would be most helpful in establishing or excluding a possible diagnosis?

(A) Thought form
(B) Thought content
(C) Continuous performance testing (CPT)
(D) Recall of four words after 5 minutes
(E) Serial subtraction

ANSWERS AND EXPLANATIONS

1. The answer is B [III; IV A 1]. Short-term memory dysfunction often accompanies intoxication, mania, and withdrawal syndrome because of diminished activity of the reticular activating system (RAS). A critical first step in the ability to initiate storage of new information is the activity of the brain stem and pontine RAS. Diminished ascending RAS input will affect the level of consciousness and reduce the level of alertness as well as the level of attention and concentration.

2. The answer is B [Figure 13-8]. Negative results on a toxicology blood screen would help to confirm a diagnosis of mania by ruling out substance abuse, the signs of which can mimic mania. The patient in question is behaving in a typical manic fashion, although a medical disorder may also cause these findings.

3. The answer is A [IV D 1 b (2)]. Delirium is the most appropriate diagnosis of those given at this point, although the details provided are sketchy. Delirium is frequently characterized by abnormalities of thought form and memory.

4. The answer is C [IV D 1 b (2)]. Long-acting cold capsules usually have anticholinergic properties, which can easily cause a toxic delirious state when taken in excess.

5. The answer is D [IV D 2]. Psychotic disorder not otherwise specified is the diagnosis that best fits this clinical situation. Although paranoid delusions often occur in dementia, this patient has age-normal memory function and abstracting ability. These findings eliminate this diagnosis. The patient is concerned about a threat, but she has no criteria for an anxiety disorder. Because she has no history of schizophrenia, the residual diagnosis is excluded. Delirium cannot be diagnosed without changes in the patient's level of consciousness, attention, and concentration.

6. The answer is C [IV D 3 b (1) (b) (i)–(iv)]. Disorientation is an unusual finding in depression and suggests another diagnosis. Somatic delusions are common, however. Difficulty in concentration, which often occurs because of preoccupation with morbid topics, can cause poor performance on continuous performance testing (CPT) and serial seven subtraction. Lack of insight is usually seen in depressed patients, who view their situation as hopeless.

7. The answer is D [IV D 3 b (2) (c)]. Recall of four words after 5 minutes is the component of the mental status examination listed that is most likely to aid in the diagnosis. A dementing process can begin with apraxia or aphasia without evidence of cerebrovascular infarction. The patient's problems might reflect apraxia or even a decline in work function caused by an early stage of dementia. The finding of difficulty in short-term memory suggests dementia. However, if short-term memory skills are excellent, further neurologic evaluation is indicated.

Chapter 14

Psychological Assessment and Psychometric Evaluation

Robert L. Jenkins
Janell Schweickert

I. **INTRODUCTION. Psychological assessment is a process of gathering information and answering questions about human behavior.** It involves the integration of data from the patient history and from medical and psychiatric examinations with those obtained from the **psychometric evaluation.** The psychological assessment is usually conducted by a clinical psychologist who is trained in normal and abnormal behavior and in psychometric evaluation.

A. **Psychological assessment**

1. **Advantages.** Psychological assessment is a complementary extension of the psychiatric examination. It provides detailed information about behavioral, cognitive, and emotional functioning. This information is important for diagnosis, treatment, and rehabilitative planning. Advantages of psychological assessment include:

   a. **Access to information** that would be unavailable through history taking and interviewing

   b. **Rapid availability of information** that might otherwise be obtained only after weeks, months, or years of treatment

   c. **Additional source of new or confirmatory information** that contributes to the differential diagnosis, facilitates an understanding of the patient's behavior and dynamics, and addresses specific questions raised by the psychiatric evaluation or during treatment

   d. **Objective and quantifiable information** about the patient from the collection of data under standardized and replicable conditions and comparison with normative data

2. **Indications.** Psychological assessments are performed for **specific indications,** not routinely. These assessments require a significant expenditure of professional and patient resources, and they should therefore be used only when there are specific questions, problems, or purposes to be addressed (Table 14-1). Psychological assessment should be considered under the following circumstances:

   a. To evaluate a psychiatric patient for whom **diagnosis** or other important issues are not clear

   b. To evaluate a patient with **brain injury** or dysfunction (e.g., to assist in treatment and rehabilitation planning)

   c. To evaluate a patient with **vague symptoms** that are difficult to substantiate with standard psychiatric, neurologic, or medical examinations. This assessment can often discriminate organic and functional impairment.

   d. To determine a **baseline level** of functioning so that future improvement or deterioration can be monitored

TABLE 14-1. Reasons for Referral for Psychological Assessment

To obtain descriptive information about a patient
To enhance understanding of psychological dynamics
To evaluate areas of behavioral, cognitive, and emotional functioning to assist in diagnosis
To aid in decision making (e.g., competency, academic placement, suicide risk)
For treatment and discharge planning
To establish baseline performance
For prognostic and predictive purposes
To evaluate functional and organic components of behavior

   e. To assess changes in behavioral, cognitive, or emotional functioning in patients who are involved in **litigation**
   f. To answer questions about a patient's **behavioral functioning** (e.g., impulse control, motivation, social maturity), **cognitive ability** (e.g., intellectual functioning, academic achievement, neurobehavioral impairment), **vocational issues** (e.g., career decisions, vocational rehabilitation), or **emotional and personality factors** (e.g., psychological conflicts and dynamics, suicide potential, reality testing)

3. Components. Psychological assessment includes a review of **background information** (e.g., medical chart, physician assessments, family interviews), a **patient interview,** and a **psychometric evaluation.**
   a. The **patient interview** is similar to the traditional psychiatric diagnostic examination, but areas of concern are emphasized. The purposes and techniques of interviewing are discussed in Chapter 12.
   b. The **psychometric evaluation** consists of one or more test procedures.

B. **Psychometric evaluation.** This evaluation is also known as **psychological testing**. It comprises a set of test techniques by which a sample of behavior is **elicited, observed, recorded, scored,** and **interpreted.**

   1. Psychometric evaluation is based on three important measurement principles: standardization, reliability, and validity (Table 14-2). All test procedures should be evaluated as to the degree to which they meet these principles.
      a. Standardization requires the collection of adequate norms and the development of uniform procedures for test administration and scoring. Standardization permits the interpretation of a test score within an appropriate context.
         (1) Normative data must be obtained from an **adequate sample from a population that is representative** of those for whom the test will be used.
         (2) Administration and scoring procedures should be uniform, replicable, and specified in detail. Therefore, every patient is examined in exactly the same manner and under the same conditions as those in the normative sample. When this type of standardization is achieved, variations in test scores are caused by patient characteristics rather than differences in presentation and scoring of the test.
      b. Reliability in psychometric evaluation is the consistency and accuracy of a test. Reliability is not expected to be perfect because human traits may change over time **(true variance),** and this change affects the consistency of test scores. Factors that are unrelated or unintentionally related to the trait being measured also affect the accuracy of a test **(error variance).** Reliability is expressed as a type of correlation coefficient: coefficients of .70, and preferably .80, or greater are adequate for test instruments in clinical use. There are four main types of reliability.

TABLE 14-2. Principles of the Psychometric Examination

Standardization
   Uniform, replicable procedures and a normative database that is representative of the population for whom the test will be used

Reliability
   Stability and accuracy of measurements over time (test–retest reliability), across different versions of the same measure (alternate-forms reliability), between scorers (interscorer reliability), or among test items (internal consistency reliability)

Validity
   Degree to which a test measures what it is intended to measure; may be based on correlation of the measure with other tests or criteria (criterion or empirical validity), degree to which experts or test users agree that test items are appropriate to the test purpose (content validity), and relation of the test measure to other variables that are theoretically similar to it (construct validity)

(1) Test–retest reliability is used to evaluate the stability of test scores over time. This type of reliability is important when a test is administered on more than one occasion.

(2) Alternate-forms reliability is used to establish the comparability among one or more versions of the same test. This type of reliability is important when multiple versions of a test are used, such as in situations that require repeated or frequent administration.

(3) Interscorer reliability is consistency among individuals scoring the test. This type of reliability is important for tests that are scored according to subjective criteria (e.g., adequacy of proverb interpretation, degree of distortion in a drawing).

(4) Internal consistency reliability is an estimate of the degree to which test scores on one or more segments of a test are correlated with each other or with the test as a whole. It is used to determine the consistency of test items in measures of homogeneous or unidimensional traits and to assess the degree to which a test result may be influenced by measurement of a fluctuating trait. As the degree of internal consistency reliability increases, so do the precision of measurement and the reliability of the test as a whole.

c. Establishing validity is the **most important aspect of test development**. A test is valid only to the degree that it measures what it is intended to measure. A test can be well standardized and highly reliable, but without demonstrated validity, the results may be misleading or meaningless. Adequate standardization and reliability are necessary, but they are not sufficient for establishing validity. There are several categories of validity.

(1) Criterion-based or empirical validity is determined by correlating the scores on the test in question with the scores on another measure or criterion that accurately represents the variable that the test measures. Criterion-based validity is important. Its most common application is the development of instruments for diagnostic and prognostic uses. There are two types of criterion-based or empirical validity.

(a) Predictive validity is established by determining the correlation of the measure with some criterion that is measured in the future [e.g., correlating Medical College Admissions Test (MCAT) scores with performance in medical school].

(b) Concurrent validity is the association of test performance with the performance of an existing criterion (e.g., correlating the results from a new test to diagnose schizophrenia with those of a known criterion, such as the Schedule of Affective Disorders and Schizophrenia).

(2) Content validity is present when experts determine that test content and scores correspond with the variables to be measured. **Face validity,** which is similar, is present when the item content **appears to measure** what the test is designed to measure. Face validity is determined by the test user or consumer rather than by experts.

(3) Construct validity addresses the various meanings and possible interpretations of test scores in relation to their underlying theoretical constructs. Evaluation of construct validity is a complex process that may include determining how closely the measurement of the test variable converges, or correlates, with theoretically similar variables or how clearly the measure can be discriminated from dissimilar variables. Additional aspects of construct validity involve determining the factor structure, sensitivity, and specificity of the instrument.

2. Psychological tests can be categorized and classified along several dimensions (see also II).

a. Tests can be classified according to their **content and purpose.**

(1) Intelligence tests assess current functioning and potential for adaptive behavior. They are used for educational planning, placement, and remediation; vocational counseling; personnel selection; and for psychodiagnostic purposes. Intelligence tests sample cognitive abilities.

    (2) Achievement tests assess mastery of acquired information, usually through schooling. Achievement tests are used for educational placement and for diagnosis of learning disabilities. They often are used in combination with intelligence and neuropsychological tests.

    (3) Developmental tests assess basic skills that are acquired through maturation and general learning. These tests are usually used for young children.

    (4) Tests that assess personality and mood state show the patient's **current mood state or enduring personality traits**. These tests are often used for diagnosis and treatment planning in psychotherapy.

    (5) Vocational tests assess the patient's interests, attitudes, and aptitudes to aid the patient in making occupational decisions.

    (6) Neuropsychological assessment uses routine and specialized cognitive and personality tests to determine the presence, scope, and implications of **neurobehavioral impairment** (brain dysfunction).

  b. Psychological tests also differ according to the process of the assessment procedure.

    (1) Individual and group tests. Group tests are administered to more than one person at a time and are time efficient. Individually administered tests are less time efficient, but provide a better understanding of the patient as an individual.

    (2) Objective and projective tests

      (a) Objective tests are highly standardized for administration, scoring, and interpretation. They are usually structured in format. Clearly identifiable correct answers exist. True–false and multiple-choice tests are usually considered objective because all response possibilities are clear and scorers can agree on the result.

      (b) Projective tests are less structured and allow greater freedom for the expression of individual ideas. These tests are based on the **projective hypothesis**. This hypothesis suggests that an individual who is given little structure and ambiguous stimuli will impose internal structure on the interpretation of the stimuli. The patient's interpretation will reveal (**project**) unconscious issues, conflicts, and aspects of personality and cognitive style. Projective tests have been criticized for their lack of objectivity and reliability. However, recently, John Exner has increased the objectivity of the most famous projective test, the Rorschach test, without compromising the advantages of its projective format.

    (3) Tests of potential ability versus typical performance. Tests of **potential ability** focus on measuring an individual's **maximum performance**. Tests of **typical performance** assess not what the patient can do, but what he typically does. Tests of potential ability often measure cognitive capacities or specific aptitudes and abilities, whereas tests of typical performance usually assess aspects of personality, cognitive style, and observable behavior.

    (4) Behavioral assessment techniques minimize inference and emphasize observable, quantifiable measures. These techniques include structured interviews, self-report checklists, logs for self-monitoring, naturalistic observation, and role playing. These techniques offer strong content validity and are useful for problem identification, treatment planning, and treatment monitoring.

II.   **SPECIFIC PSYCHOLOGICAL TESTS.** Many instruments are available. This section describes some commonly used tests, their goals, and the process of assessment. Table 14-3 lists many popular psychological tests.

A.   **Tests of intellectual ability.** Intelligence is an abstract concept that is viewed by psychologists as a composite of cognitively mediated abilities that are important to adaptive interaction with the physical, social, and psychological environment. These abilities include the capacity to acquire, store, access, and manipulate information; the ability to learn from experience; insight; abstract reasoning; the capacity to adapt to new situations; and

TABLE 14-3. Frequently Used Psychological Tests

Intelligence tests
  Wechsler Adult Intelligence Scale-Revised
  Wechsler Intelligence Scale for Children-
    Third Edition
  Wechsler Preschool and Primary Scale of
    Intelligence-Revised
  Stanford-Binet Scale, Fourth Edition

Achievement tests
  Wide Range Achievement Test 3
  Peabody Individual Achievement Test
  Woodcock-Johnson Psychoeducational Battery
  Iowa Tests of Educational Development
  Stanford Achievement Test
  California Achievement Tests

Tests of personality, mood state, and behavior
  Minnesota Multiphasic Personality Inventory
    (MMPI, MMPI-2, MMPI-A)
  Rorschach Test
  Thematic Apperception Test
  Sentence Completion Tests
  Projective Drawings (Draw-a-Person, House-
    Tree-Person, and Kinetic Family Drawing)
  Millon Clinical Multiaxial Inventory II
  Millon Adolescent Personality Inventory
  Myers-Briggs Type Indicator
  16 Personality Factor Inventory
  Beck Depression Inventory

  Children's Depression Inventory
  Geriatric Depression Inventory
  Symptom Checklist 90
  Affect Balance Scale
  Child Behavior Checklist
  Michigan Alcoholism Screening Test

Vocational tests
  Strong Vocational Interest Inventory
  Campbell Interest and Skill Survey
  Kuder Interest Inventories
  Career Assessment Inventory
  16 Personality Factor Career
    Development Profile

Neuropsychological tests
  Halstead-Reitan Neuropsychological
    Test Battery
  Luria-Nebraska Neuropsychological
    Test Battery
  Bender Visual-Motor Gestalt Test
  California Verbal Learning Test
  Aphasia Screening Examination
  Boston Naming Test
  Symbol Digit Modalities Test
  Trail Making Test
  Rey-Osterrieth Complex Figure Test
  Wechsler Memory Scale-Revised
  Wisconsin Card Sorting Test

the ability to focus and sustain direction in activities. Measured intelligence is usually stable after adolescence, and test–retest reliability is high, even in young children. **Intelligence quotient (IQ) is not static,** however, and may change considerably in children over a period of years. Whereas adult intellectual capacity is almost universally assessed by the **Wechsler Adult Intelligence Scale-Revised (WAIS-R),** a number of tests are used for children. Almost all tests of intelligence rely on objective measures.

  1. **WAIS-R.** This scale is the adult version of a series of tests that were developed by David Wechsler beginning in 1939. This version of the test was restandardized in 1981.
      a. **Description.** The WAIS-R is used for patients 16 years of age and older. Normative data are available up to the age of 74 years. The test consists of 11 subtests that assess **verbal, visual, and perceptuomotor abilities**. The **Verbal IQ** is based on six subtests that assess verbal information, verbal reasoning, auditory attention, and memory. The **Performance IQ** is derived from five subtests that assess perceptual accuracy, organization, and manipulatory skill. Table 14-4 lists the subtests. Standardization of the WAIS-R is excellent, and its reliability and validity are high.
      b. **Interpretation.** As with all tools used in psychological assessment, interpretation is rarely based on one score. Usually, a battery of tests is administered. Test results are considered in the context of patient history and level of adaptive functioning. Academic and cultural history are significant factors in the interpretation of the results of IQ tests. When other relevant factors are considered, many types of information may be derived from the WAIS-R.
          (1) **Verbal, Performance, and Full-Scale IQs** are derived from the subtest scores and represented on a standard scale with a theoretical mean of 100 and a standard deviation of 15.
              (a) **The Full-Scale IQ** summarizes a patient's performance on all of the subtests

TABLE 14-4. Wechsler Adult Intelligence Scale-Revised Subtests, Intelligence Quotient Indices, and Interpretations

Verbal subtests	
Information	Taps general fund of information and past learning
Digit span	Tests auditory attention and immediate memory
Vocabulary	Assesses depth and breadth of vocabulary
Arithmetic	Assesses immediate memory, freedom from distractibility, and mental arithmetic reasoning
Comprehension	Explores understanding of common sense information, practical problem solving, and abstract reasoning
Similarities	Evaluates ability to see relationships between objects or concepts
Performance subtests	
Picture completion	Assesses ability to detect logical inconsistencies and missing details in pictures of familiar objects
Picture arrangement	Requires evaluation of subtle social cues in a series of stimuli and organization of the stimuli into a meaningful story
Block design	Tests visual capacity to analyze abstract designs and requires spatial–constructional ability to reconstruct the designs with blocks
Object assembly	Taps perceptual organization and manipulation of puzzle-like pieces into familiar, but initially unknown, objects
Digit symbol	Tests psychomotor coordination by requiring rapid copying of symbols
Intelligence quotient (IQ) indices	
Verbal IQ	Reflects an individual's level of performance relative to the performance of others of similar age in areas of verbal information and reasoning, and attention and concentration
Performance IQ	Indicates level of function in visual perceptual organization and psychomotor and manipulatory abilties
Full-Scale IQ	Reflects overall potential for adaptive functioning

compared with a standardization sample drawn from people of similar age. IQ ranges and the corresponding percentiles are shown in Table 14-5. Because the Full-Scale IQ is a composite score, it provides little information about a patient's specific cognitive abilities.

(b) After the IQs are obtained, the **disparity between the Verbal and Performance IQs** is evaluated. Statistically large differences may be caused by academic background, socioenvironmental factors, type of disorder, learning disabilities, or lateralized brain dysfunction.

(2) **Subtest scores** are interpreted individually and compared with age-stratified normative data. They are also examined for variability between and within the subtests. This process can identify a patient's relative strengths and weaknesses. Variability in scores may be caused by the patient's adaptive skills, underlying personality, and emotional factors, or by particular types and loci of brain dysfunction.

(3) **Individual responses** are examined. No normative data are available for the standardized interpretation (as opposed to scoring) of individual responses. However, these responses may still be a rich source of pathological indicators. Verbal subtests may elicit responses that show thought process and content as

TABLE 14-5. Intelligence Quotient Ranges and Theoretical Percentile Distribution

Intelligence Quotient	Descriptor	Approximate Percentage (Percentile Range)
≥ 130	Very superior	2% (98–100)
120–129	Superior	7% (91–98)
110–119	High average	16% (75–90)
90–109	Average	50% (25–75)
80–89	Low average	16% (10–25)
70–79	Borderline	7% (2–9)
< 70	Mentally retarded	2% (0–2)

Adapted with permission from Wechsler D: *Wechsler Adult Intelligence Scale-Revised.* San Antonio, The Psychological Corporation, 1981, p 28.

well as disturbances in language function. Performance on subtests that require a high degree of perceptual accuracy show a patient's ability to organize the world and maintain contact with reality.

2. **Other tests of intellectual ability** listed below are usually used to test children. Some of these tests are also used to evaluate impaired adults.

   a. **The Wechsler Intelligence Scale for Children-Third Edition (WISC-III).** The WISC-III is used for children 6 to 16 years old. The subtests are similar to those on the WAIS-R, but with age-appropriate materials and adaptations. The WISC-III also includes supplementary subtests that further assess cognitive abilities. Full-Scale, Verbal, and Performance IQs are derived from the subtest scores. Reliability and validity are comparable to those of the WAIS-R, and the principles for interpretation are similar.

   b. **The Wechsler Preschool and Primary Scale of Intelligence-Revised** was developed for use with children 3 to 7¼ years old. This test follows the same general form as the other Wechsler scales, and the interpretive approach is similar.

   c. **The Stanford-Binet Scale, Fourth Edition (1986)** is the most recent version of the original Binet Scale. The original test was developed in 1905. It is considered the first formal test of intelligence. The test produces four cognitive scores: verbal reasoning, quantitative reasoning, abstract and visual reasoning, and short-term memory. Interpretation is also based on normative data gathered from a range of age groups.

B. **Achievement tests.** Measures of achievement evaluate information and skills that are part of specific instruction. Therefore, these tests do not necessarily assess aptitude or predict performance. These tests are used widely in educational systems and also in counseling and industry. They may determine a patient's level of achievement more precisely than an interview. Standardization of achievement tests is usually good, reliability is high, and validity is acceptable.

1. **The Wide Range Achievement Test 3** is often used in psychological assessment. This test assesses competence in **reading, written spelling, and arithmetic**. It has been standardized for ages 5 to 75 years. Subtest scores can be converted to grade equivalents, percentile ranks, and standard scores.

2. **Group-administered achievement tests** include **Iowa Tests of Educational Development, the Stanford Achievement Test, and the California Achievement Tests**.

3. **Individually administered achievement tests** include **the Peabody Individual Achievement Test and the Woodcock-Johnson Psychoeducational Battery**.

C. **Tests of mood state and personality functioning**

1. **The Minnesota Multiphasic Personality Inventory (MMPI, MMPI-2)** is widely used. This objective, self-report test provides diagnostic and clinical information about psychiatric and medical patients. The MMPI was developed in 1940, and the original

norms are still used in many settings. Updated norms are available, however, and the revised and restandardized MMPI-2 was introduced in 1989. Another version of the test, the MMPI-A, is designed for use with adolescent patients.

a. Description. The MMPI is used for **diagnosis, evaluation of current emotional state, assessment of response to treatment and treatment outcome, forensic evaluation, and general assessment of personality functioning**. It is frequently used to verify the diagnosis of malingering (see Chapter 15 X) and to evaluate patients with chronic pain. It consists of almost **600 true–false statements**.

b. Scoring. The responses are scored along primary clinical scales and three validity scales that indicate response style (Table 14-6). Many special scales have been developed for the MMPI tests to address specific aspects of mood or personality functioning (e.g., anxiety scale, MacAndrew alcoholism scale, bizarre mentation). The **reliability** of the MMPI **is modest** and variable, but it has been **extensively validated**.

TABLE 14-6. The Minnesota Multiphasic Personality Inventory (MMPI and MMPI-2)

Scale	Abbreviation	Number	Interpretation of Elevation*
Validity			
Lie scale	L	. . .	Denial of common faults and shortcomings; naive defensiveness
Frequency scale	F	. . .	Endorsement of rare or statistically unusual items; faking bad; cry for help; psychosis
Correction scale	K	. . .	Denial of inadequacy; sophisticated defensiveness
Clinical			
Hypochondriasis	Hs	1	Degree of concern about somatic functioning
Depression	D	2	Cognitive, emotional, behavioral, and physiologic correlates of depression
Hysteria	Hy	3	Denial; high need for affection; somatization; egocentric, manipulative, demanding traits
Psychopathic deviate	Pd	4	Impulsiveness; low frustration tolerance and poor social adjustment; problems with authority
Masculinity–femininity	M-F	5	Pattern of interest and attitudes more typical of the opposite sex
Paranoia	Pa	6	Suspiciousness; hypersensitivity; rigidity; possible delusions
Psychasthenia	Pt	7	Anxiety, worry, fears, and self-doubt; personal distress
Schizophrenia	Sc	8	Social and emotional alienation; unusual and idiosyncratic thoughts; bizarre experiences; possible hallucinations
Mania	Ma	9	Ineffective hyperactivity; agitation; restlessness; irritability; no tolerance for delay; expansiveness
Social introversion	Si	0	Shyness; withdrawal; social ineptness; social anxiety

*Simplifications of interpretations that can be associated with a significant elevation. Findings may also be interpreted if scores are significantly diminished.

c. **Interpretation**
   (1) **Demographic factors** such as age, socioeconomic status, career choice, and education are considered.
   (2) **Scoring.** Raw scores on each scale are converted to **T scores,** which have a mean of 50 and a standard deviation (SD) of 10. The three **validity scales** are analyzed to verify that the profile is interpretable and to assess response characteristics such as defensiveness and exaggeration of symptoms. The profile of the clinical scales is examined and interpreted. For the MMPI, a significant finding is a score that differs from the mean of 50 by 2 SDs. A difference of 1.5 SD is significant for the MMPI-2.
   (3) The **configuration of the profile** is compared with established profile patterns, which are known as code types.

2. **The Rorschach inkblot test.** The Rorschach technique is considered the major **projective** test of personality assessment. Originally developed around 1920 by a psychiatrist, Hermann Rorschach, the test is the subject of several thousand publications. There are many formats for administering and scoring the Rorschach test, but most practitioners use the objective method developed by John Exner and known as the **Comprehensive System**. This method is highly standardized and has acceptable reliability and validity.
   a. **Description.** The Rorschach test is used to assess **reality testing, personality dynamics and organization, and cognitive style**. It consists of 10 cards or plates, each containing a bilaterally symmetric inkblot design. Five of the cards contain designs of black, white, and gray; five cards have designs that include color. The patient is shown each card individually and asked "What might this be?" The responses to all 10 cards are collected in this free association stage. During the inquiry stage, the patient reviews the inkblots and identifies which characteristics of the blots were used to formulate the responses. Data are collected in a standardized manner so that outside influence is not imposed on the patient's responses.
   b. **Interpretation.**
   (1) **Quantitative.** The responses are scored quantitatively for such characteristics as number, location, adherence to the form characteristics in the blots, perception of movement and dimensionality, use of color and shading characteristics, language in which the response is phrased, and content of the percept. Some basic scoring categories and their interpretations are described in Table 14-7. Interpretation relies on calculated indices and formulas, and extensive norms exist for interpreting the data (collected from nonpatient children ages 5–16 and from adult male and female patients and nonpatients).
   (2) **Qualitative.** After the **quantitative interpretation,** most clinicians examine the data **qualitatively** to analyze the responses for repetitive content and themes, unusual responses and logic, and the sequential characteristics of the responses. Through this process, the responses may yield much information, including the patient's thought form and content, unconscious processes, psychological defenses, suicidal ideation, and interpersonal style.

3. **The Thematic Apperception Test (TAT).** The TAT was developed in the early 1940s by Henry Murray as a way to evaluate a patient's **unconscious drives, emotions, and conflicts**. The test is **projective,** but the stimuli have more structure than those of the Rorschach test. Although objective scoring is possible, most clinicians use subjective interpretation. Reliability and validity are questionable, but this test is widely used. In the context of a complete psychometric assessment, it may contribute considerably to the clinical understanding of the patient. Similar tests exist for children (e.g., **Children's Apperception Test**).
   a. **Description.** The TAT is usually used to assess issues of content rather than the structure or process of personality functioning. The test addresses **psychological needs and conflicts, aspects of interpersonal functioning,** and the **ability to use fantasy and imagination**. It consists of one blank card and thirty cards that depict one or more persons whose activities and feelings are ambiguous. The tone and context of the depicted situations are ambiguous as well. The stimuli on the cards raise specific

TABLE 14-7. Major Scoring Categories of the Rorschach Test

Category	Meaning
Location of response	Responses are scored as to whether the percept encompasses the whole blot, large details, small details, or white spaces; location provides information on how an individual approaches the world intellectually (e.g., attempting to organize various elements into a whole or focusing on practical or even unusual details)
Movement	Subdivided into major categories of human movement, animal movement, and inanimate movement; responses are associated with inner fantasy, impulses, and imagination
Form	Responses determined only by shape are scored; form relates to the perceptual and intellectual control of the individual; interpretation is modified by form quality and percentage of form responses
Color	Responses determined by chromatic and achromatic characteristics are scored, taking into account the degree to which form is present; responses with color determinants reflect emotional responsiveness and individual's control of affective stimulation
Shading	Percepts involving shading as primary determinants are believed to reflect awareness and methods of addressing affectional needs
Form dimension	Perception of depth, distance, or dimension is an important characteristic; responses relate to awareness and experience of anxiety

issues (e.g., father–son relationships, suicidal thoughts), and different cards are chosen for each patient. Typically, 10 to 20 cards are used. The **patient is asked to create a story about each picture** by describing what is happening, what led up to the situation, what the characters are thinking and feeling, and how the situation concludes.

   b. **Interpretation.** Several scoring and interpretive systems exist, but most clinicians use a qualitative scoring method. They attempt to identify the character with whom the patient identifies. Then they evaluate the story in terms of the needs and pressures that affect the behavior of the character. Consistent themes may be identified, and interpersonal relationships are examined.

4. **Sentence completion tests (incomplete sentences).** These tests are an economical means of surveying a patient's **thoughts, feelings, motivations, and behaviors** along a number of important psychological dimensions. Many forms of the test are available, and most are tailored to a specific age group (e.g., school-age children, adolescents, adults). These tests contain **sentence stems** that the patient is asked to complete. Instructions vary with the specific version of the test. For some versions, the patient is asked to complete each stem with the first thought that comes to mind. For another version, the patient is asked to complete the stems in a way that shows how she truly feels. The test items address fears, desires, fantasies, aspirations, relationships, self-concept, and frustrations. The task has obvious structure, but it contains **projective** elements as well. Interpretation is usually based on a simple inspection of the items, and the results are used to augment other clinical and test data. The test has high face validity. These tests may also contribute to a neuropsychological evaluation because they provide a lengthy sample of handwriting and written expression.

5. **Projective drawings** include **Draw-a-Person, House-Tree-Person, Draw-a-Family, and Kinetic Family Drawings**. The patient is asked to complete one or more drawings. The reliability and validity of these tests are questionable. Standard guidelines are available for the interpretation of drawings, but many clinicians do not use them. The results are considered a symbolic representation of unconscious aspects of a patient's psychological structure and functioning. Therefore, the test is **projective**. Children's drawings are often evaluated for their age appropriateness; in this context, the test assesses personality characteristics and developmental progress.

6. **The Millon Clinical Multiaxial Inventory II** was standardized for patients seeking treatment in mental health systems. This **objective** test stresses emotional and interpersonal difficulties. The results are interpreted in terms of clinical characteristics that are associated with personality disorders.

7. **The Beck Depression Inventory** is a widely used screening device that assesses the behavioral, cognitive, affective, and physiologic components of depression. It is a self-report measure. Similar inventories are used for children **(Children's Depression Inventory)** and elderly patients **(Geriatric Depression Inventory),** and to assess anxiety.

8. **The Sixteen Personality Factor Inventory** addresses nonpathological aspects of personality functioning. Interpretation may emphasize clinical issues, career development considerations, or marital concerns.

9. **The Myers-Briggs Type Indicator** is a measure of personality dispositions and preferences based on the theories of Carl Jung. The results can be used for individual, family, and marital counseling; educational and career guidance; and organizational issues and management development.

10. **The Child Behavior Checklist** is administered to parents and teachers of children under assessment. Ratings of the presence and frequency of appropriate and inappropriate behaviors are evaluated according to a standardized collection of profiles.

D. Vocational tests are not commonly used in medical settings.

1. **The Strong Vocational Interest Inventory** and **the Campbell Interest and Skill Survey** assess the interest patterns of respondents and compare them with the interest patterns of people who are successfully employed in certain fields. These tests are used for educational or professional counseling.

2. **Personality tests,** such as the Myers-Briggs Type Indicator and the Sixteen Personality Factor Inventory, also have vocational implications.

E. Neuropsychological assessment. The use of psychological tests to evaluate brain injury and dysfunction is an increasingly sophisticated and practical specialty of psychology. The neuropsychological evaluation may involve either a comprehensive examination or a specific assessment of cognitive, emotional, and adaptive behaviors with standardized tests that evaluate the condition of the brain. The tests provide diagnostic, descriptive, and prognostic information and involve no risk to the patient. Although the accuracy of neuropsychological assessment in discriminating normal individuals from those who are organically impaired may be as high as 90%, such assessments are less successful in differentiating individuals with brain dysfunction from those with chronic psychiatric disorders. The effectiveness of these tests is enhanced when patient history is considered and mood and personality measures are included in the assessment.

1. **The Halstead-Reitan Neuropsychological Test Battery (HRB)** is a well-known neuropsychological battery. It originated in the work of Ward Halstead in the 1940s, and was largely developed and researched by Halstead's student, Ralph Reitan, beginning in the 1950s. It is available in forms for young children 5 to 8 years of age as the Reitan-Indiana Neuropsychological Test Battery for Children, older children 9 to 14 years of age, and older adolescents and adults 15 years of age and older.
   a. **Description.** The HRB consists of five tests, but the battery is usually supplemented by other tests, such as the age-appropriate Wechsler Intelligence Scale. Table 14-8

describes the primary tests of the HRB and several of the ancillary tests. The validity of the HRB is high, and its reliability is adequate.

  b. Interpretation. The results of the HRB are interpreted with four methods of inference. The five primary tests of the HRB are used to calculate an **impairment index** that reflects the patient's degree of overall impairment in neuropsychological functioning. Test results are also analyzed for differences between task performance by the left and right sides of the body. The pattern of results is then evaluated for consistency in impairment across tasks that rely on specific sensory–motor modalities or cognitive abilities that are mediated by particular regions of the brain. Finally, the

TABLE 14-8. Halstead-Reitan Neuropsychological Test Battery (HRB)*

Test	Description
Primary	
Category Test	Test of abstraction, conceptual reasoning, and concept learning that uses visually presented stimuli organized into 7 subtests; the most sensitive measure in the HRB of the effects of brain dysfunction
Tactual Performance Test	Blindfolded patients place 10 geometric forms into a form board; the patient then draws from memory a diagram of the board and forms; task requires tactual–spatial analysis, constructional ability, novel problem solving, and cognitive visualization; sensitive to general brain dysfunction; the best measure of lateralized cortical dysfunction in the HRB
Seashore Rhythm Test	Consists of pairs of sequentially presented rhythmic patterns; the patient indicates whether the patterns in each pair are the same or different; requires auditory attention and tracking, and nonverbal auditory discrimination
Speech Sounds Perception Test	Nonsense words are presented from an audiotape; speech perception and matching of phonemes to graphemes are examined
Finger Oscillation Test	As a measure of fine motor control and psychomotor speed, the patient taps a key on 5 consecutive 10-second trials with the index finger of each hand
Impairment Index	Consists of the percentage of the 7 measures from the 5 above tests that fall in the impaired range; index of 0.5 or greater indicates neuropsychological impairment
Ancillary	
Trail Making Test	Part A consists of 25 circles randomly distributed on the paper and numbered 1 to 25; patient draws lines connecting them in numerical sequence; Part B consists of circles with either numbers or letters, which the patient connects in sequence while alternating between numbers and letters; these tests require visual searching, motor speed, simple sequence planning, and flexibility in thinking
Aphasia Screening Test	Samples expressive and receptive language capacity and language-mediated skills
Sensory Perceptual Examination	Includes tasks of bilateral simultaneous stimulation in visual, auditory, and tactile modalities; finger localization; fingertip number writing; tactile form recognition; and visual field confrontation
Lateral Dominance Examination	Provides measures of hand strength, and eye and foot dominance

*Primary and frequently used ancillary tests.

results are analyzed for pathognomonic signs, which indicate brain dysfunction (e.g., certain aphasic errors).

2. **The Luria-Nebraska Neuropsychological Battery (LNNB)** was developed by Charles Golden and colleagues in the mid-1970s. It is based on the theory and clinical techniques of the late A. R. Luria, a famous Russian neuropsychologist. Both adult and child versions are available.

   a. **Description.** The LNNB is designed to be administered to patients who are 15 years old and older. **The Luria-Nebraska Battery-Children's Revision** is designed for use with children 8 to 12 years old. Depending on which form of the test is used, the battery includes 11 or 12 **clinical scales** that evaluate motor function, rhythm, tactile function, visual–spatial ability, receptive speech, expressive speech, writing, reading skills, arithmetic ability, memory, and intellectual process. The battery also yields eight **localization scales** (e.g., left frontal) and five **summary scales** that describe aspects of neuropsychological impairment. Most reliability and validity measures are adequate. However, the battery has been criticized as having inadequate documentation of construct validity and using unreliable methods.

   b. **Interpretation.** Item scores are tallied on their respective scales and plotted on a T-score distribution to yield a **profile**. The scorer notes how many scales fall 1 and 2 SDs above the baseline (adjusted for age and education) to determine the probability of brain dysfunction. The pattern of elevations and the localization scales identify the **locus of the dysfunction**. A qualitative analysis is performed to enhance the understanding of the patient's strengths and weaknesses.

3. **Individualized neuropsychological batteries.** Most neuropsychologists use a **basic battery of tests** for most patients and then select **additional tests** based on individualized criteria. This method provides a general assessment of cognitive processes, expands on the standard mental status examination, and permits in-depth study of specific referral questions. All batteries should include measures to assess general intellectual ability, attention, concentration, memory, language, spatial analytic and manipulatory ability, practical and abstract problem-solving ability, conceptual ability, and flexibility in thinking. Multiple measures of specific areas of functioning provide the most reliable results. Mood and personality variables should also be examined. Most individualized batteries include an intelligence test, such as the WAIS-R, because it covers a range of cognitive abilities and provides one measure of adaptive functioning. The MMPI or MMPI-2 is often included as a personality measure and a psychopathology screen. Psychologists also use tests that are included in other batteries, such as the Trail Making Test or Finger Tapping from the Halstead-Reitan Battery supplemental tests. Other tests that are often included in individualized neuropsychological batteries are described briefly.

   a. **The Bender Visual-Motor Gestalt Test** requires patients to copy nine line drawings. Some examiners immediately follow this test with a recall trial in which the patient draws as many items as possible from memory. Although this test was used for many years to screen for brain dysfunction, it is not sensitive in this respect. When this test is combined with the Canter Background Interference Procedure (BIP), however, it is a more effective neuropsychological screening instrument. The BIP requires patients to copy the Bender designs on a sheet of paper filled with intersecting sinusoidal lines. Inordinate difficulty on this task, relative to the standard Bender administration, is interpreted as evidence of organic dysfunction.

   b. **The California Verbal Learning Test** is a repeated-trial word-learning task that is useful for assessing rate of learning, immediate and short-term memory, learning strategies, and interference effects.

   c. **The Rey-Osterrieth Complex Figure Test** assesses visuospatial constructional ability and visual memory. It compares the ability of a patient to copy a complex line drawing and then reproduce it after a 30-minute delay.

   d. **The Wechsler Memory Scale-Revised (1987)** assesses attention and concentration, recall of current and past information, immediate and 30-minute-delayed memory for verbal and visual stimuli, and associative learning. The results are summarized with composite standard scores similar to those computed by the Wechsler intelligence scales. The mean is 100, and the SD is 15. The test provides a general index of memory functioning as well as specific indices for verbal and visual memory, attention and concentration, and delayed recall.

e. **The Wisconsin Card Sorting Test** is used extensively in clinical practice and research. The test assesses abstract and conceptual reasoning as patients learn to sort cards into categories. Flexibility in thinking is also evaluated when the sorting category shifts, unannounced to the patient. The patient must detect the shift and determine the new sorting category using only feedback about whether a specific response is correct. This task is believed to be an effective method of assessing **frontal lobe functioning**.

III. ANALYSIS AND REPORTING OF TEST DATA

A. Analysis and integration of test results

1. **Patterns of test data.** A single score or result on a psychological or neuropsychological test is rarely considered. Rather, test data are examined for patterns, and findings are considered in the context of other test results and the patient's behavior and history.

2. **Test data provide extended mental status information.** Psychological tests emphasize personality adjustment and disorder, thought process and content, and personality style. Neuropsychological tests emphasize the assessment of cognitively mediated abilities. Together, they provide an extended evaluation of mental status.

3. **Race and ethnicity, age, intelligence, education, and current circumstances** (e.g., occupation, living arrangements) are considered part of the interpretive process.

B. Reporting of results

1. **Interpretation, integration, and reporting of the information** are performed by a clinical psychologist. Administration and scoring of psychological tests may be performed by a trained technician (psychometrist).

2. **A written summary of assessment should be provided.** The report may be specific or broad, depending on the questions to be addressed. Referral questions should be as specific as possible.
   a. **Content of reports.** Reports usually contain the purpose of the examination, background information, test procedures, and a description of patient status and behavior during the examination, in addition to test results and interpretation.
   b. **Presentation of results.** Psychologists present results in a variety of ways. Some list scores, others discuss performance on tests and test items, and some provide only interpretation. Data that support the interpretation of test results should be included in the report.
   c. **Summary of findings.** Test reports are often concluded with a summary of the findings. This section should contain a clear response to the referral question. This response must be based on data presented in the body of the report. Recommendations are usually outlined in this section.

BIBLIOGRAPHY

Adams RL, Jenkins RL: Basic principles of the neuropsychological examination. In *Clinical Practice of Psychology.* Edited by CE Walker. New York, Pergamon, 1981.

Buros OK: *The Ninth Mental Measurements Yearbook.* Highland Park, NJ, Gryphon Press, 1985.

Exner JE Jr: *The Rorschach: A Comprehensive System. Volume I: Basic Foundations,* 2nd ed. New York, John Wiley, 1986.

Goldstein G, Hersen M (eds): *Handbook of Psychological Assessment,* 2nd ed. New York, Pergamon, 1990.

Groth-Marnat G: *Handbook of Psychological Assessment,* 2nd ed. New York, Van Nostrand, 1990.

Kline P: *The Handbook of Psychological Testing.* New York, Routledge, 1993.

Tallent N: *The Practice of Psychological Assessment.* Englewood Cliffs, NJ, Prentice-Hall, 1992.

Wechsler D: *Wechsler Adult Intelligence Scale-Revised.* San Antonio, Psychological Corporation, 1981.

Zimmerman IL, Woo-Sam JM: *Clinical Interpretation of the Wechsler Adult Intelligence Scale.* New York, Grune and Stratton, 1973.

STUDY QUESTIONS

DIRECTIONS: Each of the numbered items or incomplete statements in this section is followed by answers or by completions of the statement. Select the ONE lettered answer or completion that is BEST in each case.

1. A physician is evaluating the data from a psychological assessment of a patient whose differential diagnosis includes malingering (intentional production of false or grossly exaggerated symptoms). The data presented in the psychological report do not present a consistent picture. Which one characteristic of a test might cause the physician to discount its results in favor of other tests?

(A) High face validity
(B) A test–retest reliability of .70
(C) High empirical validity
(D) An alternate-forms reliability of .80
(E) A high degree of standardization

2. A 50-year-old patient and a 30-year-old patient each obtain a full-scale Wechsler Adult Intelligence Scale-Revised (WAIS-R) intelligence quotient (IQ) of 115. Which conclusion is most valid?

(A) They have similar styles of thinking
(B) They will probably perform equally well in any given work situation
(C) They both show above average abilities compared with others of similar age
(D) They both had above average performance in school

3. The most important property of a psychological test for determining a psychiatric diagnosis is

(A) standardization
(B) reliability
(C) generalization
(D) validity
(E) specificity

4. A 5-year-old patient and a 25-year-old patient undergo intelligence testing with tests that have similar measures of reliability. Which of the following statements is true?

(A) The score of the 5-year-old patient will be less consistent over the next 10 years
(B) The score of the 25-year-old patient will be less consistent over the next 10 years
(C) Both will have equally consistent scores
(D) Intelligence tests have notably low reliability
(E) Intelligence tests have notably low validity

5. Which of the following statements about psychometric testing is accurate?

(A) Achievement tests provide excellent measures of innate ability and have high predictive validity
(B) Reliability is the establishment of reproducible guidelines for administration and scoring of psychometric tests
(C) The manner in which a psychometric test is administered has interpretive import
(D) Psychologists will not include a test as part of an assessment unless it has proven validity, reliability, and standardization

Questions 6–8

Based on the following case, select the correct answer to each question.

A 30-year-old man is hospitalized after expressing suicidal ideation. He has a psychiatric history, but this hospitalization is his first psychiatric contact in 10 years. He denies substance abuse, and the results of drug screening are negative. Although he appears educated and intelligent, he reports holding only low-level positions. He is socially isolated and appears oppressed by negative thoughts that he will not share with the staff. He is observed talking aloud to himself. Among the differential diagnoses considered are obsessive-compulsive disorder and schizophrenia. The staff is uncertain of his level of reality testing and requests a psychological assessment.

6. Which referral request would be the most appropriate?

(A) Assess the presence and degree of organic impairment
(B) Provide an expanded social history
(C) Establish the level of intellectual functioning
(D) Evaluate thought content and thought form
(E) Assess discharge readiness

7. Which test would be most informative?

(A) Wechsler Adult Intelligence Scale-Revised (WAIS-R)
(B) Wide Range Achievement Test 3
(C) Rorschach test
(D) Halstead-Reitan Battery (HRB)
(E) Myers-Briggs Type Indicator

8. Which test would likely be least informative?

(A) Wide Range Achievement Test 3
(B) Rorschach test
(C) Thematic Apperception Test (TAT)
(D) Wechsler Adult Intelligence Scale-Revised (WAIS-R)
(E) Minnesota Multiphasic Personality Inventory (MMPI)

DIRECTIONS: Each of the numbered items or incomplete statements in this section is negatively phrased, as indicated by a capitalized word such as NOT, LEAST, or EXCEPT. Select the ONE lettered answer or completion that is BEST in each case.

9. A 59-year-old man with a 6-year history of multiple sclerosis that is in remission reports to his physician that he is becoming increasingly forgetful. The forgetfulness is affecting his work. He feels depressed, believes that his multiple sclerosis symptoms are returning, and fears that he will become disabled. The physician is aware that even though the patient was divorced 15 years ago, he continues to feel harassed by his former wife. He feels guilt because two of his children have depression, and he believes that his life will never improve. His current wife is also depressed and under psychiatric care. Which of the following would NOT be an appropriate referral request?

(A) Evaluate the organic and functional contributions to this patient's symptoms
(B) Establish a baseline level of performance
(C) Perform psychological testing
(D) Determine the psychological dynamics of this patient's depression
(E) Evaluate this patient for potential suicide risk

10. Which of the following statements about personality tests is NOT correct?

(A) Objective tests may be used to assess idiosyncratic personality characteristics
(B) Standardization is less important for projective tests of personality than for tests of intelligence or aptitude
(C) Although projective tests are ambiguous and use a patient's subjective responses, they can be psychometrically valid and reliable
(D) Projective tests are based on the assumption that individuals reveal important aspects of their personality by the way in which they structure ambiguous stimuli
(E) Personality tests may address both state and trait characteristics of an individual

ANSWERS AND EXPLANATIONS

1. The answer is A [I B 1 b (1), (2), c (1) (a), (2)]. High face validity means that the test questions clearly reflect what the test is measuring. A patient who is attempting to present a false picture is aided in this effort when the face validity is high. Test–retest and alternate-forms reliability are relevant only when the results from the current evaluation are inconsistent with those from a previous examination or with those from another version of the same test. Reliability coefficients of .70 and greater are acceptable. High empirical validity and a high degree of standardization would never be considered a liability, and thus would not be an appropriate basis for discounting the results of a test.

2. The answer is C [II A 1 b (1) (a)–(b)]. This question shows how single scores can be misleading. A full-scale Weschler Adult Intelligence Scale-Revised (WAIS-R) intelligence quotient (IQ) score of 115 indicates above average performance compared with the age-matched standardization sample. In fact, an IQ score of 115 is classified as high average and places an individual in the eighty-fourth peer percentile. This composite score yields no information about styles of thinking. For example, the 50-year-old patient may perform well above average on verbally mediated tests, but only average on perceptually mediated tests. In contrast, the 30-year-old patient may perform within the superior range on the perceptually mediated tests, but slightly below average on the verbally based tests. Such contrasts also point out the error in the assumption that these patients' work performance will be similar. The composite scores of patients with disparate skills may appear deceptively similar. Success in a work situation depends in part on the skills required to perform the job and how those skills mesh with an individual's cognitive strengths and weaknesses. Although IQ may vary as a function of an individual's educational background and it may be used to predict academic potential, it is not directly related to, nor can it accurately predict, actual school performance for any individual.

3. The answer is D [I B 1 c]. Establishing validity is the most important aspect of test development. If a test purports to aid in clinical diagnosis, the diagnostic power of the test results must be established during the development of the test. Validity is established by correlating the results with an outside criterion. This correlation is referred to as the empirical validity of a test. Tests may be well standardized and reliable, but without demonstrated validity, the results may be meaningless.

4. The answer is A [I B 1 b; II A]. For a test to have high reliability, it must yield the same results as long as the characteristic to be measured remains constant. However, intelligence quotients (IQs) are not as stable in children as they are in adults. Children have remarkable developmental shifts as they mature and master important adaptive skills. This instability in measured IQ represents true variance (real change in intelligence). IQ measures should be sensitive to these developmental shifts. This type of inconsistency is different from error variance (inconsistency caused by an inaccurate or unreliable measure). Both the Wechsler Adult Intelligence Scale-Revised (WAIS-R) and the Wechsler Intelligence Scale for Children-Third Edition (WISC-III) have high reliability and validity.

5. The answer is C [I B 1 a (2), b, (3), 2 a (1)–(2); II B, C 3–4]. The type of standardization that specifies the procedures for the administration and scoring of a test has great interpretive import. The power of a psychometric evaluation lies in its ability to compare a patient's performance with that of other patients or with the patient's previous performance. Such comparisons are only valid if the test scores reflect actual psychological or neuropsychological processes and not the conditions of the evaluation. If ever standardized procedure is not followed (e.g., the psychologist adapts a test for use with a mute patient), the change should be noted in the report because it may affect the interpretation of the results. Although there is a positive correlation between past achievement and future achievement (those who have done well in the past are likely to do well in the future), achievement tests are not designed to predict future performance. They measure the degree of successful mastery of skills as opposed to any innate ability or the ease with which a patient acquires the skills. The establishment of reproducible guidelines for test administration and scoring is a property of the standardization process of test development. Interscorer reliability provides a measure of the efficacy of that standardization. Many psychologists include tests with questionable validity and reliability, or those without much standardization, in psychometric evaluations. These tests can add much to the clinical understanding of a patient, just as a physician's subjective interactions with a patient can be a rich source of information. Psychometric assessment can provide objective, quantified information when tests with good validity, reliability, and standardization are used.

6. The answer is D [I A 2 a, I B 2 a]. Psychological testing, especially with projective techniques, is an excellent way to assess thought content and process and to determine a patient's level of reality testing. The patient's level of intellectual functioning is not directly relevant to the differential diagnosis. Intelligence tests are components of most psychological test batteries because they contribute information about thought form and content, but this information is not the same as the level of intellectual functioning. Obtaining an expanded social history does not directly address the question of the patient's level of reality testing, although a more detailed history may be helpful in refining the diagnosis. In addition, although clinical psychologists routinely obtain a social history as part of a psychological assessment, it is usually not cost effective to have this history constitute the entire assessment. Assessing organic impairment is not relevant because the differential diagnosis contains only psychiatric disorders and there is no suspicion of any organic contribution. A psychological evaluation may be helpful in assessing a patient's readiness for discharge, but this is incidental to the central issue of the differential diagnosis.

7. The answer is C [II A 1, B 1, C 2 a–b, 9, E 1]. The Rorschach test is well suited for examining a patient's level of reality testing. Patient responses are examined for the degree of perceptual distortion, and thought form and content are directly examined. Although distorted thinking may be evident on parts of the Wechsler Adult Intelligence Scale-Revised (WAIS-R) [e.g., individual responses on the verbal subtests], the test was not designed to examine psychopathology. Relevant data from individual responses cannot be summarized objectively, and no normative data are available for comparison. This test is not as rich a source of reliable data as the Rorschach test for this type of investigation. The Wide Range Achievement Test 3 is an achievement test,

and is not relevant for the questions at hand. Likewise, there is no suspicion of neuropsychological dysfunction, so the Halstead-Reitan Battery (HRB) is not indicated. The Myers-Briggs Type Indicator is used to assess normal personality dispositions, not to diagnose psychopathology.

8. The answer is A [II A 1, B 1, C 1, C 2 a–b, C 3]. With the information given, there is no indication that learning about the patient's basic academic skills will further his diagnosis. The Rorschach test is a potentially excellent source of information that is of direct interest. The Thematic Apperception Test (TAT) is a projective test, and is likely to contribute to the clinical understanding of the patient's psychological composition. The Wechsler Adult Intelligence Scale-Revised (WAIS-R), although not directly designed to examine reality testing, can yield relevant information. The Minnesota Multiphasic Personality Inventory (MMPI) is often sensitive to different types of psychopathology.

9. The answer is C [I A 2]. An appropriate request conveys a specific purpose. In this case, a request to assess the organic and functional components of the patient's complaints is reasonable, given the presence of known neurologic disease and current symptoms that are consistent with a psychiatric disorder. The establishment of a baseline level of functioning is also appropriate in any patient for whom progressive deterioration is possible. The request for information about psychological dynamics is also appropriate, given the patient's history of long-standing interpersonal difficulty, intrapsychic conflict, and current situational stressors. Requesting additional information about the risk of self-harm in a person with depression is usually appropriate. Psychometric evaluation in the context of a psychological assessment or in addition to a psychiatric evaluation may be helpful in addressing this issue.

10. The answer is B [I A 1 d; I B 1, a (1)–(2), 2 a (4), 2 b (2) (a)–(b); II C 2]. The establishment of uniform, replicable procedures and a representative normative database are important properties for all psychometric tests. Standardization is one of the advantages of psychometric tests compared with clinical interview, mental status examination, and history taking. Objectivity in a test refers to the character of the test construction, not its uses. Objective tests have clearly defined answers or tightly defined methods for scoring answers that require subjective judgment on the part of the examiner. Thus, an objective personality test, such as the Minnesota Multiphasic Personality Inventory (MMPI), the MMPI-2, and the Millon Clinical Multiaxial Inventory II, can be a rich source of information about an individual's personality. It is not the ambiguous nature of projective tests that lowers their validity or reliability; rather, it is that many of them are scored or interpreted in a subjective, non-standardized manner. John Exner devised an objective scoring and interpretive system for the Rorschach test, which is the most famous and widely used projective test. Exner documented the validity and reliability of many of his variables. The assumption that individuals reveal important aspects of personality by their approach to structuring ambiguous stimuli is known as the projective hypothesis. Some personality tests provide information about an individual's current state as well as about enduring personality characteristics.

Chapter 15

Clinical Syndromes

Nancy A. Breslin

I. INTRODUCTION

A. **Defining psychopathology.** Human behavior is complex and variable, and defining the limits of normal behavior is difficult. Psychiatrists define **mental illness** as **behavior that causes the individual significant distress or causes significant dysfunction** (e.g., in the ability to work or have relationships), presuming that the behavior is not culturally appropriate (e.g., mourning a loss). Use of the terms "psychopathology" and "mental illness" does not suggest that the symptoms have no organic basis. Research shows **neurochemical and other biologic abnormalities** underlying many mental illnesses.

B. *Diagnostic and Statistical Manual of Mental Disorders (DSM).* Numerous attempts have been made to define mental disorders, but the most widely used text in the United States is the DSM. The current edition (DSM-IV) is the latest attempt to use research (phenomenology, genetics, drug response) to define individual disorders and develop valid, reliable definitions (see Chapter 6 III A). Each disorder listed in the DSM-IV is defined by a set of **criteria** that must be met to confirm the disorder and exclude other disorders. The organization and definitions used in this chapter are based on the DSM-IV. All major diagnoses from the DSM-IV are listed. Full criteria from the DSM-IV are given for some disorders; descriptions that are consistent with the DSM-IV criteria are given for most others. Many diagnostic categories included in the DSM-IV have one or more additional diagnosis (not listed here) that should be considered by the clinician. Diagnosis X, not otherwise specified, is used to describe clinical cases that clearly fit within a category but do not meet the criteria for any particular diagnosis. Diagnosis X, due to a general medical condition and/or substance induced, is used when symptoms are caused by a medical condition or the use of alcohol or another drug.

II. DISORDERS USUALLY FIRST DIAGNOSED IN INFANCY, CHILDHOOD, OR ADOLESCENCE.

Because of space limitations, only mental retardation, autism, and attention deficit hyperactivity disorder are discussed here. Disorders that occur in children that are more common in adults, such as mood disorders, anxiety disorders, and psychosis, are discussed elsewhere in this chapter. Placement of a disorder in another section does not suggest that it is absent or rare in childhood. Disorders that are commonly diagnosed in children are listed in Table 15-1.

A. **Mental retardation.** According to the DSM-IV criteria, the onset of mental retardation must occur before the age of 18 years. The patient must have both impaired functioning and an intelligence quotient (IQ) lower than 70. Mental retardation has many causes, including chromosomal abnormality (e.g., Down syndrome or the fragile X syndrome), genetic metabolic abnormality (e.g., phenylketonuria, Hurler syndrome), prenatal or perinatal anoxia, maternal drug ingestion (e.g., fetal alcohol syndrome, fetal hydantoin syndrome), trauma, infection, and malnutrition. Most cases have no obvious cause. Mental retardation affects 1% to 3% of the population, and is more common in boys. **Four degrees of retardation** are described in the DSM-IV. Milder forms are more common.

1. Mild: IQ between 50 to 55 and 70

2. Moderate: IQ between 35 to 40 and 50 to 55

TABLE 15-1. Disorders Usually First Diagnosed in Infancy, Childhood, or Adolescence

Mental retardation
Learning disorders
Motor skills disorder
Pervasive developmental disorders
 Autistic disorder
Disruptive behavior and attention-deficit disorders
 Attention deficit hyperactivity disorder
Feeding and eating disorders
Tic disorders
Communication disorders
Elimination disorders
Other disorders
 Separation anxiety disorder ("school phobia")

3. Severe: IQ between 20 to 25 and 35 to 40

4. Profound: IQ below 20 to 25

B. **Autism.** This disorder is one of a group of **pervasive developmental disorders**. A child with autism has significant impairment in social interaction, communication, and behavior. Symptoms begin before the age of 3 years. Problems include impaired eye contact, idiosyncratic or absent language, and repetitive mannerisms (e.g., hand flapping). These patients are often, but not necessarily, mentally retarded. The cause is at least partly genetic. Several other syndromes of pervasive developmental disorder occur, including **Rett syndrome, childhood disintegrative disorder,** and **Asperger's disorder**.

C. **Attention deficit hyperactivity disorder (ADHD)** is a **disruptive behavior disorder**. This category also includes **conduct disorder** and **oppositional defiant disorder**. ADHD is common in any pediatrics practice. The diagnosis requires either serious inattention (e.g., not listening, not following through, disorganization) or hyperactivity and impulsivity (e.g., fidgeting, inability to engage in quiet play, inability to wait to take a turn) severe enough to cause significant distress or functional impairment. Symptoms must begin before the age of 8 years. Paradoxically, the single most effective **treatment is stimulant medication**. Methylphenidate or D-amphetamine can improve both hyperactivity and attention problems. Cognitive–behavioral therapy involving both child and parents can also improve behavior.

III. **COGNITIVE DISORDERS. These disorders are caused by a general medical condition,** regardless of whether evaluation by the clinician identifies the etiology. Patients with these disorders are encountered by clinicians in every specialty.

A. **Delirium.** This disorder is common, although often unrecognized, among elderly hospitalized patients. However, it is seen in all age groups and in many settings. Because the symptoms of delirium indicate serious illness, morbidity and mortality rates are significant if the diagnosis is not made and the underlying problem is not corrected. **If untreated, delirium may progress to brain damage or death.**

1. **Diagnosis.** Delirium is an **acute, fluctuating** disturbance of consciousness and cognition. The DSM-IV criteria for delirium are listed in Table 15-2.

2. **Etiology.** Delirium is usually caused by either a general medical condition or drug use. **Medical conditions** that can cause delirium include hypoxia, infection [systemic or central nervous system (CNS)], head trauma, CNS tumors, electrolyte disturbance, endocrine abnormalities, liver failure, and renal failure. **Drug-induced causes** include

TABLE 15-2. DSM-IV Criteria for Delirium

A. Disturbance of consciousness (i.e., reduced clarity of awareness of the environment) with reduced ability to focus, sustain, or shift attention

B. Change in cognition (such as memory deficit, disorientation, language disturbance) or the development of a perceptual disturbance that is not better accounted for by a preexisting, established, or evolving dementia

C. The disturbance develops over a short period of time (usually hours to days) and tends to fluctuate during the course of the day

D. There is evidence from the history, physical examination, or laboratory findings of a general medical condition or substance intoxication or withdrawal judged to be etiologically related to the disturbance

---

DSM-IV = *Diagnostic and Statistical Manual of Mental Disorders,* 4th ed.
Reprinted with permission from American Psychiatric Association: *Diagnostic and Statistical Manual of Mental Disorders,* 4th ed. Washington, DC, American Psychiatric Association, 1994.

withdrawal from depressant drugs, such as alcohol and benzodiazepines, and overdosage of many drugs, such as alcohol, L-dopa, anticholinergics, and cocaine. Patients with compromised brain function (e.g., Alzheimer's disease) may respond with delirium to milder brain insult than patients without underlying disease.

3. **Treatment.** Many delirious patients are untreated because their mental symptoms are attributed to psychiatric problems or advanced age. When delirium is recognized, the clinician must **determine the cause** by performing appropriate examination and tests. The most appropriate treatment is to **correct the underlying problem** (e.g., withdrawing the causative drug, treating the sepsis with antibiotics). The symptoms of agitation and psychosis often improve with a low dose of antipsychotic medication or a benzodiazepine, but this improvement should not halt the aggressive search for the cause of the delirium.

B. **Dementia.** This disorder is common and has many causes. It may be confused with other cognitive disorders and with depression. Unlike delirium, **many causes of dementia are not reversible**. However, reversible causes should be considered and treated if found.

1. **Diagnosis.** Dementia is a **chronic syndrome** in which patients lose previously attained mental functions. In contrast, patients with mental retardation never attain complete function. The DSM-IV criteria for dementia of the Alzheimer's type are listed in Table 15-3. Many elderly patients with major depression appear demented (pseudodementia), but it is important to distinguish these individuals from those with true dementia because their mood and cognitive symptoms will often improve with antidepressant therapy.

2. **Etiology.** The most common cause of dementia is **Alzheimer's disease** (> 50% of cases), a diagnosis that can only be confirmed by a pathologist at biopsy or autopsy. Alzheimer's disease is presumed to be the cause when the diagnosis fits clinically and other explanations are excluded. **Multi-infarct dementia** is the next most common cause (approximately 10% of cases). Patients with multi-infarct dementia have a stepwise, rather than smooth, pattern of deterioration. Some of the less common causes are **treatable** (e.g., hydrocephalus, chronic CNS infection, vitamin deficiency, chronic hepatic or renal encephalopathy, thyroid disorder). Others are **untreatable** (e.g., Pick's disease, Creutzfeldt-Jakob disease).

3. **Treatment. Correction of reversible underlying conditions** is critical. For irreversible causes of dementia, the treatment is largely supportive. A safe, familiar environment is helpful. Superimposed depression should be treated. Antipsychotic medication may help patients with agitation, but it should be used judiciously. A promising development in the treatment of Alzheimer's disease is the discovery of an abnormal protein (apolipoprotein) in individuals at risk for the disease. Understanding the role of this protein may lead to advances in the diagnosis and treatment of dementia.

TABLE 15-3. DSM-IV Criteria for Dementia

Dementia of the Alzheimer's Type

A. The development of multiple cognitive deficits manifested by both:
1. memory impairment (impaired ability to learn new information or to recall previously learned information)
2. at least one of the following cognitive disturbances:
   a. aphasia (language disturbance)
   b. apraxia (impaired ability to carry out motor activities despite intact motor function)
   c. agnosia (failure to recognize or identify objects despite intact sensory function)
   d. disturbance in executive functioning (i.e., planning, organizing, sequencing, abstracting)

B. The cognitive deficits each cause significant impairment in social or occupational functioning and represent a significant decline from a previous level of functioning.

C. The course is characterized by gradual onset and continuing cognitive decline.

D. The cognitive deficits in A are not due to any of the following:
1. other central nervous system conditions that cause progressive deficits in memory and cognition (e.g., cerebrovascular disease, Parkinson's disease, Huntington's disease, subdural hematoma, normal pressure hydrocephalus, brain tumor)
2. systemic conditions that are known to cause dementia (e.g., hypothyroidism, vitamin B_{12} or folic acid deficiency, niacin deficiency, hypercalcemia, neurosyphilis, HIV infection)
3. Substance-induced conditions

E. The deficits do not occur exclusively during the course of delirium.

F. Not better accounted for by another axis I disorder (e.g., major depressive disorder, schizophrenia).

DSM-IV = *Diagnostic and Statistical Manual of Mental Disorders,* 4th ed; HIV = human immunodeficiency virus.
Reprinted with permission from American Psychiatric Association: *Diagnostic and Statistical Manual of Mental Disorders,* 4th ed. Washington, DC, American Psychiatric Association, 1994.

C. **Amnestic disorder.** Amnesia **may be anterograde** (the inability to learn new information) **or retrograde** (the loss of previously learned information). It may be caused by general medical conditions, such as head trauma, or may be substance induced, such as Korsakoff's syndrome seen in some chronic alcohol abusers. This diagnosis is not made if memory impairment occurs as a symptom of dementia or delirium.

IV. **MENTAL DISORDERS DUE TO A GENERAL MEDICAL CONDITION. Medical conditions can cause symptoms that mimic almost every psychiatric diagnosis.** Examples include mood disorders caused by thyroid conditions, personality changes sometimes seen in patients with Wilson's disease, and psychotic symptoms seen in some patients with epilepsy. Thus, if a patient has all of the symptoms of major depressive disorder, yet has hypothyroidism or is very anemic, then the appropriate diagnosis would be mood disorder due to a general medical condition. The treatment would be correction of the underlying problem. It is not necessary to list all of the medical conditions that can cause psychiatric symptoms, but clinicians must be aware that mental disorders can be caused by medical conditions. Therefore, they should **evaluate psychiatric patients medically as well as psychiatrically,** even when there is a history of mental illness.

V. **SUBSTANCE-RELATED DISORDERS.** These disorders are common; **a lifetime prevalence of alcohol abuse or dependence is approximately 13%, and that of other drug abuse or dependence is estimated at 6%.** Affected individuals often are not diagnosed. Some physicians are reluctant to discuss substance abuse with their patients, and many patients deny abuse.

A. **Substance abuse.** The DSM-IV characterizes substance abuse as "a maladaptive pattern of substance use leading to clinically significant impairment or distress. . . ." The diagnosis requires one of four symptoms, including failure to function at home or work or use of the substance in hazardous situations.

B. **Substance dependence.** This diagnosis is more serious than substance abuse, and is the diagnosis that is made if the criteria for both are otherwise met. The diagnosis requires three of seven listed symptoms, including tolerance (e.g., the need to take more drug to achieve the desired effect), withdrawal, taking more drug than intended, persistent desire to decrease drug use, and persistent use despite the knowledge that drug use has caused the patient physical or psychological problems.

C. **Intoxication.** This diagnosis describes maladaptive behavior or mental changes that are reversible and are related to the recent ingestion of a substance. Examples include ataxia and impaired judgment seen with alcohol intoxication and agitation and psychosis seen with phencyclidine (PCP) intoxication. Specific intoxication syndromes are shown in Table 15-4.

D. **Withdrawal.** Withdrawal is the term for a substance-specific syndrome that causes significant distress or functional impairment when the substance is discontinued. Examples include delirium tremens induced by alcohol withdrawal and depression and oversleeping induced by stimulant withdrawal (e.g., amphetamines, cocaine). Specific withdrawal syndromes are shown in Table 15-4.

E. **Acute syndromes.** Other time-limited mental disorders are seen during the intoxication and withdrawal phases of substance use. The criteria are the same as those found elsewhere in the DSM-IV. For example, a diagnosis of cocaine delirium would require that the criteria for delirium be met while the patient is intoxicated with cocaine. Not every substance causes every syndrome. Table 15-4 shows the syndromes for each substance.

F. **Persisting syndromes.** These syndromes are less common than acute syndromes, but their persistence is a serious problem. The dementia that can follow chronic alcohol use is probably the syndrome seen most often by clinicians. Alcohol-induced amnesia, which is seen in Korsakoff's syndrome, can be caused by a failure to detect or treat Wernicke's encephalopathy. Wernicke's encephalopathy is a triad of opthalmoplegia, confusion, and ataxia related to thiamine deficiency. It may be precipitated in hospitals by administering carbohydrate loads to alcoholic patients without providing thiamine supplements. Table 15-4 shows the persisting syndromes seen with various substances.

G. **Treatment of substance abuse.** Treatment of drug and alcohol abuse takes place in many settings and with varying approaches, but standard elements include the following:

1. **Safe detoxification.** Some drugs, particularly alcohol and sedative hypnotics, have potentially serious complications of detoxification. These complications include delirium tremens and seizures. Patients with strong physiologic dependence on these drugs should have their vital signs and behavior monitored during detoxification to avoid serious illness or death.

2. **Evaluation for comorbidity.** Many patients with substance abuse have associated **medical problems** that require treatment. Substance abuse is also common in patients with other **psychiatric disorders,** such as anxiety, mood, and personality disorders. Because these syndromes can be caused by the substance itself, most clinicians do not treat accompanying psychiatric disorders (e.g., adding an antidepressant medication) until the patient has a period of abstinence and undergoes reevaluation.

3. **Therapy.** Group or individual therapy is necessary to counter denial and provide support. The Alcoholics Anonymous program can be used alone or in combination with other substance treatment programs.

4. **Substance-specific treatments.** Some substances have specific pharmacologic treatments, including disulfiram for alcohol abuse and methadone for narcotic abuse (see Chapter 3 IX B 4, D 2).

TABLE 15-4. Substance-related Disorders

Substance	Intoxication Syndrome	Withdrawal Syndrome	Other Disorders
Alcohol	Inappropriate behavior, labile mood, impaired judgment, slurred speech, unsteady gait, nystagmus	Autonomic hyperactivity, tremor, insomnia, hallucinations, agitation, seizures	Persisting: dementia, amnesia; acute: delirium, psychosis; mood, anxiety, sexual, or sleep disorder
Amphetamines	Euphoria, hypervigilance, tension, impaired judgment, dilated pupils, perspiration or chills, cardiac arrhythmia, confusion, illusions, hallucinations	Dysphoria, fatigue, sleep disturbance, increased appetite	Acute: delirium, psychosis; mood, anxiety, sexual, or sleep disorder
Caffeine	Restlessness, insomnia, flushing, diuresis, rambling thoughts, tachycardia	. . .	Acute: anxiety or sleep disorder
Cannabis (marijuana)	Impaired coordination or judgment, euphoria, anxiety, increased appetite, dry mouth, illusions, hallucinations	. . .	Acute: delirium, psychosis, anxiety disorder
Cocaine	See amphetamines	See amphetamines	See amphetamines
Hallucinogens	Anxiety, depression, paranoia, impaired judgment, perceptual changes when awake and alert, dilated pupils, sweating, palpitations, tremors, blurred vision	. . .	Persisting: flashback; acute: delirium; psychosis; mood or anxiety disorder
Inhalants	Assaultiveness, apathy, impaired judgment, dizziness, nystagmus, incoordination, lethargy, tremor, weakness	. . .	Persisting: dementia; acute: delirium, psychosis; mood or anxiety disorder
Nicotine	. . .	Dysphoria, insomnia, irritability, anxiety, difficulty concentrating, increased appetite	. . .
Opioids	Euphoria followed by apathy; dysphoria, impaired judgment, pupillary constriction, drowsiness, slurred speech, impaired attention and memory	Dysphoria, nausea, muscle aches, rhinorrhea, diarrhea, insomnia	Acute: delirium, psychosis; mood, sleep, or sexual disorder
Phencyclidine (PCP)	Belligerence, impulsiveness, agitation, impaired judgment, nystagmus, hypertension, numbness, ataxia, dysarthria, rigidity, seizures	. . .	Acute: delirium, psychosis, mood or anxiety disorder
Sedatives, hypnotics, or anxiolytics	See alcohol	See alcohol	See alcohol

Adapted with permission from American Psychiatric Association: *Diagnostic and Statistical Manual of Mental Disorders,* 4th ed. Washington, DC, American Psychiatric Association, 1994.

VI. **PSYCHOTIC DISORDERS. Psychosis is the inability to test reality.** It includes such symptoms as hallucinations (e.g., hearing voices, seeing things that are not present), delusions (fixed, false beliefs), and disorganized patterns of thought and speech (see Chapter 8). Psychosis also occurs in association with other disorders, particularly delirium, mood disorders, and substance-related disorders.

A. **Schizophrenia.** This illness strikes approximately 1% of the population. The incidence is approximately the same in men and women. Onset usually occurs in late adolescence or early adulthood. The illness causes acute episodes of significant psychosis and chronic dysfunction, even with appropriate treatment. The mortality rate from suicide and medical illness is much higher in schizophrenic patients than in the general population.

    1. Diagnosis. The DSM-IV uses both **longitudinal** (course of illness) and **cross-sectional** (symptoms seen during a particular episode) features for the diagnosis of schizophrenia. The criteria are listed in Table 15-5. Significant brain changes occur in many patients with schizophrenia. These changes include enlarged ventricles on magnetic resonance imaging (MRI) and changes in frontal cortex blood flow patterns on single-photon emission computer tomography (SPECT). However, these tests are not sensitive or specific enough to be used in the routine diagnosis of schizophrenia.

TABLE 15-5. DSM-IV Criteria for Schizophrenia

> A. Characteristic symptoms. At least two of the following, each present for a significant portion of time during a 1-month period (or less if successfully treated):
> 1. delusions
> 2. hallucinations
> 3. disorganized speech (e.g., frequent derailment or incoherence)
> 4. grossly disorganized or catatonic behavior
> 5. negative symptoms (i.e., affective flattening, alogia, or avolition)
> Note: only one A symptom is required if delusions are bizarre or hallucinations consist of a voice keeping a running commentary on the person's behavior or thoughts, or two or more voices conversing with each other.
>
> B. Social/occupational dysfunction. For a significant portion of the time since the onset of the disturbance, one or more major areas of functioning such as work, interpersonal relations, or self-care is markedly below the level achieved prior to the onset (or when the onset is in childhood or adolescence, failure to achieve expected level of interpersonal, academic, or occupational achievement).
>
> C. Duration. Continuous signs of the disturbance persist for at least 6 months. This 6-month period must include at least 1 month (or less if successfully treated) of symptoms that meet criterion A (i.e., active phase symptoms) and may include periods of prodromal or residual symptoms. During these prodromal or residual periods, the signs of the disturbance may be manifested by only negative symptoms or two or more symptoms listed in criterion A present in an attenuated form (e.g., odd beliefs, unusual perceptual experiences).
>
> D. Schizoaffective and mood disorder exclusion. Schizoaffective disorder and mood disorder with psychotic features have been ruled out because either (1) no major depressive or manic episodes have occurred concurrently with the active phase symptoms; or (2) if mood episodes have occurred during active phase symptoms, their total duration has been brief relative to the duration of the active and residual periods.
>
> E. Substance/general medical condition exclusion. The disturbance is not due to the direct effects of a substance (e.g., drugs of abuse, medication) or a general medical condition.

DSM-IV = *Diagnostic and Statistical Manual of Mental Disorders,* 4th ed.
Reprinted with permission from American Psychiatric Association: *Diagnostic and Statistical Manual of Mental Disorders,* 4th ed. Washington, DC, American Psychiatric Association, 1994.

2. **Etiology.** Schizophrenia research finds evidence of dysfunction in the mesolimbic dopamine system and possibly the frontal and temporal cortices. However, the cause of such dysfunction is not known. The following are among the etiologies that have been proposed.

    a. **Genetics.** The concordance rate for schizophrenia is higher in monozygotic than in dizygotic twins, and the illness is seen in the biologic relatives of adopted patients. Thus a genetic component is likely. However, the finding that monozygotic twins have only about 50% concordance suggests the role of environmental factors. These factors are not yet understood.

    b. **Prenatal or perinatal injury.** Some research suggests that a variety of pregnancy-related problems, including maternal exposure to certain viruses and problems with labor and delivery, are associated with the development of schizophrenia.

3. **Treatment.** Patients are often hospitalized during acute psychotic episodes. Patients with schizophrenia usually respond well to treatment with antipsychotic drugs (see Chapter 3). Supportive therapy for the patient and family and occupational therapy for the patient can be helpful. Outside of the hospital, most patients with schizophrenia require maintenance medication as well as social support, such as special housing, day hospital treatment, supportive therapy, and vocational rehabilitation.

B. **Schizophreniform disorder.** Some patients have an illness that resembles schizophrenia, but remits (including any residual symptoms) within 6 months.

C. **Schizoaffective disorder.** Patients with this disorder have periods of concurrent psychosis and mood (affective) disorder (either mania or major depression) as well as periods of hallucinations or delusions that last for at least 2 weeks without prominent mood symptoms. The latter criterion distinguishes these patients from those diagnosed with mood disorder with psychotic features. This distinction is important because the overall prognosis for patients with schizoaffective disorder is usually worse than that for patients with mood disorder. The treatment may also differ.

D. **Delusional disorder.** An individual with delusional disorder has a fixed, false belief about a possible real-life situation (e.g., a patient thinks that the government is monitoring his behavior). The patient may act on the belief, but otherwise exhibits no psychotic behavior. A bizarre delusion (e.g., a patient believes that aliens control her movements) requires another diagnosis.

E. **Brief psychotic disorder.** A patient with this disorder has as few as one psychotic symptom and recovers within 1 month. The illness is not caused by drug use, a general medical condition, or another mental illness.

F. **Shared psychotic disorder.** This condition is also known as folie à deux. This diagnosis describes a patient who did not originally have a psychotic disorder, but developed a shared delusion because of close contact with a psychotic person, such as a parent or spouse.

VII. **MOOD DISORDERS.** There are many moods other than elation and depression, but in the DSM-IV, the classification mood disorders describes disorders along the manic–depressive axis. Table 15-6 compares the mood disorders.

A. **Depressive disorders.** Everyone experiences depression, but this diagnosis is limited to patients who have sadness or apathy that significantly interferes with functioning. Major depression is a common illness, with a lifetime prevalence of approximately 6% (higher in women). Manic episodes occur in approximately 1% of individuals at some time. Both

TABLE 15-6. Differentiation of Mood Disorders

Diagnosis	Major Depressive Episode	Milder Depression	Mania	Hypomania
Major depressive disorder	+	±	−	−
Dysthymic disorder	−*	+	−	−
Bipolar I disorder	±	±	+	±
Bipolar II disorder	+	±	−	+
Cyclothymia	−	+	−†	+

+ = This syndrome must be present to make the diagnosis; − = This syndrome must be absent to make the diagnosis; ± = This syndrome may be present or absent.
*A major depressive episode must not occur during the first 2 years of the illness.
†A manic episode must not occur during the first 2 years of the illness.

major depressive disorder and bipolar disorder **occur with or without psychotic features** (e.g., hallucinations, delusions). Patients with psychotic features are more likely to require hospitalization and treatment with antipsychotic medication or electroconvulsive therapy (ECT). Mood disorders are often recurrent.

1. Major depressive disorder

　　a. Diagnosis. A patient with major depressive disorder experiences an episode of significant distress or functional impairment that lasts for **at least 2 weeks**. The patient also has seriously depressed mood or significantly decreased interest in activities and at least three or four other physical or mental symptoms of depression. The DSM-IV criteria for major depressive episode are listed in Table 15-7.

　　b. Treatment. Major depressive disorder is treatable, with 70% to 80% of patients responding to medication and a perhaps higher percentage responding to a combination of medication and psychotherapy. Hospitalization is needed initially for some patients, particularly those who are suicidal. Most depressed patients are treated by family practitioners or internists. In some cases, these physicians prescribe inappropriately low dosages of medication, which can reduce efficacy. These physicians also may not have the time to offer patients needed support. Patients with severe symptoms may respond to combinations of medication, ECT, or augmenting drugs.

2. Dysthymic disorder. This disorder is milder than major depressive disorder, but it is significant because it lasts at least 2 years.

B. **Bipolar disorders.** This classification can be confusing because the term bipolar is usually used to describe patients who experience mania, even if they never experience depression (the other pole). The DSM-IV criteria for **mania** are shown in Table 15-8. **Hypomania** is similar to mania except that the duration is as brief as 4 days, and the episode is not severe enough to require hospitalization or to cause significant functional impairment.

1. Bipolar I and bipolar II disorders

　　a. Diagnosis. A patient with bipolar I disorder has at least one manic episode, with or without a major depressive episode. A patient with bipolar II disorder has at least one major depressive episode and at least one hypomanic episode. A manic episode confirms the diagnosis of bipolar I disorder. As with major depression, **psychosis may or may not be present**.

　　b. Treatment. Patients who experience manic episodes are often hospitalized for their own safety. **Lithium** is the first-line medication for mania. It is also used to treat the depression associated with bipolar illness. **Carbamazepine and valproate** are often effective when lithium therapy fails or is not well tolerated. Because these drugs take effect in approximately 1 week, mania is often initially treated with either antipsychotic drugs or benzodiazepines. These agents are tapered as the lithium takes effect. Unlike patients with schizophrenia, many patients with bipolar illness are socially and occupationally functional when medication is maintained. However, noncompliance and relapse are common.

TABLE 15-7. DSM-IV Criteria for Major Depressive Episode

A. At least five of the following symptoms have been present during the same 2-week period and represent a change from previous functioning; at least one of the symptoms is either (1) depressed mood or (2) loss of interest or pleasure.

  1. Depressed mood most of the day, nearly every day, as indicated by either subjective report (e.g., feels sad or empty) or observation made by others (e.g., appears tearful); in children and adolescents, can be irritable mood
  2. Markedly diminished interest or pleasure in all, or almost all, activities most of the day, nearly every day (as indicated either by subjective account or observation made by others)
  3. Significant weight loss or weight gain when not dieting (e.g., more than 5% of body weight in a month), or decrease or increase in appetite nearly every day; in children, consider failure to make expected weight gains
  4. Insomnia or hypersomnia nearly every day
  5. Psychomotor agitation or retardation nearly every day (observable by others, not merely subjective feelings of restlessness or being slowed down)
  6. Fatigue or loss of energy nearly every day
  7. Feelings of worthlessness or excessive or inappropriate guilt (which may be delusional) nearly every day (not merely self-reproach or guilt about being sick)
  8. Diminished ability to think or concentrate, or indecisiveness, nearly every day (either by subjective account or as observed by others)
  9. Recurrent thoughts of death (not just fear of dying); recurrent suicidal ideation without a specific plan; or a suicide attempt or a specific plan for committing suicide

B. The symptoms cause clinically significant distress or impairment in social, occupational, or other important areas of functioning.

C. The symptoms are not due to the direct effects of a substance (e.g., drugs of abuse, medication) or a general medical condition (e.g., hypothyroidism).

D. The symptoms are not better accounted for by bereavement (i.e., after the loss of a loved one, the symptoms persist for longer than 2 months or are characterized by marked functional impairment, morbid preoccupation with worthlessness, suicidal ideation, psychotic symptoms, or psychomotor retardation).

DSM-IV = *Diagnostic and Statistical Manual of Mental Disorders,* 4th ed.
Reprinted with permission from American Psychiatric Association: *Diagnostic and Statistical Manual of Mental Disorders,* 4th ed. Washington, DC, American Psychiatric Association, 1994.

 2. **Cyclothymia.** This disorder lasts at least 2 years and involves episodes of hypomania and depressed mood. If the depressed mood meets the criteria for major depressive episode, then the diagnosis is bipolar II disorder.

VIII. **ANXIETY DISORDERS.** These disorders are the most common psychiatric disorders, with a lifetime prevalence of approximately 15%. Some anxiety disorders cause severe morbidity (e.g., agoraphobia, obsessive-compulsive disorder), and some (e.g., panic disorder) are confused with cardiac disease or other medical problems, so correct diagnosis is important.

A. **Panic disorder**

 1. **Diagnosis.** The diagnosis of panic disorder requires the presence of panic attacks that are **recurrent,** are **unexpected,** are not caused by a medical problem or substance use, and are followed by a period of distress or dysfunction. Panic attacks usually last 5 to 10 minutes. They involve intense fear or discomfort as well as physical symptoms such as palpitations, sweating, chest pain, shortness of breath, nausea, and numbness. It is

TABLE 15-8. DSM-IV Criteria for a Manic Episode

A. A distinct period of abnormally and persistently elevated, expansive, or irritable mood, lasting at least one week (or any duration if hospitalization is necessary)

B. During the period of mood disturbance, at least three of the following symptoms have persisted (four if the mood is only irritable) and have been present to a significant degree:

1. inflated self-esteem or grandiosity
2. decreased need for sleep (e.g., feels rested after only 3 hours of sleep)
3. more talkative than usual or pressure to keep talking
4. flight of ideas or subjective experience that thoughts are racing
5. distractibility (i.e., attention too easily drawn to unimportant or irrelevant external stimuli)
6. increase in goal-directed activity (e.g., socially, at work or school, or sexually) or psychomotor agitation
7. excessive involvement in pleasurable activities that have a high potential for painful consequences (e.g., the person engages in unrestrained buying sprees, sexual indiscretions, or foolish business investments)

C. The mood disturbance is sufficiently severe to cause marked impairment in the occupational functioning or in usual social activities or relationships with others or to necessitate hospitalization to prevent harm to self or others, or there are psychotic features

D. The symptoms are not due to the direct effects of a substance (e.g., drugs of abuse, medication) or a general medical condition (e.g., hyperthyroidism)

Note: Manic episodes that are clearly precipitated by somatic antidepressant treatment (e.g., medication, electroconvulsive therapy, light therapy) should not count toward a diagnosis of bipolar I disorder.

DSM-IV = *Diagnostic and Statistical Manual of Mental Disorders,* 4th ed.
Reprinted with permission from American Psychiatric Association: *Diagnostic and Statistical Manual of Mental Disorders,* 4th ed. Washington, DC, American Psychiatric Association, 1994.

important to note that panic attacks can occur with anxiety disorders other than panic disorder. Some patients with panic disorder also have agoraphobia.

2. **Treatment.** Tricyclic antidepressants, monoamine oxidase (MAO) inhibitors, and benzodiazepines (particularly alprazolam) are used to treat patients with panic disorder with or without agoraphobia. Relaxation training is a nonpharmacologic approach to treatment.

B. **Agoraphobia** ("fear of the market place"). This disorder is often a complication of panic disorder, but it may occur by itself.

1. **Diagnosis.** Patients with this disorder have strong fears of some situations outside the home (e.g., being in a crowd, traveling by bus or train). Often, the patient fears that he will be unable to escape or will do something embarrassing (e.g., have a panic attack). As a result, the patient does not leave home, leaves home only with a companion, or experiences severe distress when away from home. Some people with agoraphobia never leave home.

2. **Treatment.** Lasting improvement can be achieved with a behavioral technique known as in vivo exposure. With this treatment, the patient is exposed to the feared situation in the presence of a supportive therapist. Not all patients respond completely to this intervention.

C. **Specific phobia.** Patients with this disorder become fearful in specific situations, such as when flying or in the presence of certain animals (e.g., snakes). To differentiate this disorder from delusional disorders, the patient must recognize that the fear is excessive or irrational. Panic attacks may occur in response to the stimulus. Treatment is similar to that for agoraphobia.

D. **Social phobia.** This disorder is similar to specific phobia, but the patient fears a social situation (e.g., giving a lecture, attending a party). Panic attacks may occur in response to the social situation. Treatment can be behavioral, as with agoraphobia, or pharmacologic. The patient takes a benzodiazepine to inhibit anxiety or a β-blocker to inhibit tachycardia and tremulousness before each performance. MAO inhibitors also have proved useful.

E. **Obsessive-compulsive disorder.** This disorder should not be confused with obsessive-compulsive personality disorder (see Chapter 11 IV B 3 c).

1. **Diagnosis.** Patients with this diagnosis experience obsessions and/or compulsions. **Obsessions are recurrent, intrusive thoughts** that are distressing to the patient. The patient attempts to suppress, or neutralize, these thoughts. **Compulsions are repetitive behaviors** (e.g., hand washing) **or mental acts** (e.g., repeating words or numbers silently) that are often done to neutralize an obsessive thought. The patient may believe that the repetitive behaviors will prevent an unwanted occurrence. To differentiate obsessive-compulsive disorder from psychosis, the patient must realize that the thoughts or behaviors are irrational. To make the diagnosis, these symptoms must be distressing or time consuming, or must interfere with the ability of the individual to function.

2. **Treatment.** Patients may respond to treatment with **serotonergic antidepressant medication** (e.g., clomipramine, fluoxetine) or to **behavioral therapy.** For example, if a patient with a compulsion to wash his hands repeatedly after touching doorknobs is asked to touch one and is prevented from washing his hands, his level of anxiety may decrease.

F. **Posttraumatic stress disorder (PTSD).** This diagnosis is often associated with veterans, but it is also seen in individuals who have witnessed a murder or experienced another traumatic event.

1. **Diagnosis.** Individuals with this disorder have experienced or witnessed a life-threatening event and responded with fear or horror; reexperience the event (e.g., nightmares, flashbacks, intrusive thoughts); attempt to avoid thoughts or situations associated with the event, and experience a degree of numbing; and experience increased arousal, such as insomnia, irritability, or trouble concentrating. The symptoms last at least 1 month.

2. **Treatment.** Patients who experience recurrent threats need protection. When the threatening experience is over, treatment includes support and psychotherapy. The therapy is often time limited. Antidepressant and antianxiety medication also are useful.

G. **Generalized anxiety disorder.** Patients with this disorder worry excessively. As a result, they experience significant distress or difficulty functioning. Accompanying physical symptoms may include insomnia, fatigue, and muscle tension. Relaxation therapy produces modest results. Benzodiazepines are effective in some patients.

IX. **SOMATOFORM DISORDERS.** These disorders are important to physicians of all specialties, because affected patients have mental disorders that present with physical symptoms. Most people occasionally experience a mental state with accompanying physical symptoms (e.g., upset stomach when anxious), but somatoform disorders tend to be chronic and disabling.

A. **Somatization disorder.** Patients with this disorder have **chronic, diffuse physical symptoms** that are not explained by a medical condition. Patients seek treatment for the physical symptoms, and function may be impaired. The patient has at least four pain symptoms, two gastrointestinal symptoms, one sexual symptom, and one pseudoneurologic symptom (e.g., double vision, weakness, deafness) at some point. Group therapy and prophylactic visits to a primary care physician are helpful, and avoiding unnecessary medical procedures is important.

B. **Conversion disorder.** Patients with this disorder have **motor or sensory symptoms** (e.g., paralysis, deafness) that cannot be explained by a medical condition. The symptoms appear to be caused by emotional conflict or stress. Unlike malingering and factitious disorder, the symptoms are **not intentionally produced**. Treatment may include support, suggestions that the symptoms will remit, and insight-oriented therapy.

C. **Hypochondriasis.** A patient with this disorder experiences physical symptoms and becomes preoccupied with the belief that she has a serious illness. This belief persists after the patient receives appropriate evaluation and reassurance. The belief causes significant distress or dysfunction and persists for at least 6 months. If the belief becomes delusional (a subtle distinction at times), then the diagnosis of delusional disorder is made. Treatment involves education, suggestion, and a good alliance with a physician.

D. **Body dysmorphic disorder.** This disorder is similar to hypochondriasis except that, rather than a serious illness, the patient believes that he has a seriously defective appearance. For example, a woman is distressed by the belief that the pores on her nose are too large. She seeks treatment and limits her social contacts for this reason.

E. **Pain disorder associated with psychological factors.** This disorder is similar to conversion disorder, except that the symptom is pain rather than motor or other sensory symptoms. The disorder may be chronic, and it may lead to inappropriate tests and treatments. Treatment includes detoxification from narcotic analgesics, which are often prescribed despite their lack of efficacy; physical rehabilitation; and cognitive–behavioral therapy, including relaxation therapy and evaluation for sources of secondary gain (e.g., a man who had back pain that was attributed to stress during divorce proceedings now has the secondary gain of not having to go to work or pay alimony because of his "disability").

X. **FACTITIOUS DISORDER.** This disorder is difficult to understand because patients feign or even induce illness. For example, a patient may add a drop of blood to a urine sample to fake a kidney ailment. These patients appear to have a **psychological need to be regarded as ill** and to receive care, even if treatment involves surgery or painful tests. This disorder must be distinguished from **malingering,** which is not considered a mental illness. Malingerers deliberately feign symptoms for an external, alterior (nonpsychological) reason, such as to avoid work, obtain a prescription for narcotics, or win a lawsuit.

XI. **DISSOCIATIVE DISORDERS.** These disorders are controversial. Some clinicians see many cases. Other clinicians claim that dissociation is iatrogenic or indicates another mental problem, such as a severe personality disorder. However, accumulating evidence in the clinical and neuroscience literature supports the presence of this group of disorders. These disorders include bizarre symptoms, and they are often represented (not necessarily accurately) in movies and the press. The diagnosis of a dissociative disorder is not made if the symptoms are caused by drug ingestion (e.g., alcoholic blackouts) or a general medical condition (e.g., temporal lobe epilepsy).

A. **Dissociative amnesia.** Individuals with this disorder have amnesia for important personal information.

B. **Dissociative fugue.** A patient with this disorder suddenly travels away and cannot recall her past. The patient may be confused about self-identity or assume a new identity.

C. **Dissociative identity disorder (multiple personality disorder).** A patient with this disorder has two or more distinct identities or personality states that control his actions. The "host" personality, who may present to a physician, is aware of "lost time," but may not know what occurs during that time and may be embarrassed to discuss it. For example, a patient may have injuries but not know how they occurred, or may give an implausible explanation. Most patients with this disorder experienced **severe childhood trauma,** such as sexual or physical abuse.

D. **Depersonalization disorder.** A patient with this disorder has feelings of detachment from body or mind; however, reality testing remains intact. The symptoms of depersonalization cause the patient significant distress or functional impairment.

XII. **SEXUAL AND GENDER IDENTITY DISORDERS.** These disorders are described in Chapter 9.

XIII. **EATING DISORDERS.** Patients with eating disorders often will present to a physician with related physical problems (e.g., bowel dysfunction because of chronic laxative abuse, parotid gland inflammation, or tooth decay caused by self-induced vomiting).

A. **Anorexia nervosa**

1. **Diagnosis.** This disorder is usually seen in teenage girls and young women. These patients have low body weight and a **fear of becoming fat**. Many have a **distorted body image**. Self-starvation leads to amenorrhea (cessation of menstruation), which is another criterion for the disorder. Binge eating or purging (self-induced vomiting or the use of laxatives) may occur.

2. **Treatment.** Medical complications that must be evaluated include leukopenia, electrolyte imbalance, endocrine disturbance, and osteoporosis. Depression commonly accompanies starvation, and usually responds to **weight gain,** which should be **gradual**. Behavioral therapy, such as reinforcement of weight gain, is helpful, as is family therapy. After the patient gains weight, individual and group psychotherapy is important.

B. **Bulimia nervosa**

1. **Diagnosis.** Patients with bulimia engage in **recurrent binge eating** (consuming an excessive amount of food in a short period, with an accompanying sense of lack of control over the eating) and **purging** or other compensating behaviors, such as excessive exercise. The DSM-IV criteria require that both binge eating and the compensatory behavior occur (on average) twice each week for at least 3 months. Medical complications include tooth erosion, electrolyte imbalance, parotid gland swelling, and gastrointestinal disorders.

2. **Treatment.** Therapy for bulimia includes nutritional instruction, individual or group psychotherapy, family involvement, and antidepressant medication.

XIV. **SLEEP DISORDERS.** There are several approaches to diagnosing sleep disorders. The DSM-IV divides sleep disorders into **primary and secondary disorders**. Primary sleep disorders include dyssomnias and parasomnias. Secondary sleep disorders include those that are caused by another mental disorder, a general medical condition, or substance use. Dyssomnias and parasomnias are described briefly (also see Chapter 2 III A).

A. **Dyssomnias.** Patients with dyssomnias have difficulty initiating or maintaining sleep or with the sleep cycle. The diagnosis is made after patient history and evaluation have excluded medical, drug-induced, and other psychiatric explanations (e.g., insomnia as a symptom of major depressive disorder).

1. **Primary insomnia.** A patient with primary insomnia has trouble falling asleep or staying asleep. The problem lasts at least 1 month. This trouble causes significant distress or functional impairment.

2. **Primary hypersomnia.** Patients with this disorder experience excessive sleepiness for at least 1 month which leads to distress or dysfunction.

3. **Narcolepsy.** Patients with narcolepsy have irresistible daytime sleep attacks (even while talking or driving), cataplexy (sudden loss of muscle tone when awake), and almost immediate onset of rapid eye movement (REM) activity upon falling asleep.

4. **Breathing-related sleep disorder.** Several breathing disorders, such as sleep apnea, can cause insomnia or hypersomnia.

5. **Circadian rhythm sleep disorder.** This disorder represents a mismatch between an individual's sleep–wake cycle and his environment. This condition is seen with some types of shift work and in individuals who experience frequent jet lag. The diagnosis is made only if the patient experiences significant distress or functional impairment.

B. Parasomnias. These disorders occur during either REM or non-REM sleep phases.

1. **Nightmare disorder.** Patients who have frequent nightmares can experience significant distress or functional problems. Because dreaming occurs during REM sleep, nightmares usually occur in the latter part of the night.

2. **Sleep terror disorder.** This disorder is usually seen in children. Patients recurrently awaken from sleep in a panicked state (e.g., screaming, tachycardia). Sleep terrors differ from nightmares in that they do not follow a dream, the person is unresponsive to comfort from others, and the person does not remember the episode. Sleep terrors occur during deep, non-REM sleep, usually early in the night.

3. **Sleepwalking disorder.** This disorder occurs during non-REM sleep, usually early in the night. It occurs predominantly in children. The person is difficult to awaken while walking, and does not remember the episode.

XV. IMPULSE CONTROL DISORDERS

A. Intermittent explosive disorder. Patients with this disorder experience periods of destructive aggression that are out of proportion to the precipitating stress and are not caused by another psychiatric condition (e.g., psychosis, antisocial personality disorder) or drug use.

B. Kleptomania. Patients with this disorder steal to release building tension rather than for monetary gain or vengeance.

C. Pyromania. Patients with this disorder set fires to release tension rather than for external reasons, such as for money or vengeance.

D. Pathological gambling. Patients with this disorder are preoccupied with gambling. They often attempt unsuccessfully to stop gambling, lie or commit crime to enable gambling, jeopardize personal relationships and employment, and gamble with increasing amounts of money.

E. Trichotillomania. Patients with this disorder compulsively pull their hair to the point of hair loss. This disorder may be related to obsessive-compulsive disorder, and may respond to similar treatment.

XVI. **ADJUSTMENT DISORDER.** Any individual may experience emotional symptoms in response to stress, but in some people, the symptoms become clinically significant. Patients with adjustment disorder experience anxiety, depression, behavioral problems, or a mixture of symptoms that are either distressing or cause dysfunction. Symptoms start within 3 months of a stressor and last no more than 6 months after the stress is over. The symptoms are not caused by bereavement and do not meet the criteria for another mental disorder. For example, while his wife is being treated for cancer, a man experiences distress and misses many days at work. He feels well within 1 month of his wife's recovery.

XVII. **PERSONALITY DISORDERS.** Some individuals exhibit personality features that are **chronically maladaptive** and interfere with such functions as the ability to work or to sustain meaningful relationships. These disorders may occur alone or may co-exist with other mental disorders, such as depression or substance abuse. The symptoms of the various disorders overlap, and few patients exhibit a "pure" personality disorder. The DSM-IV describes 10 personality disorders (see Chapter 11 IV). Identifying one or more of these disorders in a patient can help the clinician to understand the behavior of the patient and provide appropriate treatment. Behavior that suggests a personality disorder begins by early adulthood and occurs in a variety of contexts.

XVIII. **CONCLUSION.** Every physician will encounter patients who exhibit mental symptoms that cause significant distress or dysfunction. The identification of particular disorders will help the clinician to better understand patients, predict problems, and provide appropriate treatment or referral.

BIBLIOGRAPHY

American Psychiatric Association: *Diagnostic and Statistical Manual of Mental Disorders,* 4th ed. Washington, DC, American Psychiatric Association, 1994.

American Psychiatric Association: *Treatments of Psychiatric Disorders: A Task Force Report of the American Psychiatric Association.* Washington, DC, American Psychiatric Association, 1989.

STUDY QUESTIONS

DIRECTIONS: Each of the numbered items or incomplete statements in this section is followed by answers or by completions of the statement. Select the ONE lettered answer or completion that is BEST in each case.

1. Which of the following statements about dementia is true?

(A) Multi-infarct dementia is the most common form of dementia

(B) Pick's disease and Creutzfeldt-Jakob disease are treatable causes of dementia

(C) Hydrocephalus and thyroid disorders are treatable causes of dementia

(D) Alzheimer's disease can be diagnosed only by positron emission tomography (PET) scan

(E) Dementia and delirium are mutually exclusive diagnoses

2. A 17-year-old girl comes to a clinic for evaluation of amenorrhea. The patient is 5 feet, 8 inches tall, and weighs 92 pounds. If the correct diagnosis is anorexia nervosa, then your evaluation is likely to show all of the following findings EXCEPT

(A) she has the symptoms of major depressive disorder

(B) she has significant tooth damage from self-induced vomiting

(C) she feels fat and wants to lose weight

(D) results of a battery of laboratory tests are normal

(E) she feels the need to use laxatives daily

DIRECTIONS: Each of the numbered items or incomplete statements in this section is negatively phrased, as indicated by a capitalized word such as NOT, LEAST, or EXCEPT. Select the ONE lettered answer or completion that is BEST in each case.

3. Each of the following statements is correct regarding the similarities and differences between schizophrenia and bipolar mood disorder EXCEPT

(A) schizophrenia and manic episodes both have a lifetime prevalence of approximately 1%

(B) patients with both disorders may require treatment with antipsychotic medication at times

(C) between episodes, patients with schizophrenia usually show significant functional impairment, whereas many patients with bipolar mood disorder return to their normal level of functioning

(D) hallucinations are seen in patients with schizophrenia, but never in bipolar mood disorder

(E) first-line maintenance medication treatment for schizophrenia is antipsychotics, and for bipolar mood disorder, it is lithium

4. Each of the following statements is true regarding major depressive disorder EXCEPT

(A) major depressive disorder has a lifetime prevalence of approximately 6%

(B) approximately 70% to 80% of patients with major depressive disorder respond to appropriate treatment with antidepressant medication

(C) an individual must have significant depressive symptoms for 2 months to meet the criteria for major depressive disorder

(D) most patients with major depressive disorder are treated by primary care physicians rather than psychiatrists

(E) for a patient who is experiencing a major depressive episode, a history of manic episode changes the diagnosis from major depressive disorder to bipolar mood disorder

DIRECTIONS: Each set of matching questions in this section consists of a list of four to twenty-six lettered options (some of which may be in figures) followed by several numbered items. For each numbered item, select the ONE lettered option that is most closely associated with it. To avoid spending too much time on matching sets with large numbers of options, it is generally advisable to begin each set by reading the list of options. Then, for each item in the set, try to generate the correct answer and locate it in the option list, rather than evaluating each option individually. Each lettered option may be selected once, more than once, or not at all.

Questions 5–7

For each set of symptoms, select the substance-related disorder in which it is commonly seen.

(A) Alcohol intoxication
(B) Amphetamine intoxication
(C) Hallucinogen intoxication
(D) Opioid intoxication
(E) Phencyclidine (PCP) intoxication

5. Euphoria, hypervigilance, dilated pupils, and cardiac arrhythmia

6. Apathy, pupillary constriction, drowsiness, slurred speech

7. Labile mood, slurred speech, unsteady gait, nystagmus

Questions 8–10

For each case example, select the most appropriate diagnosis.

(A) Panic disorder
(B) Agoraphobia
(C) Social phobia
(D) Obsessive-compulsive disorder
(E) Posttraumatic stress disorder

8. A 23-year-old law student comes to a clinic at the request of her father. She states that each time she is called on in class, she feels flushed, dizzy, sick, and tremulous, and is fearful of embarrassing herself. Because this situation is so distressing, she is considering withdrawing from law school.

9. A 40-year-old, anxious man mentions during an examination that he has just lost his job. On questioning, he reluctantly admits that he had been increasingly late for work because it takes him hours to get ready each morning. He knows that it sounds crazy, but his shoelaces must be tied in a special way. He sometimes reknots his necktie 40 to 50 times, because if his grooming is not perfect, he worries that something bad will happen and that it will be his fault.

10. A 35-year-old woman makes an appointment to request sleeping pills. On questioning, she states that she was seriously injured in a car accident 4 months ago. Another passenger was badly injured as well. Since the accident, she has had insomnia and nightmares, cannot ride in a car, and cannot stop thinking about the accident.

![decorative] **ANSWERS AND EXPLANATIONS**

1. The answer is C [III B]. Hydrocephalus and thyroid disorders must be considered in the evaluation of a patient with dementia because both conditions are potentially reversible. Pick's disease and Creutzfeldt-Jakob disease are not treatable. Alzheimer's disease, which is the most common form of dementia, can be definitively diagnosed only by a pathologist. Dementia and delirium can occur in the same patient, although diagnosing dementia in a patient who is delirious is difficult without a thorough history.

2. The answer is D [XIII A]. Significant depressive symptoms are common in patients with anorexia nervosa, as are self-induced vomiting and the use of laxatives. The vomiting can lead to tooth erosion and swollen parotid glands, and chronic laxative abuse can cause gastrointestinal complications. Feeling fat despite being significantly underweight is a feature of anorexia nervosa. This patient's laboratory test results probably would not be normal. Starvation and vomiting usually cause leukopenia and electrolyte and endocrine disturbances.

3. The answer is D [VI A; VII B]. Patients with major depressive disorder or bipolar mood disorder can have periods of psychosis, including hallucinations and delusions, during episodes of mood disturbance. This similarity between the two disorders can make diagnosis difficult if the patient is being seen for the first time and the background history is not available.

4. The answer is C [VII A]. The criteria for major depressive disorder require that at least five symptoms of depression be present for 2 weeks, rather than 2 months. Symptoms include depressed mood, loss of interest in activities, weight loss, insomnia, fatigue, and suicidal ideation.

5–7. The answers are: 5-B, 6-D, 7-A [Table 15-4]. Other features of amphetamine intoxication, which resembles cocaine intoxication, are impaired judgment, perspiration or chills, confusion, illusions, and hallucinations.

Opioid intoxication causes initial euphoria, but the user then becomes apathetic and dysphoric. Impaired attention and memory are also seen.

Phencyclidine (PCP) intoxication shares the symptoms of unsteady gait and nystagmus with alcohol intoxication. However, with PCP intoxication, belligerence, impulsiveness, and agitation are characteristic behavior, whereas labile mood and slurred speech are seen with alcohol intoxication.

8–10. The answers are: 8-C [VIII D], **9-D** [VIII E], **10-E** [VIII F]. The student appears to be having recurrent panic attacks when she is asked to perform in class. Therefore, she has social phobia. The diagnosis could be confirmed by verifying that she has never had an unexpected panic attack, which would suggest panic disorder, and that the episodes are not caused by drug ingestion or a general medical condition.

This man engages in compulsive behavior (e.g., tying his shoelaces and necktie in impossibly perfect ways) as a way of preventing something bad from happening. He recognizes that the behavior is irrational, yet it has been so time consuming that he has lost his job.

This woman shows symptoms of posttraumatic stress disorder in response to a serious car accident. She reexperiences the event through nightmares and intrusive thoughts, avoids riding in cars, and has insomnia, which is associated with increased arousal.

Chapter 16

Ethics in Medicine

Bradley Lewis
David DeGrazia

I. **INTRODUCTION.** The ethical concerns of medical care have been an integral part of western medicine since its inception. However, it was not until the late 1960s and early 1970s that medical ethics emerged as a distinct area of academic and professional interest. Various factors contributed to the emergence of this field, including an explosion of new technologies and procedures (e.g., organ transplants, recombinant DNA technology), social concern about human abuses (e.g., Nazi medical atrocities), and a sharp increase since the 1960s in the percentage of the gross national product dedicated to health care. Questions about the goals of medical care, the moral obligation of the physician to the patient and to society, and the extent to which a physician may allow quality of life considerations to affect medical decision making are addressed in this growing field of interest.

A. **The Hippocratic tradition** provides the foundation for many ethical principles in contemporary western medicine. It begins with a group of medical writings known as the Hippocratic corpus, which probably dates from the fourth century B.C. The **Hippocratic oath** commences a long tradition of medical ethics whose core principle is that **a physician is morally obliged to benefit the patient and to protect the patient from harm** in accordance with the physician's best judgment. The oath makes no mention of the importance of patient autonomy or of balancing the physician's duty to the patient with duties to the rest of society. Some believe that mainstream American medicine departed from the Hippocratic tradition with the approval of the 1980 version of the **American Medical Association (AMA) Principles of Medical Ethics**. These principles acknowledge the patient's rights (autonomy) and the physician's responsibility to society and not exclusively to the patient (justice). They also recognize the judgment of the patient and others in addition to the physician.

B. **Scope of medical ethics**

1. **Social issues.** Medical ethics extends beyond the physician–patient relationship to include social issues that become increasingly important as the cost of care rises inexorably and affects other aspects of social life. Questions about the allocation of limited resources and the balance between medical and other societal needs are important issues in medical ethics.

2. **Legal issues.** Ethical issues also affect the legal field. The legal system often settles disputes involving fundamental ethical issues (e.g., informed consent, termination of care, surrogate motherhood).

3. **Psychiatric and behavioral medicine issues**
   a. The rights of incompetent individuals
   b. The justification of involuntary psychiatric hospitalization
   c. The development and application of mind-altering and behavior-modifying technologies
   d. Decisions about death and dying (e.g., morality of suicide)

C. **Definitions**

1. **Values are objects, actions, or states** (e.g., happiness), **or the beliefs or attitudes concerning them and their desirability**. For every value, there is a corresponding principle that requires the promotion of that value (e.g., respect for life).

2. **Ethics is the study of the general nature of moral obligation and specific moral choices.** Ethics involves an exploration of values and principles. In determining whether a judgment, choice, rule, or principle is moral versus, for example, legal, political, or religious, scholars in ethics apply various criteria.
   a. Moral action guides often are considered **supreme** (i.e., to override other types of considerations, such as legal concerns).
   b. They are generally considered **universalizable** (i.e., generalizable to similar cases).
   c. They usually concern the welfare of other individuals.

3. **Morality** has several meanings.
   a. In academic settings, the term is typically used interchangeably with ethics.
   b. However, morality also has a meaning closely connected to the word **mores, or a particular set of moral attitudes, beliefs, and customs**. In this sense, different cultures, or even different philosophers or theologians, may have different moralities.
   c. **Morality also refers to the moral system that is considered objectively correct** (e.g., Morality requires all persons to be treated with respect).

II. THE CHARACTER OF ETHICAL CONFLICT

A. Types of conflict

1. **Conflict occurs when individuals have different values or principles.** For example, physicians consider the preservation of life one of their most important goals, so life is one of their values. However, a Jehovah's Witness who needs a blood transfusion may regard freedom from blood products such an important value that it precludes transfusions, even when they are necessary to stay alive.

2. Individuals who agree on a basic value or principle may have **different conceptions of the value or principle**. For example, Aristotelians and medieval theologians agreed that happiness, or human flourishing, was the fundamental value (and goal) of humankind, but the former conceived of this goal as something to be achieved in this life, whereas the latter conceived of it as being achieved in an afterlife.

3. It is possible to agree on a certain value or principle and even on a particular conception of it, yet disagree as to what **means** will best bring about the value or fulfill the principle. This disagreement is not an ethical conflict. For example, an oncologist and a patient with cancer may agree on the value of minimizing suffering. However, one might believe that the increased dosage of a particular narcotic analgesic would be an effective means to reduce suffering, whereas the other might believe that the analgesic would lead to greater suffering because of the narcotic side effects.

4. Conflicts also occur when individuals agree on more than one value or principle, but disagree as to their **relative weight or priority**. For example, two physicians might agree on the principle of confidentiality and the principle of preventing harm. However, if a patient states an intention to maintain a sexual relationship with her lover, despite being infected with human immunodeficiency virus (HIV), one physician may believe that preventing harm takes priority and favor disclosing the danger to that person or the police, whereas the other may favor respecting the patient's confidentiality.

B. Addressing conflicts.
Differences in values, conceptions, or means can create ethical conflicts in medicine. Decisions are often made informally within the physician–patient relationship, sometimes with family involvement, without the use of institutional mechanisms (e.g., government policy, professional codes, hospital ethics committees).

1. Conflicts are often influenced by factors other than ethical considerations. For example, the political convictions of the community in which a hospital is located may influence care (e.g., by affecting how the relative importance of life and quality of life are seen). Economic factors may also affect health care delivery, for example, when an intensive care unit is budgeted too few beds to meet current need.

2. Health professionals must recognize ethical issues when they arise, distinguish them from other factors, and attempt to resolve them in terms of the theories, principles, and rules that constitute the basis of sound ethical reasoning.

III. GENERAL ETHICAL THEORY.

The most conspicuous source of systematic thinking in contemporary medical ethics may be the ethical theories developed by western **secular moral philosophers**. Medical ethics is a modern branch of moral philosophy, or ethics, that is concerned with moral problems that arise in medical practice, policy, and research. Because medical ethics is a component of the discipline of ethics, it turns to general ethical theories and principles for guidance.

A. **Utilitarianism states that the right action is that which brings about the greatest possible good.** Thus, utilitarian theories are distinguished by what they consider good (value theories) and by their broad strategies for maximizing good. All versions of utilitarianism share the feature of defining moral rightness entirely in terms of the **consequences** of an action, as opposed to the type of action (e.g., a lie) or the character or intentions of the person involved.

1. Value theories
  a. **Hedonism,** defended by the classic utilitarians Bentham and Mill, **is the view that a good consequence is pleasure.** This theory encompasses pleasure of all types, including refined pleasures, such as reading great literature, performing charitable acts, and friendship.
  b. **Pluralism holds that good consequences are derived from several intrinsically valuable pursuits.** Different theorists value different pursuits, including friendship, beauty, knowledge, love, and health.
  c. **Preference utilitarianism states that individuals should maximize the satisfaction of their preferences or desires.** This theory sometimes plays a role in health policy analysis and in decisions about the just allocation of resources.

2. Approaches to maximizing good consequences
  a. **Act utilitarianism** applies the idea of maximizing good consequences to **specific acts** in specific circumstances. For example, a dermatologist might weigh the psychological benefits of cosmetic surgery for a particular patient against the burdens of great financial expenditure and the trauma of undergoing surgery. Act utilitarians take a comparatively case-by-case approach to deciding which action maximizes good consequences.
  b. **Rule utilitarianism** applies the idea of maximizing good consequences to **general practices,** not to specific acts. For example, rather than asking, "Would it maximize good consequences to allow this severely handicapped baby to die?," this approach would ask, "Would it maximize good consequences to have a regular practice of allowing babies to die in certain circumstances?"

B. **Deontology.** Deontologists hold that **an act is right insofar as it complies with some overriding** (nonutilitarian) **principle of obligation.** Therefore, a **type of action** (e.g., killing, torture) is considered right or wrong. There are many deontological theories, and most consider consequences to some extent. However, they do not justify principles and actions exclusively in terms of consequences.

1. Features of deontological theories
  a. Deontologists believe that individuals have diverse duties, some of which are the result of **special relationships** (e.g., physician–patient, parent–child, debtor–creditor). For example, a parent should provide for a child's welfare, not because doing so maximizes good consequences overall, but simply because this obligation is part of being a parent. Utilitarians, on the other hand, ignore special relationships.
  b. Deontologists hold that utilitarianism cannot adequately address the fact that **past actions can lead to current obligations**. For example, they argue that the act of

making a promise or of injuring someone obliges the individual to keep the promise or to offer compensation, respectively. The basis for such an obligation is not that promise keeping or compensation maximizes good consequences.

   c. Deontologists typically insist on the moral importance of the **motives and character** of an agent, apart from the consequences of its actions. For example, if a surgeon always carefully explains to patients the risks and benefits of a surgical procedure, as well as the alternatives, but does so only to win praise from colleagues and avoid malpractice suits, in this view there is nothing praiseworthy about such actions.

   d. Contemporary deontological theories often take the form of **rights theories**. According to these theories, each individual has certain moral claims (e.g., to life, liberty, some minimal standard of welfare) that cannot be overridden by utilitarian appeals to the consequences of specific actions. For instance, Rawls (see III B 2 d) argues that, regardless of whether it is justified on utilitarian grounds, slavery violates the right to liberty and is therefore wrong.

2. **Deontological theories**

   a. The most prominent deontological theory is that of **Kant,** who held that an act is praiseworthy only if it is performed, not from self-interest or because of its actual consequences, but because of a sense of duty. Duty can be determined by the application of Kant's **categorical imperative,** which has three formulations. The second formulation is the most relevant for medicine: "So act as to treat humanity, whether in your own person or in that of any other, in every case as an end and never as merely a means only." Kant also held that an act is a duty only if it is addressed by a rule that is universally valid and therefore rational. For example, breaking promises is always wrong because, if everyone followed a rule of breaking promises, no one would take promises seriously, and the institution of promise keeping would be destroyed.

   b. A less rigid deontological theory that considers consequences is that of **Ross.** According to Ross, the right action, or an individual's **actual duty,** is determined by examining the respective weights or competing **prima facie duties** (e.g., promise keeping, reparation for past injuries), which are known by moral intuition. Prima facie duties are binding, but can be overridden by other prima facie duties in cases of conflict. For example, a physician who could benefit one patient by breaking a promise to a second whom she had promised to see first must consider the two prima facie duties and decide which seems more important under the circumstances.

   c. **Rawls's theory of justice,** which applies to **social institutions,** not individual actions, is a recent deontological theory.

      (1) Rawls argues that certain principles of justice are validated by imagining what principles would be selected by free and equal persons in a hypothetical bargaining situation. Social contractors are imagined to select principles in the absence of knowledge (e.g., about talents, wealth, health, place in society) that could bias their view. Equal access to health care is often argued from a Rawlsian perspective. Unbiased social contractors would likely choose equal access because health is a prerequisite to opportunity in a free society.

      (2) According to Rawls, the contractors would agree that everyone should be permitted the greatest amount of liberty that is compatible with everyone's having it equally. They would also agree that, once equal liberty is ensured, unequal distribution of primary social goods (e.g., income) is permitted only if there is fair opportunity and everyone benefits from allowing the inequality. Thus, entrepreneurs might be allowed to receive great economic rewards, but only if this arrangement improved opportunities and working conditions for the least advantaged.

   d. **Robert Nozick's** version of **libertarianism** is a second deontological theory of justice. Libertarian justice is guaranteed by the results of free and fair exchanges in the marketplace. According to this view, Rawlsian and utilitarian redistributions of goods are unjust because they require certain individuals to benefit others (e.g., through taxation). This theory views liberty as the only genuine right. For example, the only just system of health care allocation is one in which health insurance is voluntarily purchased at the individual's initiative.

C. **Virtue theory** regards the primary ethical category as character, focusing on the question "What should I be?" Recent attention to virtue theory signals the reemergence of the type of ethical theory proposed by Plato and Aristotle.

1. Virtue theorists consider judgments about a person's character traits, disposition, and motives more important than judgments about actions. For example, if a cardiologist makes a technical or judgmental error that leads to further medical complications, this theory questions whether the error was caused by **negligence** or a **bad attitude** or was an **innocent mistake**.

2. Virtue theorists also believe that rules and principles, which tend to be complex or to conflict frequently, are not useful in practice. For example, in a medical emergency, it is better for a physician to be able to rely on deeply ingrained character traits (e.g., prudence, benevolence, truthfulness) than to attempt to consult abstract rules of action. However, for each virtue, there is usually a corresponding principle (e.g., benevolence corresponds to beneficence).

IV. **MAJOR ETHICAL PRINCIPLES.** Ethical decision making is often a difficult and stressful task. Physicians must address complex issues and deal with uncertainties. In clinical situations, there often is not time to consult ethical theories, and ethical theories are usually not specific enough to provide guidance for specific cases. For these reasons, medical ethics relies heavily on ethical principles: respect for autonomy, beneficence, nonmaleficence, and justice. These principles are endorsed by all of the ethical theories. They are also comprehensive enough to provide an analytic framework for individual cases. Unfortunately, ethical principles often conflict. For example, a physician may be able to benefit a patient with a procedure, but the patient may not want to undergo the procedure. As a result, there is a conflict between beneficence and respect for autonomy.

A. **Autonomy is the capacity for a person to be self-governing:** to be able to deliberate on possible courses of action, form a plan, and act on the basis of these deliberations.

1. **Respect for autonomy** is the principle that **autonomous, and therefore competent, individuals should be allowed to determine their own course of action** for reasons that are their own, and not imposed by another. This principle is relevant to the practice of **informed consent**.

2. Respect for autonomy demands more than freedom from external constraints. Individuals should not be intimidated, manipulated, or psychologically pressured. In addition, individuals should not be lied to or denied information that is directly relevant to their decisions.

B. **Beneficence is the obligation to promote the welfare of others.** In medicine, beneficence involves the obligation to take active steps to promote health and prevent or remove harmful conditions. This principle is relevant on both an individual level (e.g., caring for a patient) and a social level (e.g., considering institutional structures and their benefits for society).

C. **Nonmaleficence is the principle that an individual should not harm others.** Many medical ethicists distinguish nonmaleficence from beneficence to emphasize that it is negative in character (i.e., it requires that an individual not do something). In most cases, the obligation not to harm others is greater than the obligation to benefit them. Nonmaleficence is relevant on both an individual and a social level.

D. **Justice concerns the distribution of benefits and burdens.** According to this principle, each individual must receive a fair share of available goods and services as well as necessary burdens (e.g., taxes). Theories of justice have different conceptions of what constitutes a fair share. For example, a **fair share** may be defined as equal distribution of benefits (strict egalitarianism); distribution according to need (socialism); whatever distribution maximizes benefits overall (utilitarianism); or whatever distribution results from free exchanges among individuals (libertarianism).

V. FUNDAMENTAL ISSUES AND CONTROVERSIES IN MEDICAL ETHICS

A. The physician–patient relationship

1. **Ethical models.** Chapter 11 describes four models of the physician–patient relationship: paternalistic, informative, interpretive, and deliberative. The paternalistic approach and the models of patient autonomy can be described from an ethical perspective.
   a. **Paternalism** is the model that arose from the Hippocratic tradition and its emphasis on beneficence. It occurs when a clinician interferes with the action or decision making of a patient for the patient's benefit. Paternalism once commonly characterized the physician–patient relationship; now it is reserved for specific unusual situations (e.g., psychiatric detention).
      (1) **Strong paternalism** interferes with the freedom of a substantially autonomous, competent person. An example is psychiatric detention of a patient who knows that she has a mental disorder and understands the treatment options, but refuses inpatient treatment. Because this patient is capable of giving informed consent, there is a definite conflict between beneficence and respect for autonomy.
      (2) **Weak paternalism** interferes with the freedom of a person who is not substantially autonomous. An example is psychiatric detention of a patient who has bipolar disorder and is involved in potentially self-damaging behavior, but does not understand that he has a psychiatric problem. In this case, beneficence is relevant, but respect for autonomy is not.
      (3) When a person with a psychiatric disorder is detained, not for her benefit but to **protect others,** the detention is not paternalistic. As with paternalistic detention, beneficence is either favored over respect for autonomy or is the only relevant principle. When a patient is detained to protect others, beneficence is directed to the people who are protected.
   b. **Autonomy model.** Although paternalism is sometimes appropriate, there is an emerging consensus for an autonomy model in most situations. This model involves shared decision making. The physician brings medical knowledge and suggestions, and the patient brings knowledge of his interests and values. In an attempt to balance the sometimes conflicting principles of beneficence, autonomy, and justice, this model favors autonomy in the case of competent adult patients, who are presumed to have a right to self-determination.

2. **Managing medical information**
   a. **Truth telling.** The physician's obligation of truth telling derives from the principle of respect for patient autonomy. Many physicians, however, still view truthfulness through the Hippocratic tradition of beneficence. As such, they may consider it ethical to withhold information (e.g., a diagnosis of cancer) if the information might be upsetting and potentially harmful to a patient's fragile condition. A similar justification is sometimes used with deception (e.g., placebo medication) or even lying (e.g., telling a patient a false diagnosis). The contrasting view is that intentional suppression of relevant information violates a patient's right to autonomy and therefore the fundamental obligations of the physician. The solution may be to **consider truth telling a strong prima facie duty** that can be overridden only in unusual situations.
   b. **Informed consent.** Before a physician performs a medical procedure on a competent patient, the physician must obtain the patient's informed consent. This consent is obtained after the physician and patient make a joint decision about the treatment. Joint decision making requires the physician to disclose relevant information about alternative procedures and their effects to a competent patient. The patient

must comprehend the information before he can voluntarily enter into an agreement with the physician about a course of treatment. Because these conditions address the patient's ability to make informed and voluntary decisions for himself, they involve respect for autonomy. In certain situations, informed consent may be bypassed.

(1) Occasionally, a competent patient declines information and prefers to have the physician make a medical decision (e.g., whether to initiate chemotherapy). In this case, the appropriate course of action is debatable. A defensible course is to honor the patient's wish not to be given further information, thereby respecting the patient's autonomy, and considering this wish a waiver of informed consent.

(2) In an **emergency** the physician may assume that the patient would want to have her life saved. After the emergency passes, the requirement for informed consent returns.

(3) **Implied consent** is given for routine procedures in which there is minimal risk to the patient (e.g., taking blood pressure).

(4) On rare occasions a physician believes that informing the patient may cause the patient serious and identifiable harm. When this argument is legitimate, **informed consent may be bypassed through therapeutic privilege**. This exception is subject to paternalistic abuse, however, and should not be evoked without serious and identifiable harm. For example, concern that the patient will become anxious or depressed is not adequate to evoke therapeutic privilege.

c. Confidentiality is important in medicine because of the disclosure of sensitive information by patients. Although truth telling and informed consent are new topics in medical ethics, confidentiality has been a fundamental part of the physician–patient relationship since the Hippocratic oath: "Whatever I see or hear, professionally or privately, which ought not to be divulged, I will keep secret and tell no one."

(1) Respect for confidentiality can be justified by appeal to either respect for autonomy or nonmaleficence because breaches of confidentiality damage the trust that permits a strong physician–patient relationship.

(2) Despite the importance of confidentiality, beneficence to society or to another person sometimes takes priority. For example, when a patient announces an intention to kill a specific person, the physician is required by law to protect that person. This protection often involves warning the person or the appropriate authorities. This issue was addressed in the California Supreme Court case *Tarasoff v. Regents of the University of California.*

3. Decision making

a. Refusal of medical treatment. Recent court decisions generally support the right of competent patients to refuse medical interventions, even when such refusal is likely to lead to death. For these court decisions and the physicians who respect them, respect for autonomy outweighs beneficence in this context. Some states permit involuntary detention of individuals who appear to be substantially dangerous to themselves because of mental illness, even if these individuals are competent to give informed consent. These states paternalistically place beneficence above respect for autonomy in these cases.

b. Deciding for others. Some of the most difficult cases in medical ethics involve choosing what is best for incompetent patients (e.g., children, mentally retarded adults). Surrogate decision making is necessary for these patients.

(1) **Competence** is a legal term; therefore, only a judge has the authority to declare an individual legally incompetent. The declaration of incompetence centers on whether a person basically understands the treatment issues involved. A person who is mentally ill, or demented, may be competent to refuse medical treatment if she understands the treatment that is offered and the risks associated with refusing the treatment. Incompetence is defined in terms of specific situations (e.g., an individual may be competent to make medical decisions for himself but incompetent to manage his finances).

(2) When a person is incompetent to decide, a surrogate decision maker is chosen. Usually, a member of the patient's family is chosen; occasionally, a court-ordered guardian is used. If the patient was formerly competent, the surrogate decision maker attempts to assess the wishes of the patient by consulting formal statements (e.g., living will, medical advance directive, patient values history) or informal statements (e.g., letters, expressed religious convictions). If these sources are not available, or if the patient was never competent, then the surrogate must decide based on what an average person's best interests would be under similar circumstances.

(3) Occasionally, there is a conflict between the decision of the surrogate and the patient's apparent best interests. For example, a father may refuse life-sustaining treatment for his child because of his faith in the Christian Science tradition. If the father were deciding for himself, and were competent, autonomy would take precedence, and he would be able to refuse treatment. However, because the child cannot deliberate and decide alone, it is reasonable to follow a policy of beneficence and attempt to secure the welfare of the child (e.g., appointing a guardian other than the father). This approach is particularly important when the medical decision is essential to the life of the child.

c. **Living wills.** In many states, competent adults are permitted to sign living wills. This directive authorizes physicians to withhold or discontinue artificial life support if the patient is terminally ill and incompetent. Another option is a **durable power of attorney,** in which an individual names a person to act in her behalf in a similar situation. Some argue that a durable power of attorney affords more flexibility than a living will in addressing novel and unexpected situations near the end of life.

(1) These options became increasingly important with the passage of the United States **Patient Self-determination Act** in 1991. This act requires health care facilities that receive federal funding to provide patients with written information about relevant state laws regarding their rights to refuse or discontinue treatment.

(2) It is no longer widely believed that patients benefit from the greatest application of technology. Patients have a right to refuse treatment, even at the end of life, and many physicians recognize that helping patients to achieve a **natural death** or a **death with dignity** may involve psychological and social assistance as much as technical assistance.

B. | **Issues near the end of life**

1. **Defining death.** Before the availability of artificial life support, a person was considered dead when his breathing and heartbeat stopped. With artificial respiration, a person can continue to breath and his heart can continue to beat without input from the brain.

a. In 1968, Harvard Medical School issued a report recommending changing the definition of death to include a greater focus on the brain. Their approach, which is widely adopted, uses a **whole brain death standard**. The criteria for brain death require complete and irreversible cessation of all brain functions, cortical and brain stem.

b. Some critics of this approach argue that the standard should be **neocortical death,** or **higher brain death,** rather than whole brain death. The continuing uncertainty involves patients who lose all cognitive functioning and are irreversibly unconscious, but retain brain stem functioning.

2. **Euthanasia**

a. Euthanasia comes from the Greek words for "good death" or "easy death." Euthanasia is either painlessly causing death or deliberately not acting to prevent death as a result of natural causes in terminally ill patients. Two important distinctions must be made in discussing euthanasia.

(1) A distinction is made between **active and passive euthanasia**. This distinction is also referred to as the distinction between **killing** and **letting someone die**.

(2) A distinction is made between **voluntary and nonvoluntary euthanasia**.

b. It is much more difficult to support active euthanasia (killing) than passive euthanasia (letting someone die).

(1) In the Cruzan case, the United States Supreme Court ruled that all means of life-prolonging medical treatment, including, in this case, a feeding tube, could be withdrawn, even though the patient was not terminally ill.

(2) The AMA supports the view that active euthanasia, even **when performed** for humane reasons, is always **morally wrong**.

(3) Critics of this view, such as the Americans Against Human Suffering and the Hemlock Society, frequently cite the Dutch alternative approach, in which a competent patient may request active euthanasia.

C. Medical technology and research

1. Reproductive and genetic technologies

a. In vitro fertilization is a process whereby mature eggs are removed from the ovarian follicle, fertilized, allowed to begin division in the laboratory, and replaced in the uterus. If the fertilized egg attaches to the uterus, fetal development will proceed as in natural fertilization. Some argue that allowing in vitro fertilization technology creates a "slippery slope." For example, if it is possible to throw away embryos that are not implanted, what will prevent researchers from raising embryos and fetuses in the laboratory as research subjects or organ donors? This possibility raises serious autonomy and nonmaleficence issues from the point of view of the potential infant. Critics of these arguments believe that it is possible to develop new standards for emerging technologies without losing control of sensible decision making. This approach allows for the beneficent advantages offered by new technologies.

b. Surrogate motherhood is another new reproductive modality in which one woman is paid to bear a child for another. In the famous Baby M case, the surrogate mother changed her mind about giving up the child after the birth. The controversy surrounding the case led some to conclude that surrogacy is always wrong.

(1) A typical argument, based on the principle of autonomy or on Kant's categorical imperative, is that the child is not being treated as an end in itself by the surrogate mother, but rather as a means to obtain financial gain. In addition, surrogacy raises social concerns (e.g., the practice might exploit financially disadvantaged women).

(2) Others argue that regulation can minimize the potential harms of surrogacy without infringing on the freedom of persons who wish to pursue this reproductive technology.

c. Human genetics. Controversy surrounds the increasing knowledge of the mechanisms of inheritance and genetic change. The issues concern the extent to which this knowledge should be used in **genetic intervention** (e.g., screening, prenatal diagnosis, abortion), **therapy,** and **research**.

(1) Genetic intervention and therapy are similar to other new medical technologies. Many argue that regulating procedures can be developed to allow the use of these technologies while the principles of autonomy and beneficence are respected. However, others argue that genetic research is different because it can alter the genetic composition of populations of organisms, potentially violating the principle of nonmaleficence.

(2) Genetic manipulation may result in biohazards. From a justice perspective, there is concern about how much uncertainty society should risk or critics of genetic research should assume.

(3) In 1989, the United States Congress approved 31 million dollars to initiate the **Human Genome Project,** which involves hundreds of scientists and scores of laboratories. Ethical questions in this area will have increasing importance.

2. Medical research

a. Human research. It is useful to contrast human research with medical therapy. Whereas therapy involves well-established procedures that are performed for the benefit of individuals or groups, research involves scientific activities that are designed to contribute to generalizable knowledge. There are two types of human medical research: **clinical research,** in which research is combined with therapy or prevention and has potential direct benefit to the subjects (e.g., random drug trials), and **nonclinical research,** which is not intended to provide direct benefit to the subjects (e.g., healthy volunteers involved in new drug metabolism studies).

(1) Nonclinical research is more difficult to defend, especially in view of the traditional patient-benefit and nonmaleficence principles of medicine.

(2) Arguments for both types of human research appeal to the principles of benefi-cence (i.e., substantial social benefit gained from research) and justice (i.e., un-fairness of prohibiting research when current patients benefit from research on past volunteers).

b. **Animal research.** Most literature on animal research refers to nonhuman mammals (e.g., monkeys, dogs, rats). Two issues are especially important in analyzing the ethi-cal issues of animal research: the **consequences of the research and the moral sta-tus of animals**.

   (1) Arguments in favor of animal research generally rely on the principle of benefi-cence (e.g., good consequences for humans can be achieved with animal re-search). The argument is stronger when certain good medical consequences for humans can be achieved only through animal research.

   (2) Arguments for the moral status of animals typically appeal to the animal's sensi-tivity to pain; capacity for consciousness, or mental awareness; and capacity for other mental states (e.g., beliefs, desires). According to this argument, if animals have moral status, they should be treated according to the principles of benefi-cence, nonmaleficence, and justice.

D. **Health care allocation**

1. **Microallocation** refers to distribution decisions that directly affect individuals (e.g., one heart donor is available, but there are six people in need). The ethical issue is deter-mining how these resources should be allocated.

   a. A **utilitarian** approach attempts to determine the consequences of saving one person rather than another. For example, one issue is which patient is more likely to con-tribute to the general welfare of society. Another issue is which policy (e.g., giving resources to those with greatest need) has the most utility.

   b. According to the second formulation of Kant's categorical imperative, each person has equal worth and dignity. From that perspective, a random approach or a first-come, first-served approach might be appropriate.

2. **Macroallocation** refers to distribution decisions that affect large groups of individuals. It often applies theories of justice.

   a. The **free market** approach to distribution is supported by Robert Nozick and a liber-tarian theory of justice. According to this theory, all individuals should be free to enter into and withdraw from economic contracts, including medical contracts, in accordance with their desires.

   b. However, there is increasing support for the belief that all individuals are entitled to a **decent minimum** of health care. According to this standard, adequate, as opposed to maximum, health care is a condition of equal opportunity, similar to adequate education and protection from crime, in a free market society. Arguments for a de-cent minimum frequently appeal to Rawls's theory of justice.

BIBLIOGRAPHY

Ackerman T, Strong C: *A Casebook of Medical Ethics.* New York, Oxford University Press, 1989.

Arras J, Rhoden N: *Ethical Issues in Modern Medicine,* 3rd ed. Mountain View, CA, Mayfield, 1989.

Beauchamp T, Childress J: *Principles of Biomedical Ethics,* 3rd ed. New York, Oxford University Press, 1989.

Beauchamp T, Walters L: *Contemporary Issues in Bioethics,* 3rd ed. Belmont, CA, Wadsworth, 1989.

Macklin R: *Mortal Choices.* Boston, Houghton Mifflin, 1987.

Munson R: *Intervention and Reflection: Basic Issues in Medical Ethics,* 4th ed. Belmont, CA, Wadsworth, 1992.

Perlin T: *Clinical Medical Ethics: Cases in Practice.* Boston, Little, Brown, 1992.

STUDY QUESTIONS

DIRECTIONS: Each of the numbered items or incomplete statements in this section is followed by answers or by completions of the statement. Select the ONE lettered answer or completion that is BEST in each case.

1. According to modern medical ethics, which principle does the Hippocratic tradition emphasize?

(A) Autonomy
(B) Utilitarianism
(C) Paternalism
(D) Beneficence
(E) Responsibility

Questions 2–3

A 45-year-old single white man who is a United States senator is admitted to the hospital. He has irreversible heart failure and needs a heart transplant. His long-term physician argues that the senator should be placed at the top of the transplant waiting list because he is important to the vital interests of the state that he represents.

2. What ethical theory supports this argument?

(A) Virtue theory
(B) Rights theory
(C) Utilitarianism
(D) Egalitarianism
(E) Libertarianism

3. The senator's case is presented to the hospital ethics committee. One of the committee members argues that the senator should not receive preferential treatment because all human life has dignity and profound worth. What ethical theory supports this argument?

(A) Virtue theory
(B) Rights theory
(C) Utilitarianism
(D) Libertarianism
(E) None of the above

4. "It's Over, Debbie," is an anonymous account published in the *Journal of the American Medical Association* that describes a physician who decides, without consulting anyone, to administer a lethal injection to a suffering patient with cancer. What ethical principles might this action violate?

(A) Justice and beneficence
(B) Autonomy and nonmaleficence
(C) Rights and virtue
(D) Truth telling and informed consent
(E) Paternalism and respect

5. The physician's obligation for truth telling is grounded in what ethical principle?

(A) Virtue
(B) Rights
(C) Autonomy
(D) Egalitarianism
(E) Libertarianism

Questions 6–7

A 21-year-old single white man comes to the emergency room with a stab wound to his abdomen. He is alert and coherent, but he refuses to allow the medical team to evaluate him, insisting that he must leave the emergency room to "get the guy back." He understands that if the wound goes untreated, he may experience severe consequences, even death, because of infection and internal hemorrhaging.

6. Should the medical team allow the patient to refuse treatment?

(A) No, because he is a danger to others
(B) Yes, because anyone who refuses treatment should be allowed to do so
(C) No, because he may suffer severe consequences if he is not treated
(D) Yes, because he is competent to refuse treatment
(E) Yes, because he is in the emergency room rather than in the hospital

7. While the medical team is deciding how to proceed, the patient runs from the emergency room yelling, "That lowlife brother of mine is a dead man. I'm going to blow him to bits!" Does the medical team have any responsibility to the patient's brother?

(A) No, because the brother stabbed the patient first
(B) Yes, the medical team is obliged to protect the brother by warning him and the police
(C) No, because the information given to the medical team is protected by confidentiality rights
(D) No, because the medical team does not know whether the patient has a gun
(E) Yes, if the brother is harmed, the medical team must treat him without charge

Questions 8–10

At 4:00 A.M., a patient enters a hospital emergency room in a drunken stupor. A physician attempts to arouse him, but his only response is a request for another round. His friends state that the patient fell and hit his head while they were attempting to help him into a car. During the examination, the patient awakens and says that he is ready to go home. The physician attempts to reason with him, but he is adamant, and it is clear that the only way to keep him from leaving will be to restrain him.

8. At this point, what ethical principles are in conflict?

(A) Virtue and rights
(B) Informed consent and competence
(C) Strong paternalism and weak paternalism
(D) Nonmaleficence and justice
(E) Beneficence and autonomy

9. The physician decides to retain the patient for further evaluation. Again he becomes lethargic, and this time, he is incontinent. The physician is concerned that the patient may have a subdural hematoma, and believes that an emergency computed tomography (CT) scan should be obtained. What should the physician do?

(A) Wait until the patient awakens, and ask for informed consent
(B) Attempt to call his nearest relative to obtain informed consent
(C) Ask his friends for informed consent
(D) Proceed with the CT scan because it is an emergency situation and the risks of the procedure are minimal
(E) Assume therapeutic privilege and forgo informed consent

10. The results of the CT scan are normal, but the physician believes that the patient should stay in the hospital for further observation. Once again, he is awake and demanding to leave the hospital. What factor would be most important in determining whether the patient is competent to refuse treatment?

(A) Whether he is oriented to person, place, and time
(B) Whether he can count backward by seven and name recent United States presidents
(C) Whether his blood alcohol level is in the intoxicated range
(D) Whether he is actively hallucinating or delusional
(E) Whether he understands his medical condition, the recommendations, and the risks associated with refusing to follow them

Questions 11–12

A 72-year-old widowed white woman has metastatic breast cancer. Her physicians inform her that the condition is fatal and that she has only a few months to live. Because she wants a dignified death, she decides to enter a hospice. After 1 month in the hospice, her pain is so unbearable that she asks her physician to give her a lethal intravenous drip of phenobarbital.

11. What does the American Medical Association (AMA) recommend in this situation?

(A) Because the patient makes a voluntary request for euthanasia, the AMA would recommend that the physician comply
(B) The AMA would recommend that the physician obtain a psychiatric consultation to exclude depression before complying, despite the voluntary request
(C) The AMA holds that active euthanasia is always morally wrong
(D) The patient's request for euthanasia constitutes passive euthanasia; therefore, the AMA would support it
(E) The AMA would recommend that the physician determine whether the patient is competent to decide before complying

12. If pneumonia developed before the physician decided how to proceed, and the patient changed her request to being allowed to die without antibiotics, what should the physician do?

(A) The situation has not changed; the AMA holds that passive euthanasia is also morally wrong
(B) If the patient is competent, she has a right to passive euthanasia in this case
(C) Because antibiotics are such a routine treatment, the patient cannot request passive euthanasia in this situation
(D) The patient is not competent to make this request because an individual is never competent to request death
(E) The patient should be given antidepressants

13. In the debate over animal research, what two issues are particularly important?

(A) Whether the animal is about to die and whether there is no other way to obtain the information
(B) The degree of pain involved in the research and the amount of pain medication given
(C) Whether the animal is already sick and whether the research may help the animal medically
(D) Whether the animal has even been a pet and whether the former owner is informed
(E) The consequences of the research and the moral status of the animal

14. Arguments that a decent minimum of health care should be available for all frequently appeal to which theory of justice?

(A) Utilitarian
(B) Rawlsian
(C) Libertarian
(D) Virtue theory

ANSWERS AND EXPLANATIONS

1. The answer is D [I A]. The Hippocratic oath commences a long tradition of medical ethics whose core principle is that a physician is morally obliged to benefit the patient and protect the patient from harm in accordance with the physician's best judgment. Paternalism also grows out of the Hippocratic tradition, but it is not an ethical principle. Utilitarianism and responsibility are not ethical principles. Autonomy is an ethical principle which was not emphasized in the Hippocratic tradition.

2. The answer is C [III A]. Utilitarianism bases moral decisions on an effort to maximize good consequences. In the case of the senator, it could be argued that more good consequences would result if he were to regain health than if another individual regained health. None of the other theories listed base moral decisions on consequences.

3. The answer is B [III B 1 d]. Rights theory is a common contemporary form of deontological theory. According to rights theory, each individual has moral claims that cannot be overridden by utilitarian appeals to good consequences. Virtue theory supports action based on well cultivated virtues rather than a duty to individuals moral claims. Libertarianism is concerned with a duty to the moral claim of individual freedom, but it would be difficult to support the committee member's argument with a focus on freedom.

4. The answer is B [IV A–C]. Autonomy is respect for the self-regarding decisions of others, and nonmaleficence is avoiding harm to others. An argument could be made that the action violates beneficence as well. Justice, rights, virtue, decency, informed consent, paternalism, and respect are not ethical principles.

5. The answer is C [V A 2 a]. Truth telling is based on the principle of respecting patient autonomy. Virtue, rights, egalitarianism, and libertarianism are not ethical principles.

6. The answer is D [IV A 1]. The patient understands his medical condition and the risks of refusing treatment. Therefore, he is competent to refuse treatment. According to the principle of autonomy, patients who are competent may refuse treatment, even in life and death situations. Concerns over the patient's dangerousness should not enter into decisions about medical treatment. Patients who are not competent may not be able to refuse treatment. The patient understands the possible consequences of refusing treatment and has decided to accept them. The issues would be similar if the situation had occurred in the hospital.

7. The answer is B [V A 2 c (2)]. Since the ruling of *Tarasoff v. Regents of the University of California,* physicians have the responsibility to make reasonable efforts to protect third parties when a patient announces an intention to harm specific persons. Who stabbed whom first and payment for the brother's care are irrelevant issues. Confidentiality rights are outweighed when a patient intends harm to others. Without information about the patient's access to a gun, the medical team has reason to be concerned for the safety of the patient's brother.

8. The answer is E [IV A–B]. Beneficence is promoting the welfare of others, and autonomy is respecting their self-determining decisions. The only other ethical principle listed is nonmaleficence, which is not in conflict in this situation.

9. The answer is D [V A 2 b (2)]. In an extreme emergency situation, informed consent may be bypassed. Therapeutic privilege may be used to bypass informed consent on rare occasions because the physician fears that informing the patient will cause serious and identifiable harm, but this situation is not relevant to this case.

10. The answer is E [V A 3 b (1)]. Competence is always defined in terms of specific issues. In this case, competence depends on the patient's understanding of the treatment that is offered and the risks associated with refusing treatment. The other aspects of the physical and mental examinations are relevant, but they are not the most important criteria for competence.

11. The answer is C [V B 2 b (2)]. The AMA does not support active euthanasia, even with competent patients. In the Dutch system, a competent patient can obtain voluntary active euthanasia. Passive euthanasia is letting a patient die without providing treatment.

12. The answer is B [V B 2 b (1)]. A patient who is competent and adequately informed has the right to refuse treatment at the end of life as well as at any other time.

13. The answer is E [V C 2 b (1)–(2)]. The debate over animal research involves a conflict between the good consequences that can be obtained by the research and whether animals have moral status, and thus should be treated according to ethical principles.

14. The answer is B [V D 2 b]. John Rawls's theory of justice argues that social arrangements made by hypothetical unbiased participants would include provisions for the disadvantaged because any of the participants might be in that situation. Although they could be made compatible, utilitarianism and virtue theory are infrequently associated with the argument for decent minimum of health care. Libertarianism is incompatible with a decent minimum perspective because of its focus on individual freedom.

Chapter 17

The Health Care System

Richard F. Southby
Kala Ladenheim
Philip S. Birnbaum
Warren Greenberg

I. HEALTH CARE DELIVERY IN THE UNITED STATES

A. History and structure

1. **Health care professionals**
   a. **Physicians**
      (1) **History of the medical profession in the United States**
         (a) **Entrance into the medical profession** in colonial America was chiefly through **apprenticeship**. Allopathic practitioners competed with others, including eclectics, homeopaths, and naturopaths.
         (b) **Medical education** in the colonies followed the Scottish model of university-based education, rather than the English model of hospital-based medical schools. The first medical school in the American colonies was founded in 1756 at the College of Philadelphia, which later became the University of Pennsylvania. By 1776, only 5% of medical practitioners held medical degrees.
         (c) Until the middle of the nineteenth century, physicians competed for the sale of their services. **Licensing was not required** by state or federal government. Entrance to medical school was easy, and many schools were for-profit institutions. The annual income of physicians was among the lowest for all professional groups.
      (2) **Foundation of organized medicine.** After the establishment of the **American Medical Association (AMA)** in 1847, licensure of physicians became mandatory. The **Flexner Report in 1910** called for closing "diploma mill" medical schools and strengthening their curricula by including medical education in the university setting. The number of medical schools decreased from 162 in 1910 to 69 in 1944, with a corresponding reduction in the number of students. By the mid-1950s, there were approximately 8000 first-year medical students, only 1500 more than in 1910.
      (3) **Government role**
         (a) By 1950, the expansion of **National Institutes of Health (NIH)** extramural research provided impetus and support for the development of preclinical medical faculties and facilities.
         (b) **The Health Professionals Educational Assistance Act of 1963** provided substantial federal support for undergraduate medical training. Grants to medical schools provided funds for new construction and renovations. First-year enrollments increased from approximately 9000 students in 1965 to more than 18,000 in 1982. The physician-to-population ratio is expected to increase from 152 physicians per 100,000 population in 1970 to 240 physicians per 100,000 population in the year 2000. Currently, there are more than 400,000 physicians in the United States.
      (4) **Specialization versus primary care.** Before World War II, approximately 80% of physicians were general practitioners and 20% were specialists. Since then, the ratio has reversed. With rapid advances in medical knowledge and technology, urban growth, the development of large hospitals, the availability of health insurance, and increased demands for care, the trend toward specialization and

subspecialization has accelerated during the last 30 years. The high proportion of specialists is believed to contribute to high medical costs, and the government has recently sought ways to reverse the trend by improving reimbursement for primary care and encouraging managed care.

   (5) Supply and distribution. Despite the recent increase in the number of practicing physicians, medically underserved areas persist. These areas typically include inner cities and rural areas. Specific groups, such as ethnic minorities, persons with chronic mental illness, and the homeless, also tend to be underserved. Federal and state programs to repay student loans or to pay the medical education costs for physicians who practice in underserved areas provide essential personnel in many areas. However, these programs rarely provide impetus for physicians to remain in the underserved areas once their loans are repaid.

  b. Other health care providers

   (1) During the twentieth century, the **ratio of physicians to associated health care personnel** (e.g., registered nurses, psychiatric social workers, physical therapists) has changed dramatically. In 1900, the ratio of physicians to associated health care workers was 1:1. The current ratio is 1:20. As with physicians, there are **cycles of shortage and surplus** in these professions. These cycles are exacerbated by lengthy training. The nursing supply is typically cyclic. An increase in unfilled registered nurse positions in acute care facilities in the mid-1980s focused public interest on nursing duties, career patterns, educational requirements, and salary structure. Currently, many regions are experiencing surpluses of nurses in acute care.

   (2) Independent and dependent practitioners. Health providers are defined according to the degree to which they can practice without outside authorization or supervision. These distinctions are often marked by the ability to obtain independent reimbursement for care. There are struggles over status and responsibility among practitioners at each of these levels.

    (a) Definitions. Physicians, chiropractors, dentists, and optometrists are examples of **independent practitioners** who can legally provide specific services without outside supervision or authorization. **Dependent practitioners** provide defined services—often within a legally defined **scope of practice**—under the supervision or authorization of independent practitioners, although they often work with a high degree of independence. Dependent practitioners include pharmacists, nurses, and physical and occupational therapists.

    (b) Midlevel practitioners. Physician assistants and nurse practitioners act as physician extenders in settings that include remote rural clinics, hospitals, health maintenance organizations (HMOs), group practices, and underserved urban areas. Physician assistants work under direct physician supervision. Nurse practitioners, including nurse-midwives, are often licensed to practice independently within limits.

    (c) Nurses. Nurses are the largest group of providers. The profession developed as an occupation supportive of physicians. Levels of professional training and responsibility range from licensed practical nurses to independent practitioners with doctoral degrees. Specialization among nurses is increasing (e.g., nurse-anesthetist). Duties range from direct patient care to strictly administrative responsibilities.

   (3) Alternative care givers. The theory of **therapeutic nihilism** questions the efficacy of much medical care. Many people use alternative therapy (e.g., chiropractic, acupuncture, nutritional therapy) and self-care. The family continues to be the single most important source of care for persons with chronic conditions.

   (4) Patient care teams. The patient-focused care team model, which may involve nurses, social workers, and others, developed in the context of care for chronically ill patients. Some universities have experimented with joint education of physicians and other providers to encourage the development of such teams.

2. Institutional providers
  a. Hospitals
   (1) Establishment of public hospitals. Cities in colonial America established institutions in the mid-1770s for feeding, sheltering, and quarantining the mentally and chronically physically ill, the disabled, and those with contagious diseases. Medical care was only a peripheral function of most of these institutions, and the quality of life that they provided made them a feared rather than a sought-after source of support.
   (2) Establishment of voluntary hospitals. At approximately the same time, usually under the impetus of European-trained physicians, voluntary hospitals were founded in Philadelphia, Boston, and New York. These hospitals were dependent largely on local philanthropy. Because of the quality of care, paying patients also sought treatment in these hospitals and were admitted along with indigents, who had been the sole clients of the publicly operated hospitals.
   (3) Later developments. By 1900, there were approximately 4000 hospitals in the United States, with a combined capacity of approximately 400,000 beds. Developments in medical science and technology—from infection control and anesthesia to radiology—combined with advances in the training of physicians, nurses, and other health personnel to complete the transformation of the hospital.
   (4) Government role. The Hill-Burton program, which started in 1946, provided funds to many communities, particularly rural areas, to increase the number of hospital beds and to attract physicians to underserved areas. Currently, the federal government provides transitional funds to help many of the same hospitals convert to subacute medical centers or link with larger hospitals to form networks.
   (5) Current status
    (a) There are now almost 7000 hospitals in the United States, with a combined capacity of more than 1 million beds. All levels of government provide direct care for specific patient groups, through the Veterans Administration system (federal) as well as through state, county, and municipal hospitals. One-third of all nongovernment hospitals belong to **multi-institutional systems** (i.e., two or more hospitals with common ownership, management, or both).
    (b) For-profit facilities, which now number approximately 1000, have emerged as a major component of the health care system. Many began as private, usually physician-owned, institutions. Struggling public and community hospitals are absorbed by these chains as well.
    (c) The number of hospitals is decreasing for the first time since the Great Depression, with small (fewer than 100 beds) and rural hospitals particularly affected. This decrease reflects a change in the efficient operating size of hospitals and an increase in patient expectations. Small hospitals cannot sustain the range of services and equipment available in larger hospitals. The American Hospital Association (AHA) and the United States Department of Health and Human Services disagree as to the number of closures and the effect of reimbursement methods on hospital closures.
   (6) Expanded services and networks. Hospitals have responded to a decline in demand for inpatient services by adding a variety of outpatient, community, and specialized services. Hospitals are also increasingly active as centers of physician–hospital organizations that contract to provide care on a capitation basis [see I B 2 c (2)].
   (7) Joint ventures. To promote closer ties between a hospital and its medical staff (the term "bonding" is frequently applied in this context), projects financed and owned jointly by physicians and hospitals have developed. Examples are physician office buildings, imaging centers, and reference laboratories. The federal government has voiced concern that joint ventures may tend to be in restraint of trade and has developed regulations that increase government involvement in the health care delivery field. One area of particular scrutiny is **physician self-referral,** in which patients are sent to physician-owned ancillary services.

b. Ambulatory care. In the 1980s, emphasis shifted from inpatient care to ambulatory care. Most patient visits still take place in physician offices, but increasingly, care is received in organized settings. These settings include clinics, HMOs, and hospital outpatient settings. **Freestanding "surgicenters," "emergicenters," and diagnostic imaging centers** now offer many services traditionally provided in hospitals. Some of this growth is the result of regulations that limit hospital charges and expansion, but do not affect other providers. In addition to reimbursement changes, new technologies and techniques make many services that once required a hospital stay possible on an ambulatory basis. Freestanding centers are increasingly being regulated on a par with hospitals. Table 17-1 lists ambulatory care settings.

c. Long-term care. Long-term care is a set of medical, social, and supportive services provided to persons who are unable to care for themselves independently as a result of chronic illness or physical or mental disability. Although these services are often associated with nursing home care for elderly persons, persons of all ages need long-term care (Table 17-2). More than 70% of long-term care takes place in homes and communities, primarily through family and informal care givers.

   (1) Long-term care is often provided by **patient-centered care teams**. Physicians are involved when conditions change, but nurses generally manage stable patients.

   (2) **Changing demographic trends.** The demand for long-term care is expected to increase over the next several decades because of rapid growth of the "old-old" (older than 85 years) population, increased survival rates at all ages for persons with severe disabilities, and changes in family structures that reduce the availability of family support.

   (3) **Changing disease patterns** contribute to the need for long-term care. The **epidemiologic transition** is marked by the rising prevalence of chronic conditions, such as cancer, heart disease, and Alzheimer's disease. Multiple chronic conditions and disabilities often interact.

   (4) The health care system evolved to provide acute care, but a shift to a **chronic care paradigm** is underway. Acquired immune deficiency syndrome (AIDS) shifted from an acute care to a chronic care model within a short time. Initially, treatment focused on the management of medical crises. Currently, care emphasizes prevention, community education, and maintenance of human immunodeficiency virus (HIV)-positive patients at home with practices that include drug and dietary therapy and community support services.

3. Organized delivery systems. The 1980s and 1990s are marked by rapid growth in organized health care delivery systems. These systems are groups of providers that are organized to provide a spectrum of care for a specific population. When financed by a capitated premium, they are known as HMOs.

TABLE 17-1. Ambulatory Care Settings

Private and group practice

Organized ambulatory care
Community-based clinics and groups
Hospital-affiliated settings
  Emergency room
  Clinic
  Walk-in ambulatory care service
  Outpatient therapy, surgery, and imaging
Freestanding centers (surgicenter, emergicenter)
Health maintenance organizations

Ancillary services
  Laboratories
  Pharmacies
  Diagnostic and imaging services

TABLE 17-2. Types of Long-Term Care

> Subacute care
> Nursing facilities
> Home and community-based care
> Case management

a. **Two perspectives.** Pressure from both government and private payers is pushing providers to join together. Two common approaches are **organized delivery systems or networks,** which emphasize creating a single coordinated system of care (e.g., group and staff HMOs, rural networks) and **managed care plans,** or health plans, which focus on a single coherent financing structure and a consistent set of medical standards **[e.g., independent practice associations (IPAs)].**

b. **Health maintenance organizations**

    (1) **History.** HMOs began in 1929, when physicians Donald Ross and H. Clifford Loos in Los Angeles and Michael Shadid in Elk City, Oklahoma, established the first prepaid health plans in the United States. The early growth of these plans was opposed by medical societies and physicians, who reacted to later growth with a combination of indifference, acquiescence, and action to create their own HMOs. In 1988, more than 31.9 million individuals were enrolled in 607 HMOs, compared with 1976, when 175 HMO systems enrolled just 6 million people.

    (2) **Government role.** The federal government has encouraged the growth of HMOs to create a more competitive health care system. HMOs benefited from the passage of the federal HMO Act of 1973, requiring certain employers to offer them as an alternative to standard insurance plans where they were available.

    (3) **HMO versus indemnity coverage**

        (a) HMO subscribers pay an annual premium to the organization in return for a prearranged package of **health care benefits** from its participating providers (Table 17-3). In contrast, **indemnity insurance** provides that, in exchange for a premium, **payments** will be made for specific services from any properly licensed provider. No assurance is made that services will be available.

        (b) For physicians, indemnity coverage permits professional autonomy and fee-for-service reimbursement. **Managed care plans** (i.e., HMOs, managed indemnity plans) involve **varying degrees of scrutiny and bureaucratic control** over practices. Many HMOs pay physicians through capitation, salary, or sharply discounted fee schedules and risk sharing. Although HMOs account for a relatively small portion of the market, managed care practices that reduce autonomy, such as **utilization review,** are now standard in most insurance plans.

    (4) **HMOs as competitive health plans.** HMOs compete with other insurance plans by offering more comprehensive care, including prophylactic services, while promising to lower costs. HMOs claim that savings are achieved through more efficient, health-oriented care because of the use of midlevel practitioners;

TABLE 17-3. Typical Benefits Offered by a Health Maintenance Organization

> Hospitalization
> Limited mental health services
> Physician services (ambulatory and inpatient)
> Preventive medicine services
> Dentist services
> Optometrist services
> Podiatrist services
> Ancillary services

controls and limits on hospitalization, consultations with specialists, and the use of advanced technology; and negotiated discounts. Some studies suggest that HMO savings may be the result of a generally healthier patient base.

(5) **Types of HMOs.** Prepaid group practices form **group model HMOs**. In **staff model HMOs,** a corporation employs salaried physicians and often owns hospitals and other facilities. **Network HMOs** are linked collections of group practices. Hospitals and affiliated physicians may form **physician–hospital organizations (PHOs)**. **IPAs** are loosely associated physicians in private practice. IPAs were the fastest growing form of HMO in the late 1980s. Staff and group model HMOs generally provide care primarily or exclusively to the members of the HMO, but physicians in network and IPA HMOs may contract with several HMOs and also take fee-for-service patients. Governance and ownership models include nonprofit organizations with community boards, physician-owned networks, and commercial for-profit plans.

c. **Other alternative delivery systems. Preferred provider organizations (PPOs) or arrangements (PPAs)** are increasingly common. These plans are discounted fee-for-service systems that offer coverage from participating providers and lower levels of coverage from providers who are outside the system. **Point-of-service (POS) plans** are a variant that involves HMOs and out-of-plan providers. Major insurers, including Blue Cross and Blue Shield plans, have entered the market by offering **triple-option** plans that offer subscribers a choice of an HMO, a PPO, or an indemnity plan.

d. **Physician issues**

(1) **Risk sharing.** Capitation requires physicians to assume some degree of financial risk for the care provided. Depending on how it is managed and the role that physicians play in the health care decisions, this approach can lead to ethical conflicts or to efficient care.

(2) **Gatekeeper primary care case management.** Primary care physician gatekeepers approve all referrals and manage and coordinate patient care.

(3) **Any willing provider.** HMOs and PPOs may be classified as **closed panel** (only care provided by selected members is covered) or **open panel**. The AMA is seeking legislation to require that managed care plans accept all practitioners that fit their profiles. These bills are opposed by HMO supporters who see them as opposing managed care.

4. **Public health**

a. **History and purpose.** Public health has developed separately from direct medical services to individuals. **Public health practitioners** are concerned with the **community**.

(1) Public health services are normally the responsibility of **government**. Starting as volunteer organizations to address specific threats to the health of the community, by the middle of the nineteenth century, these organizations had evolved into **governmental health departments** with full-time officials.

(2) Responding to the wave of immigration and to developments in technology, every state had organized some form of **health department** by 1909. Since 1935, the federal role in public health activities has increased substantially, in line with significant social, political, and economic changes.

(3) **The Surgeon General of the United States Public Health Service** has, in recent years, played a major role in defining national health issues and setting policies related to those issues (e.g., campaigns concerning smoking and health, AIDS as a public health problem).

b. **Activities.** Public health functions can be roughly divided into three areas: community health planning, which involves assessing community needs and resources; community medical care, which involves providing direct care or specific services that the community deems essential to the general welfare; and community health care, which involves providing population-based and environmental health services (Table 17-4).

TABLE 17-4. Public Health Activities

Health planning
    Community needs assessment
    Capacity regulation
    Technology management
Community medical care
    Maternal and child health
        Prenatal care
        Immunization
    Visiting nurses
    Public clinics
Community health care
    Communicable disease control
    Sanitation, restaurants, and facilities
    Health education and promotion
    Environmental health
    Epidemiology

B. **Financing.** Health services are financed through a mix of public and private sources. Government programs, primarily Medicaid and Medicare, provide 42% of all health care dollars. Private health care is purchased through a combination of insurance (35%) and out-of-pocket (22%) spending. Most private health insurance is obtained through the workplace, although the percentage of employers offering coverage is declining.

1. **Funding sources**
   a. **Evolution of health insurance.** The current system of health insurance traces its origin to sickness funds established in Germany in the late 1800s. These programs were designed to protect family income and only over time came to include the cost of medical care. Blue Cross (hospitals) and Blue Shield (physicians) plans were created by provider groups during the Depression of the 1930s in response to concerns about solvency. Health insurance became tied to the workplace during World War II, when wage freezes and labor shortages led employers to use the benefit to attract workers. The two major public programs, Medicare and Medicaid, were enacted in 1965.
   b. **Cost shifting.** Approximately 17% of Americans younger than 65 years have neither public nor private health coverage. Hospital emergency rooms may not refuse care to persons who need emergency treatment. Costs of **uncompensated care** are shifted to other payers in the form of higher charges. This cost shifting is sometimes called an **implicit tax**. **Disproportionate share programs and uncompensated care pools** help to fund hospitals that provide a high level of uncompensated care. These programs are often funded at least in part through provider taxes. In this case, an **explicit tax** is substituted for an implicit tax.
   c. **Insurance and risk.** Insurance is designed to share the future risk of health care costs. Older people and those with certain chronic conditions have a higher **anticipated risk** of spending higher amounts in a given year. Acute illnesses and injuries are **unanticipated risks**. Increasingly, people with poor health find insurance unavailable or unaffordable. **Experience-rated coverage** protects only against unanticipated risk. **Community rating** charges the same premiums for all participants, thereby treating both types of risk alike. Because this practice fulfills a social function, community rating carriers often receive special tax treatment.
      (1) **Nonprofit organizations: Blue Cross/Blue Shield and HMOs.** Blue Cross/Blue Shield plans (the two groups have merged) were once all community-rated nonprofit carriers, although many now operate as commercial carriers. They pay approximately 32% of the health insurance benefits in the private sector. They often serve as the **fiscal intermediary,** or agent, for public programs (Medicaid and Medicare). HMOs often are nonprofit as well. **Community-rated** Blue Cross/Blue

Shield plans and HMOs often serve a sicker than average population because healthier groups can obtain coverage at lower prices through commercial carriers.

(2) Commercial insurance plans. There are nearly 1000 for-profit commercial insurers in the United States. Many of these insurers also provide life insurance and pension coverage to their corporate clients. The commercial insurer share of the private sector market is approximately 40%.

(3) Self-insured plans. Rather than purchasing insurance, most large employers (covering more than one-half of all American workers) self-insure, often using **third-party administrators** to run their plans. Federal law **[Employee Retirement and Income Security Act of 1974 (ERISA)]** preempts state regulation of self-insured plans. Many firms self-insure to avoid state mandates and premium taxes.

d. Public insurance

(1) Medicare is a two-part federal program that is financed through tax revenue as part of the Social Security system. Eligible individuals include most persons 65 years of age and older and disabled individuals under specified conditions, including patients with end-stage renal disease. Part A, which is provided to all, offers four levels of care. Part B is an insurance program for physician and related services, and individuals must pay a premium that covers part of the cost of the benefit. Catastrophic coverage was added in 1989 and almost immediately repealed. Many persons purchase supplemental private insurance to pay noncovered costs, such as deductibles and drug benefits. Table 17-5 shows benefits under Medicare.

(2) Medicaid is a joint federally and state-sponsored medical assistance program for indigent persons who are receiving welfare for families with dependent children and for the indigent elderly and disabled. It pays for hospital, physician, and other services, including nursing home care and prescribed drugs. Each state defines the financial eligibility criteria and specific optional services to be covered. Costs are shared by the federal and state governments, with the federal share varying by state.

(3) Other programs and state experiments. Approximately one-half of the indigent are covered by Medicaid. State and local **general assistance medical care** programs reimburse providers directly from limited budgets. Several states have programs that provide coverage similar to Medicaid for all people whose income is below the federal poverty level. In some cases, these programs permit persons whose income is above this level to buy in to the program, often through capitated plans.

e. The uninsured. In 1992, more than 37 million United States citizens, 17% of the under-65 population, had no coverage, public or private. This group is varied. Most of the uninsured (84%) are workers or their family members, with 52% working full time. Small companies, service occupations, youth, and early retirement are associated with uninsured status. For 60 percent of the uninsured, family income is less than 200% of the federal poverty level.

TABLE 17-5. Medicare Benefits

Part A
 Inpatient hospital care
 Medically necessary care in a skilled nursing facility
 Home health care
 Hospice care

Part B
 Physician services
 Outpatient hospital care
 Diagnostic tests
 Durable medical equipment
 Ambulance service
 Other health services and supplies

f. The underinsured. For those with insufficient insurance coverage, **out-of-pocket expenditures** can be high. Cost sharing has increased in recent years, with employees asked to pay a higher share of premiums, copayments, and deductibles. The elderly now spend a greater percentage of their income on health care than before the enactment of Medicare in 1965.

2. Payment methods
   a. Cost versus price. The overall cost of health care reflects past policies that were designed to develop great capacity in facilities, technology, and personnel for health care delivery. Recent changes in payment methods that tend to affect health care use rather than capacity have only an indirect effect on the cost of health care. Price discounts and rate limits that affect part of the market have led to cost shifting and increased volume and intensity rather than overall cost control.
   b. Payments to hospitals
      (1) Before October 1983, hospitals were typically reimbursed on a **cost-incurred, or retrospective basis,** regardless of the extent of costs. Many Blue Cross plans, commercial insurers, and state Medicaid programs still reimburse hospitals in this manner. Since this date, Medicare has reimbursed hospitals through the **prospective payment system (PPS)** based on prospective prices rather than retrospective costs.
      (2) The diagnosis-related group (DRG) system is a PPS that was first used by the federal government (Medicare) and is now copied or adapted by other payers. It applies only to hospital services and not to physician services, although PPS systems for physician care and long-term care are under development at this time. Under this system, Medicare pays a set amount for each diagnosis, in conformity with the principal diagnosis specified under the DRG system, regardless of the actual cost to the hospital. The actual cost of care may be higher or lower. For example, when a patient enters a hospital after a heart attack, the hospital receives the same reimbursement regardless of the length of stay, the number of tests performed, or the severity of illness. Hospital payments are indexed to the wage base (i.e., whether the location is rural or urban) and the number of full-time residents or interns. The system has a provision for outliers, or individuals who are so ill that the cost of hospitalization would far exceed any DRG payment.
      (3) The DRG system reverses the incentives of the hospital (i.e., to expand, purchase costly equipment, provide a high intensity of services) that were reinforced by the retrospective payment system. Under the DRG system, hospitals that can reduce costs retain the difference between the actual cost of providing care and the Medicare payment.
      (4) Some states (e.g., Maryland, New York) use **all-payer hospital rate-setting systems,** which allocate total hospital costs among all payers according to a set formula. This system prevents cost shifting. Most of these programs were phased out after the federal government adopted the PPS.
      (5) Some HMOs reimburse hospitals on a **per diem basis,** and some HMOs own their hospitals, effectively operating with a global budget.
   c. Payments to physicians
      (1) Fee-for-service basis. The most common form of payment is the fee-for-service system. The price set by the physician is paid by the patient directly or by an insurance carrier on behalf of the patient. A variation on this system is **negotiated or discounted fee-for-service payment,** in which different carriers reimburse at different rates. These rates are usually set jointly by the payer and the physician. The greater the ability of the plan to assure a patient base, the deeper the discount that is likely to be sought.
      (2) Capitation basis. Physicians may also be paid on a capitation basis. A fixed sum per patient per year is assessed, regardless of the volume or intensity of the services actually provided to the patient. This method is seldom used by individual practitioners, but it is commonly used in group settings, particularly in association with HMOs. Capitation requires physicians to **assume risk,** whether for

their own services, all physician services, or all care. The greater the responsibility and risk the doctor assumes, the higher the capitation rate.

(3) Salary. As employees of an organization, salaried physicians are paid a fixed amount for a specified period to provide services to a specific population. For example, military physicians provide services to members of the armed services and their dependents.

(4) Resource-based relative value scale. Medicare reimburses physicians according to a resource-based relative value scale to set reimbursement levels for various services and specialties in relation to one another. This scale takes into account factors such as risk, cost of physician preparation, and practice-associated costs. This system includes an adjustment for anticipated changes in the volume of services as relative prices change.

II. MANAGEMENT, ECONOMICS, AND POLITICS

A. Management

1. Organization and control

a. Professional model. Society accords the medical profession and its members what is known as ascribed status on the completion of specific goals (e.g., achieving the degree of doctor of medicine, licensure to practice, board certification). Perhaps the greatest amount of autonomy given to any professional in American society is accorded to members of the medical profession. This status simultaneously gives the physician autonomy in relationships with patients and with institutional providers (e.g., hospitals) and requires that the physician maintain high levels of professional behavior and competence.

b. Professionalization of providers. Health care institutions create and sustain organizational and social climates that imbue students with professional values, attitudes, and behaviors. Senior instructors and staff members serve as role models for students throughout their professional training. This professionalization is a form of socialization into the professional role and is achieved through complex formal and informal mechanisms that may be slow to adapt to new social structures in medicine.

c. Physicians and medical bureaucracies

(1) Physician–hospital roles

(a) The **physician–hospital relation.** Physicians typically occupy positions of influence in health care institutions. This influence is based on their professional knowledge, authority, and exclusive right to practice medicine.

(b) Dependency. Hospitals depend on physicians as the source of referral for treatment and, consequently, revenue for the institution. This dependence exists regardless of whether the hospital is in any sense the employer of the physician.

(c) Distinct responsibilities. The physician and the health care institution administrator are both responsible for patient welfare. The administrator's responsibility is exercised through the operation and fiscal management of the institution. The physician's responsibility is primarily, if not solely, to the patient.

(d) Conflict. One of the consequences of this difference in areas of responsibility is conflict among physicians, other health care professionals, and administrators and members of the governing boards of institutions. Each group has different demands and expectations. Conflicts must be resolved through formal and informal mechanisms in the interests of organizational survival and development and patient care.

(2) Physician-managed care roles

(a) Corporate model. In the last two decades, physician autonomy has been challenged by government and corporate entities that seek to control costs by managing care. This "corporatization" is a significant change from the traditional physician role. At the same time, managed care plans may offer physicians greater financial security and better working conditions than they would face in private practice.

  (b) **A system in transition.** There is a great deal of variability in the roles that physicians play in managed care organizations. In group model HMOs or PHOs, physician members may play a dominant policy-setting role, or they may be reluctant participants in a bureaucratically managed enterprise in which they have little stake.

  (c) **Conflicting interests.** Physicians in HMOs may face conflicts between their role as patient advocate and their financial stake in limiting care. Some economists argue that tension between physicians and managers is desirable to assure that the patient has an advocate within the system.

2. **Quality and practice.** One outgrowth of the corporatization of medical care is a search for objective measures of quality to use in assessing the value of care, finding least-cost methods of care that are consistent with sound outcomes, and comparing physicians.

  a. **Malpractice versus bad care: Harvard Malpractice Study.**[1] Quality of care and risk of malpractice suits are not necessarily related. A study of medical care in New York identified both faulty or negligent care and malpractice suits, but found that they were generally not outcomes of the same incidents.

  b. **Continuous quality improvement and total quality management.** Hospitals and other health care organizations now use total quality management and continuous quality improvement methods to monitor and improve their operations. This customer-oriented practice uses workplace teams that cut across occupational categories to seek, identify, and recommend ways to improve patient care processes.

  c. **Credentialing and contracting.** Hospitals and health care plans are legally responsible for verifying staff credentials. One tool is the National Provider Data Base, which contains information on the litigation history of all physicians.

  d. **Standards**

    (1) **Practice patterns and peer review. Descriptive standards** compare patterns of care (e.g., numbers of procedures, diagnostic tests, and consultations). These profiles may be provided to physicians as feedback, they may be part of a peer review or administrative process designed to change patterns, or they may be used to select or reject members of a managed care plan.

    (2) **Practice protocols and utilization review. Normative standards** compare physician behavior against an absolute standard of care. The federal government is developing and disseminating information on desirable standards. The use of overly simple standards in this process is a continued source of conflict between physicians and managed care plans.

  e. **Report cards** are simplified and abstracted quality reports that are used by individual or organizational buyers. The likely standard, the **Health plan Employer Data and Information Set (HEDIS),** is being developed.

3. **Information systems.** Health care systems rely increasingly on electronic databases to collect service and billing, and even clinical information. Requirements include standardized and accurate reporting; confidentiality, including the use of unique patient identifiers; uniform reporting systems; and increased use of magnetic strips or smart cards (cards with imbedded chips or magnetic strips containing patient medical and identification information) by patients.

B. **Patients and consumers.** Patients are increasingly encouraged to see themselves as partners, not dependents, and physicians are expected to enable patients to participate as actively as possible in decisions about diagnosis and care.

1. **Becoming a patient.** An individual entering a hospital or other health care institution is expected to behave in clearly defined ways. Patients are expected to submit to the requirements of the organization (e.g., acceptance of organizational and professional authority, treatment regimens, the institution's timetable). This process of becoming a patient makes the patient dependent on the organization and its personnel.

2. **Modifying the experience.** Attempts to make this socialization process less rigid and more personal reduce the negative effects of the process on patients, assuming that the sick role is not encouraged. Patients are expected to follow the physician's direction for cure and rehabilitation so that they can leave the sick and dependent role as soon as possible.

3. **Becoming a consumer.** The erosion of professional authority is part of a general trend that engages patients as active consumers. In response to the choices available to them, patients expect the physician to invest time to help them to understand the alternatives.

4. **Choice.** Patients exercise choice in selecting plans, physicians, and treatments. They also expect to participate in choosing among therapies by seeking information about the economic implications of physician decisions. **Informed consent** and **living wills** are two points at which these discussions are necessary.

5. **Expectations of medicine are changing.**
   a. **"Medicalization."** The process of redefining conditions once considered social phenomena (e.g., alcoholism) as diseases requiring medical intervention has predominated until recently. Medicalization justifies the sick role on the part of the patient and provides a basis for ascribed authority for the physician. Actions to reduce additional national expenditures for health care may reduce medicalization, further removing individuals from the sick role and decreasing the areas over which the medical profession has authority.
   b. **Malpractice.** Expectations for a successful outcome have been fostered by increasing occasions for intervention by health care providers. The inability to fulfill these expectations consistently has led to an increase in malpractice claims, with accompanying increases in the cost of insurance. The attention paid to this aspect of health care further weakens public acceptance of physician decision making.
   c. **Physician agency versus prudent buyers.** Increasingly, employees are participating in plans that include limits on available services or providers. They expect physicians to take their economic concerns into account in suggesting care. This situation may lead to ethical dilemmas.

C. | **Politics and health care**

1. **Government or markets?** The United States favors decentralized government that exerts limited control over individuals and markets. The resultant health care delivery system is a complex mix of public and private roles. Government now funds 42% of all health care costs, but does not require coverage for the rest of the population. The United States government plays a lesser role in assuring health coverage than the government in most other countries, and it does not play a role in setting or negotiating overall rates and budgets for providers. Within the programs that it funds directly, however, it is an active and aggressive buyer that is often effectively a regulator, both because of its dominant share of the market and because other buyers often imitate it.

2. **Role of government**
   a. **The federal government** has authority for health care through the commerce and the general welfare clauses of the United States Constitution. Its largest role in health care today is financing care for certain populations, both directly and through its support of health education and the regulation and research that accompany those programs. It funds health research, the gathering and dissemination of public health information, and a number of categoric programs.
   b. **State and local governments** have authority under police powers. Traditionally, they have been responsible for regulation and licensure of providers, direct provision of services to various groups, and regulation of insurance and community public health services. They also jointly finance care for needy groups and administer a variety of federally funded programs. Most states already have enacted various types of reform, including insurance reforms and changes in Medicaid. Oregon, Washington, Hawaii, Minnesota, and Florida have begun major reforms that are designed to provide universal coverage for their citizens.

   c. Problems of federalism. The United States has a federal system of government that is deliberately designed to create tensions across the different levels of government to protect individuals from government authority. States that seek to carry out universal reforms are blocked by ERISA, Medicare, and Medicaid. National commercial interests prefer a larger federal role, whereas states seek to expand their autonomy and eliminate **unfunded mandates**.

3. Role of interest groups. Interest groups play a key role in the representative system of government in the United States. Historically, the AMA has influenced government health policy to the point that its role has been sharply criticized as protecting physician interests at the expense of the general good. Insurers, businesses, unions, and consumer groups also influence health policy. In addition to shaping laws, interest groups influence regulations and policy implementation.

   a. Regulatory capture. Providers and insurers are two industry groups whose livelihoods are at stake in the design and implementation of health policies. A common consequence of regulation in highly technical fields is **regulatory capture,** in which the regulating body takes on the values of the regulated industry. This situation is common in health planning agencies.

   b. Businesses and individuals. Consumers and buyers, including governments as buyers of health care, are becoming increasingly influential in establishing government health policies to improve access and lower costs. This influence on policies that they support and that run counter to the interests of industry groups is considered **consumer or buyer dominance**. Special interest groups that represent people with specific needs [e.g., the American Association of Retired Persons (AARP), which represents the elderly, or various disease-specific groups that support research and treatment] create political pressure to expand programs. These groups often share agendas with provider groups.

D. **Health care economics.** Economic theory is the basis for much current health policy. At the same time, economists point to many ways in which health care differs from ordinary market goods.

1. Is health care an economic good? According to a seminar paper by economist Kenneth Arrow,[2] health care differs from other economic endeavors in a number of ways (Table 17-6). Efforts to make health care respond to competitive markets focus on finding ways to correct or compensate for these differences. For instance, community rating makes insurance available for people with chronic illnesses, purchasing pools aggregate demand so that it will be predictable, and improved information about quality supports buyers. Many strategies for increasing competition focus on developing a market for insurance rather than for health care.

TABLE 17-6. Violations of Market Assumptions in Health Care

Demand is irregular and unpredictable

Providers adhere to nonmarket (collectivity oriented) norms

Uncertainty as to the quality of the product is high, and there is great inequality of information between patient and doctor

The supply of doctors is both subsidized and rationed, and the supply of medical care services is strongly influenced by social, nonmarket forces

Competition is restricted by licensure rules that limit entry

Price fixing (discrimination by income) is the norm in a structure equivalent to a collective monopoly

Insurance distorts the behavior of consumers and providers

Traditional insurance is pointless for people with chronic illness because there is a known likelihood of illness

2. **Trends in health care expenditures.** In 1950, health care expenditures in the United States were $12 billion, or 5.3% of the gross national product (GNP), or the total goods and services produced. By 1965, expenditures had grown to $42 billion, or 6.5% of the GNP. By 1988, health care expenditures reached $559 billion, or 11.6% of the GNP. In 1992, health care accounted for 14% of the GNP. It is estimated that health care costs will be 18% of the GNP and $1 trillion to $1.5 trillion in the year 2000. In 1992, the United States had its fifth consecutive year of double-digit health care inflation, with health care costs increasing at two to three times the pace of the GNP.

3. **International comparisons** show that the United States spends far more on health care than any other nation, both in real terms and as a share of national income, while failing to provide coverage for all. Federal health care spending is 15% of the budget. It is the fastest growing part of the federal budget after debt service.

4. **Health care inflation** is caused by general inflation; health care wages rising faster than the economy; other medical prices rising faster than inflation; more intensive use of medical care and expensive technologies; and changing demographic trends, including population growth, aging, and a greater incidence of disability. Observers suggest that the adoption of Medicare and Medicaid in 1965, which increased access to health care for the elderly and the indigent, respectively, as well as the widespread increase in private health insurance, have been important cost drivers. Canada adopted universal coverage at approximately the same time, but has not experienced the same level of cost increases, suggesting that a key difference is the lack of cost containment mechanisms in the United States system.

5. **Costs, prices, rationing, and efficiency.** According to economists, prices reflect the supply and demand for services and the way in which they are produced. If supply increases, prices will decrease. If demand increases, prices will also increase unless a new mechanism for providing the services is found. Price limits distort the market and lead to less efficient use of resources and decreased satisfaction. Different strategies to control costs may be understood in these terms.

   a. **Supply-side controls.** Although for most products prices decrease as availability increases, economists find that **physicians can induce demand for their services**. Doubling the number of physicians did not lead to a reduction in health care prices.[3] Commenting on this propensity, Milton Roemer[4] claimed that "a built bed is a filled bed." Limiting the supply of care givers or services is one strategy for controlling costs.

      (1) **Certificate of need** programs and other health planning activities are designed to slow capital growth, expansion of facilities, and purchase of expensive new technologies. Generally, these programs do not achieve this objective. The conservative adoption of technology in Canada is sometimes cited as an example of rationing by limiting equipment.

      (2) **Rationing** may also limit covered services. Oregon is experimenting with rationing care based on a public prioritization process. Hundreds of condition–treatment pairs were prioritized, with an emphasis on life-saving and preventive care. To provide coverage for everyone whose income is less than the poverty level, a point in the prioritized list was chosen, and only services above that point are covered.

   b. **Demand-side control.** Economists argue that health care spending is out of control in part because insurance insulates patients from the cost of care. Beginning in 1971, the Rand Corporation[5] conducted a study of the effect of cost sharing on the use of care. Findings confirmed that individuals who had to pay more used less care. Higher cost sharing is now standard in most insurance plans.

   c. **Price control.** The United States government does not impose global price controls, but uses its position as a major buyer to set prices for publicly purchased care. Other dominant buyers, such as large insurers or businesses, also demand and receive favorable rates. To compensate, costs are shifted to other payers, and total prices seem to escalate even faster because cost increases and price increases caused by cost shifting are combined.

d. Changed production function: technology. Prices may decrease without changes in supply and demand if a new means of providing a service is found. Technology is often blamed for cost inflation, but some technologies lower costs (e.g., cataract surgery, minimally invasive alternatives to cholecystectomy). Costs increase when technology is used for conditions that formerly would have received no treatment and when new techniques are overused or inappropriately used. Studies to determine the **appropriate use of technologies** are designed to limit adverse economic effects of innovation. Managed care and changed practice patterns have elements of both supply-side rationing and changed production.

III. HEALTH CARE REFORM

A. **The "three-legged stool."** Health care reform is driven by concern over lack of access to health care for the estimated 35 to 40 million uninsured Americans. Another concern is the cost of health care, which has increased much faster than the rate of inflation over the last decade. Quality, access, and cost are known as the three-legged stool because changes to the health care system must balance all three.

B. **History of reform.** Although the need for health care for the total population was recognized at the beginning of the twentieth century, attempts to pass national health insurance were unsuccessful during the New Deal era in the 1930s and after World War II. It was not until the civil rights movement of the 1960s that the concept of health care as a right won a major victory. The acceptance of this concept by large segments of society contributed to the successful passage into law of the Medicaid and Medicare programs in 1965. Later attempts under Presidents Nixon and Carter to extend coverage to all United States citizens failed.

C. **Major approaches to reform.** A range of approaches to reform are under discussion in 1994. Many of these proposals are drawn from models in other countries, and some are uniquely American. These plans vary in the extent to which government is involved as a payer and as a regulator of both coverage and costs.

1. **National health service versus national health insurance.** No proposals for national health service or socialized medicine are under debate. In **socialized medicine,** formerly found in many Eastern European countries, all health facilities are owned by the government, all health workers are government employees, and all health services are provided by the government. The British **national health service** has strong government control of health services, but includes privately owned hospitals. Physicians are paid by the government, but may also maintain private practices. **National health insurance** systems, such as Canada's Medicare, function like a single nationwide Blue Cross/Blue Shield plan, with government as the sole payer in a system that includes both fee-for-service and other payment mechanisms.

2. **Single-payer plan.** Modeled on the Canadian plan, a single-payer system provides for tax-based financing and universal health coverage. Physician payments would probably be negotiated, although capitated plans might also be part of the system. Hospital global budgets and control of technology would also be used to control costs. Advocates of this plan claim that more than 15% of health care spending is for unnecessary administrative costs that would be eliminated under this plan. Savings from this plan would therefore provide sufficient funds to cover the uninsured.

3. **Employer mandate and the play-or-pay option.** Employer mandate builds on the existing pattern of coverage by requiring all employers to provide coverage to their workers. This system is in place in Hawaii; no other state may attempt it because of ERISA. Under the "play-or-pay" option, a payroll tax is imposed on employers, who are permitted to opt out by showing that they have coverage for their workers. Small employers,

TABLE 17-7. Elements of Health Reform

Financing method
Tax treatment of health expenditures
Eligibility and coverage
Insurance reform
Information systems
Managed care
Tort reform
Antifraud, self-referral
Antitrust
Provider supply and primary care supply
Capital and technology planning

who are more likely not to provide coverage for their workers, are opposed to this approach. This plan is in place in Massachusetts and Oregon.

4. **The Clinton managed competition plan.** The Clinton proposal is a complex plan that is based on managed competition. This system is loosely modeled on the German system, with a uniquely American place for managed care plans, such as HMOs. Financing would be arranged through a mix of employer mandates and expanded public coverage. States could opt for a single-payer system instead.
   a. **Managed competition,** proposed by the Jackson Hole group,[6] creates a system to allow everyone to buy coverage under the same advantageous circumstances as large employers. It creates structures called alliances, or cooperatives, that are sometimes described as health insurance markets or shopping malls. The alliances negotiate directly with carriers.
   b. Instead of being limited to a few plans, members choose among a selection of plans based on price and value. In theory, if they are given accurate and complete information, people will choose the most efficient and effective plans, thus reducing costs while maintaining the quality of care. HMOs are expected to become dominant under this system.
   c. The Clinton proposal is criticized for both its simplifications (e.g., limiting the number of benefit structures to make comparisons possible) and its complexity, which reflects the complexity of the current health system.
   d. **Variations** on the plan would eliminate the employer mandate, allow multiple competing alliances, or limit the alliances to small employers and individuals.

5. **Individual mandate and consumer choice.** Other reform proposals would replace the current favorable tax treatment of employer health coverage with a limited deduction, tax credit, or voucher. This plan is often proposed in conjunction with an individual mandate or with tax-deductible individual medical savings accounts.

6. **Incremental reforms.** If comprehensive reform is not achieved, a plan may be approved that provides a timetable to achieve universal coverage. In states that have taken this approach, incremental reforms generally include expanding Medicaid to cover all individuals whose income is lower than the poverty level, with subsidies to the working poor and near-poor; changes designed to encourage the formation of organized delivery systems, including HMOs; insurance reform; and uniform administrative systems. There is general agreement that these changes are likely to be ingredients of any plan for reform. Common elements are listed in Table 17-7.

REFERENCES

1. Localio AR, et al: Relation between malpractice claims and adverse events due to negligence: results of the Harvard Medical Practice Study III. *N Engl J Med* 325:245–251, 1991.

2. Arrow K: Uncertainty and the welfare economics of medical care. *Am Econ Rev* 53:941–973, 1963.

3. Kovner AR (ed): *Health Care Delivery in the United States,* 4th ed. New York, Springer-Verlag, 1990, pp 272–274.

4. Roemer MI, Shain M: *Hospital Utilization Under Insurance.* American Hospital Association, 1959.

5. Newhouse JP, et al: Some interim results from a controlled trial of cost sharing in health insurance. The Rand Corporation, Santa Monica, CA, 1982.

6. Enthoven AC, Alain C: The history and principles of managed competition. *Health Aff* Suppl: 24–48, 1993.

BIBLIOGRAPHY

Fox RC: *Essays in Medical Sociology.* New York, John Wiley, 1979.

Heydebrand WV: *Hospital Bureaucracy—A Comparative Study of Organizations.* New York, Dunellen, 1973.

Kovner AR (ed): *Health Care Delivery in the United States,* 4th ed. New York, Springer-Verlag, 1990.

Litman TJ, Robins LS (eds): *Health Politics and Policy,* 2nd ed. Albany, NY, Delmar, 1991.

Raffel MW: *The U.S. Health System: Origins and Functions.* New York, John Wiley, 1984.

Roemer MI: *An Introduction to the U.S. Health Care System.* New York, Springer, 1982.

Starr P: *The Social Transformation of American Medicine.* New York, Basic Books, 1982.

Stewart PL, Cantor MG: *Varieties of Work Experience.* Cambridge, Mass., Schenkman, 1974.

Stewart PL, Cantor MG: *Varieties of Work.* Beverly Hills, CA, Sage, 1982.

Williams SJ, Torrens PR (eds): *Introduction to Health Services,* 2nd ed. New York, John Wiley, 1984.

STUDY QUESTIONS

DIRECTIONS: Each of the numbered items or incomplete statements in this section is followed by answers or by completions of the statement. Select the ONE lettered answer or completion that is BEST in each case.

1. One of the main purposes of the Hill-Burton program was to

(A) increase the number of physicians
(B) increase the number of hospital beds
(C) provide supplemental insurance for Medicare patients
(D) provide health insurance for the indigent
(E) provide a system of review of physician hospitalization practices

2. The diagnosis-related group (DRG) system was designed by Medicare and is now used by some other insurers as well. Features of this system include which one of the following?

(A) The physician in charge of an individual patient comes to prior agreement with the hospital about the length of stay
(B) The hospital is required to ensure that only the resources approved for the DRG will be used
(C) A single payment is made to cover all hospital and doctor bills for a patient's stay
(D) In general, the hospital receives a specific payment regardless of the intensity or length of care rendered to the patient
(E) Features of the hospital, such as its location or the number of resident physicians employed, are not considered in making a payment

3. The health care delivery system of the early to mid-1990s in the United States can best be described as

(A) providing an appropriate level of care to all but a very small fraction of the public
(B) a socialized system of hospital care
(C) a pluralistic system, paralleling the structure of society in general, with a variety of modes of care delivery and financing
(D) well-distributed geographically and with reasonable distribution among medical specialties
(E) consuming about the same percentage of the gross national product compared with other developed nations

4. The Medicare program is best described as

(A) an entitlement health care program for the elderly poor
(B) an insurance program for catastrophic illness-related hospital bills
(C) a direct provider for specific categorized diseases (e.g., end-stage renal disease)
(D) a form of insurance under which the federal government pays certain health care costs for the elderly and for some individuals with disabilities
(E) a national health insurance plan shared by the state and federal governments

5. An HMO is a modality for delivering health care to a specific group of enrolled patients under a premium structure, which most often can be described as

(A) providing for preventive care only
(B) requiring monthly revisions
(C) requiring significant additional payments upon hospitalization
(D) providing full financial coverage for a prescribed comprehensive benefits package
(E) providing for physician services only

6. Which of the following is an example of cost shifting?

(A) A family switches from one insurance company to one with generous mental health benefits after the daughter develops schizophrenia
(B) A large company decides to self-insure, thereby avoiding state mandates and taxes on insurance premiums
(C) A nonprofit hospital decides to set its charges at 30% above costs, so the patients with insurance will subsidize those who cannot pay
(D) An insurance company has a "preexisting condition" policy, i.e., it excludes payment (for 1 year) for care related to any illness that a patient has when joining the plan
(E) A company requires employees to make a $10 copayment for each physician visit, in the hopes of decreasing use of the plan

DIRECTIONS: Each of the numbered items or incomplete statements in this section is negatively phrased, as indicated by a capitalized word such as NOT, LEAST, or EXCEPT. Select the ONE lettered answer or completion that is BEST in each case.

7. Medicare is a federal government financial program intended to ensure health care to eligible patients. Medicare Part A (hospital insurance) coverage includes all of the following EXCEPT

(A) physician inpatient hospital visits
(B) home health care
(C) hospice care
(D) routine hospital inpatient care
(E) medically necessary care in a skilled nursing facility

8. Expenditures for health care in the United States have grown from $12 billion in 1950 to $559 billion in 1988. All of the following factors were significant contributors to the rise EXCEPT

(A) the enactment of the Medicare and Medicaid programs in 1965
(B) significant increases in both numbers and categories of health care delivery personnel (other than physicians) and their supply/demand–related wage increases
(C) the availability of private health insurance, largely as a benefit of employment
(D) the emergence of HMOs in the early 1970s
(E) the increasing average age of the American population

DIRECTIONS: The set of matching questions in this section consists of a list of four to twenty-six lettered options (some of which may be in figures) followed by several numbered items. For each numbered item, select the ONE lettered option that is most closely associated with it. To avoid spending too much time on matching sets with large numbers of options, it is generally advisable to begin each set by reading the list of options. Then, for each item in the set, try to generate the correct answer and locate it in the option list, rather than evaluating each option individually. Each lettered option may be selected once, more than once, or not at all.

Questions 9–11

Match the descriptions of models of health care reform with the names by which they are known.

(A) Employer mandate
(B) Managed competition
(C) National health service
(D) Single payor plan
(E) Individual mandate

9. In this system, which is based on the British model, the government pays doctors' salaries and all citizens are entitled to care, although individual's may elect to receive private care on a fee-for-service basis

10. This plan builds on the current system of public and private health insurance but expands coverage by requiring employers to buy insurance for all employees or to pay increased taxes

11. Under this system, all individuals would be able to choose from a number of health care alliances. The alliances would deal for discounted care from providers and try to offer low cost and high quality to attract subscribers

ANSWERS AND EXPLANATIONS

1. The answer is B [I A 2 a (4)]. The Hill-Burton program was an attempt to increase the number of hospitals and hospital beds. This program (more precisely, the Hospital Survey and Construction Act of 1946) was intended originally to ensure the availability of acute hospital facilities in rural areas. In time, this purpose was sidetracked and hospital construction, expansion, and modernization were supported nationwide by a system of grants and low-interest loans. Hospitals that received support were (and are) obligated to render specific amounts of uncompensated care to patients in designated low-income categories in keeping with a series of complex formulas. At present, it is widely considered that overbedding in many geographic areas has been an unintended result.

2. The answer is D [I B 2 b (2)]. The diagnosis-related group (DRG)–based prospective payment system that is currently being used by Medicare covers only hospital services and does not include physician services. A price is paid by Medicare to the hospital, and this price is not affected by any arrangements made by the physician, although the price is affected by the wage base of the hospital, a calculation that considers the location and the number of resident physicians. The DRG system assures the government that, regardless of the resources used by the hospital or the length of stay of the patient, the federal payment will not vary from the amount set according to the specific principal diagnosis.

3. The answer is C [I A, B]. The variety of payment and delivery models existing in health care reflect the variety available in almost all aspects of society in the United States. Such a system is not socialized in significant part and does not provide coverage to a significant segment of the population. There remain geographic areas (including both rural and urban locations) with little or no access to medical care. Compared with other industrialized societies, the United States expends a significantly greater part of its gross national product for health care. There is considered to be a poor distribution of medical specialties, despite a plethora of medical specialties, and a shortage of primary-care physicians.

4. The answer is D [I B 1 d (1)]. Medicare was designed to provide health insurance for the elderly and certain other specific groups, such as patients suffering from end-stage renal disease. Part A provides basic coverage for hospital-provided health care. Part B, for which participants must pay a premium, pays for physician services, outpatient tests, and equipment. It covers most elderly individuals, regardless of income. It is not to be confused with Medicaid, which is a medical assistance program that is directed at the indigent and is shared by the federal and state governments.

5. The answer is D [I A 3 b]. Health maintenance organizations (HMOs) are designed to provide a comprehensive health care package that emphasizes preventive care but also includes episodic hospitalization and, under many programs, additional features such as vision and dental care. Another feature of HMOs is that a single annual premium, which may be paid monthly, is the only payment required of a subscriber, and it is set for a period of 1 year.

6. The answer is C [I B 1 b]. Cost shifting, which involves raising charges for insured and other paying patients as a way of subsidizing uncompensated care, is a common phenomenon in health care. Requiring employees to make copayments when they receive care is known as cost sharing, and is designed to discourage unnecessary care. Many insurance companies have clauses that preclude payment for preexisting conditions, and this is designed to prevent patients from joining higher benefit plans only after they become ill. This practice, as well as self-insurance, is unrelated to cost shifting.

7. The answer is A [Table 17-5]. Medicare is a two-part program. Part A covers inpatient hospital care, home health care, hospice care, and medically necessary care in a skilled-nursing facility. Physician services are covered only under Part B of Medicare.

8. The answer is D [II D]. Although many factors have contributed significantly to the increase in expenditures for health care in the United States, the major cause is considered to be overall inflation. The establishment of Medicare and Medicaid expanded access to services and increased the need for greater capacity, with associated elevation of costs. Increased coverage by private insurance plans similarly provided funds for a broader range of services. Demands for health services provided by physical therapists, physician assistants, and other paraprofessionals introduced new and growing costs. On the other hand, HMOs generally are seen as effective in controlling health care costs.

9–11. The answers are: 9-C, 10-A, 11-B [III C]. Employer mandates require companies to ''play or pay,'' i.e., to pay increased taxes to subsidize government insurance, or else provide insurance to all employees (even low wage and part-time employees, who are often uninsured under the current system). Managed competition would encourage the development of large health care alliances, which would compete for subscribers by offering good quality at good prices. Britain's national health service has been proposed as another model. It uses salaried doctors and budgeted hospital payments to provide care to all citizens. Canada's single payor system differs in that doctors negotiate fees with the government, rather than being salaried. The government limits the expansion of technology and hospital spending as a way of controlling costs. Individual mandate would require the uninsured to buy health insurance, using a system of tax deductions or vouchers to help those with low incomes.

CASE STUDIES IN CLINICAL DECISION MAKING

Case 1: Abnormal Movements and Psychotic Depression

A 32-year-old man has intermittent depression for several years. One year ago, he had a severe depressive episode and a psychotic symptom, the delusion that his own evilness caused an earthquake is Asia. He responded to treatment with a serotonin reuptake-blocking antidepressant (sertraline) and a dopamine-blocking antipsychotic drug (haloperidol). He now has abnormal movements: his face, hands, and shoulders twitch involuntarily. He can control these twitches briefly if he concentrates but they return and are becoming more bothersome. He also has trouble with his memory.

QUESTIONS

1. *Which brain structures might be involved in this patient's abnormal movements?*

2. *How might the treatment of his depression relate to his current symptoms?*

3. *What else might be causing his symptoms?*

DISCUSSION

This patient's abnormal movements suggest a problem with the basal ganglia. This problem might stem from his treatment with haloperidol. The effectiveness of this drug as an antipsychotic agent is thought to arise from its blockade of dopamine receptors in the limbic system. However, it blocks dopamine receptors in other parts of the brain as well. Blockade of dopamine receptors in the basal ganglia can cause symptoms that resemble Parkinson's disease, such as stiffness and shuffling gait. If dopamine-blocking drugs are taken for several months or longer, however, the dopamine system attempts to readjust to the blockade, and the postsynaptic receptors in the striatum become supersensitive. This sensitivity can result in abnormal movements and is thought to play a role in tardive dyskinesia ("late-onset abnormal movements"), which this patient may have.

However, there are other possible explanations. Because his movements are bilateral, a focal problem, such as a tumor or stroke, is unlikely. However, a number of disorders affect the basal ganglia bilaterally. Fahr's disease, in which there is idiopathic calcification of the basal ganglia, can produce parkinsonian symptoms, apathy, psychosis, and dementia in adulthood. Wilson's disease, a rare autosomal recessive disorder in which abnormal copper deposits are found in the liver and brain, can produce abnormal movements (characteristically a flapping movement of extended wrists), psychosis, depression, dementia, and emotional lability. In patient's with Wilson's disease, Kayser-Fleischer rings are seen in the iris. Onset occurs in adolescence or adulthood. Huntington's chorea is an inherited disorder (autosomal dominant) that involves atrophy of the caudate. It usually begins to affect people in early to midadulthood. Although choreiform (twitchy) movements are a characteristic symptom, many patients experience depression or psychosis. Dementia and personality changes are usually seen as well.

The patient's eyes are normal. He does not have parkinsonian symptoms nor does he exhibit the flapping seen with Wilson's disease. His family history is unknown because he was adopted. The physician decides to evaluate the patient for Huntington's chorea.

QUESTIONS

4. What further testing would be appropriate?

5. Would structural or functional imaging provide more useful information?

Genetic tests for Huntington's chorea that use linkage analysis have been an important breakthrough. These tests are useful only if the patient has living relatives with and without the disease who can be tested to determine the linkage pattern for the particular family. Such testing would not be helpful for an adopted patient.

Because atrophy of the caudate nucleus is seen in patients with Huntington's chorea, structural imaging would help to determine whether this condition is causing these symptoms. Normally, the caudate nucleus is seen bulging into the lateral ventricles on either computed tomography (CT) or magnetic resonance imaging (MRI) scan, giving a "butterfly" appearance to the ventricles. Individuals with Huntington's chorea, however, have ventricles that resemble round eyes. Functional imaging, such as positron emission tomography (PET) or single-photon emission computer tomography (SPECT) scans, would not be as helpful because the resolution is lower and a detailed view of the caudate anatomy is needed for the diagnosis.

Case 2: Disorientation in a Patient with Schizophrenia

A 30-year-old man with a 12-year history of chronic undifferentiated schizophrenia presents to the emergency room with a sudden onset of high fever, extreme muscular rigidity, and disorientation.

QUESTIONS

1. What are possible causes of the patient's signs and symptoms?

2. What diagnostic studies are urgently indicated?

DISCUSSION

High fever and disorientation suggest an infectious process that involves the central nervous system (CNS). Rigidity suggests dysfunction of the extrapyramidal motor system. The fact that the patient has schizophrenia suggests that he might be taking antipsychotic drugs. Overdose with these agents can cause signs and symptoms of anticholinergic toxicity, including delirium, as well as seizures, hypotension, and cardiac arrhythmias. Extrapyramidal symptoms can be associated with overdose, but extreme muscular rigidity is usually not associated. In addition, hypothermia, rather than fever, would be expected.

In addition to routine blood work (to look for an elevated white blood cell count, electrolyte abnormalities, and toxic ingestion), a lumbar puncture allows examination of the cerebrospinal fluid for signs of CNS infection.

The laboratory results are inconsistent with infection. A possible diagnosis that is consistent with the findings in this patient is the neuroleptic malignant syndrome. This rare condition is associated with the use of antipsychotic drugs; however, it does not seem to be related to the duration of treatment or the dosage of the medication.

QUESTIONS

3. What other signs and symptoms would you expect to find?

4. What is the treatment of this disorder?

DISCUSSION

Neuroleptic malignant syndrome is a medical emergency. In addition to fever, rigidity, and confusion, signs of the syndrome include abnormalities in autonomic function, such as hypertension and tachycardia. Because of the muscular symptoms, elevated levels of serum creatinine phosphokinase are also noted.

Immediate intervention should include hospitalization and supportive measures. Antipsychotic medications should be discontinued. Anticholinergic medications may worsen the confusional state. Sedatives, such as barbiturates, should be avoided because they could further cloud consciousness. Because the disorder is associated with drugs that cause dopamine blockade, dopaminergic agents, such as bromocriptine, are often used.

Case 3: Feelings of Worthlessness in an Otherwise Healthy Patient

A 35-year-old obese taxi driver presents with a 2-month history of decreased energy level, increased sleep, poor motivation, frequent crying spells, and feelings of worthlessness and guilt. The patient is in good physical health and denies previous psychiatric problems. His mother died 4 months ago.

QUESTIONS

1. What would an appropriate initial medical workup include?

2. What other information would be important to obtain from the patient?

DISCUSSION

An appropriate workup would involve thorough physical and neurologic examinations, a complete blood count, and a general chemical profile that includes liver function studies, electrolyte status, and thyroid function tests. The thyroid tests are necessary because subclinical thyroid problems, usually hypothyroidism, may be present and contribute to the clinical picture.

Suicidal ideation and plans on the patient's part must be explored. The presence of manic symptoms must be determined, as well as the presence of other psychotic symptoms.

The medical workup and the additional information gathered from the patient lead to a diagnosis of major depression.

QUESTIONS

3. How would the physician discuss the diagnosis with the patient?

4. What types of therapy are available to this patient?

DISCUSSION

Depression is a common psychiatric problem that is often undiagnosed and therefore untreated. Approximately one person in six will have at least one episode of major depression in her lifetime. Women are at higher risk for depression than are men.

It is important for the physician to reassure the patient that his illness is common and treatable. It is important to stress, particularly to the patient without a previous history of psychiatric illness, that the patient is not crazy and his illness is not due to personal weakness. A discussion of the better prognostic signs (i.e., sudden onset, a major precipitant, lack of suicidal ideation, a good family and social support system, and the absence of alcohol and drug abuse) should also help the patient accept the diagnosis.

Pharmacotherapy is effective and, with the advent of the newer antidepressants, is associated with fewer side effects than the older medications. Psychotherapy is very helpful in mild to moderate cases of depression, especially cognitive and interpersonal therapies. There should be an attempt to strengthen the patient's family and social support networks. Vocational training might be warranted at times.

Case 4: Tantrums in a 4-Year-Old

A woman comes to a family practice office because she is having trouble with her 4-year-old son. He frequently throws tantrums. When he has a tantrum, she offers him a cookie, and he often calms down. However, the frequency of tantrums is increasing.

QUESTION

1. What type of learning is the boy exhibiting, and how is it working?

DISCUSSION

The boy is demonstrating operant conditioning, which is a type of instrumental conditioning. The boy's tantrums are being reinforced because he is given a reward (cookie) every time they occur. Reinforcing such behavior leads to an increase in frequency.

QUESTIONS

2. What advice should be given to the mother?

3. What schedule of reinforcement would be involved?

DISCUSSION

The mother should stop reinforcing the behavior. She should stop offering the cookies and ignore the tantrums. When a behavior is not reinforced, extinction of the behavior eventually occurs.

The woman is curious about one other matter. Her son is a messy eater, and he always drops cookie crumbs on the floor. The family dog then eats the crumbs. The woman noticed recently that when her son has a tantrum, the dog begins to drool. She wonders why.

QUESTIONS

4. *What type of learning is the dog exhibiting?*

5. *What stimuli and responses are involved?*

DISCUSSION

The dog is learning through classical conditioning. Eating cookie crumbs (unconditioned stimulus) normally causes the dog to salivate (unconditioned reflex). Over time, the sound of the boy's tantrum (conditioned stimulus) is repeatedly paired with cookie crumbs. Although this sound does not normally cause salivation in a dog, after many associations, the dog develops a drooling response to the tantrum alone (conditioned reflex).

Case 5: Designing a Clinical Study

A clinician observes that several patients who drank a particular herbal tea experienced relief from their depression. The clinician wants to design a study to determine if the tea is truly effective.

QUESTIONS

1. *What is the first step in conducting such a study?*

2. *How should the study be designed?*

DISCUSSION

First, the clinician conceptualizes a specific research design, which includes choosing the independent variable (herbal tea as treatment) and the dependent variable (depression). The clinician realizes that it is important to perform a true experiment, using random assignment and double-blind, placebo-controlled methods, to evaluate the effectiveness of the tea. He next writes up a research proposal and consent form and submits it to his institutional review board (IRB) for approval. After suggesting a few changes, the IRB approves the protocol and gives the clinician permission to begin his study. The clinician then asks the next 30 patients who appear depressed if they would like to participate in his study. Eighteen patients agree to participate.

The clinician uses a standard scale to rate the patients' symptoms of depression at baseline. The patients are then randomly assigned to two different groups. Nine patients are given a tea purchased from the supermarket to drink daily for the same period. The tea bags are disguised and coded by another doctor so that neither the clinician nor the patients know which patients are receiving the herbal tea. Using the same rating scale, the clinician assesses the severity of each patient's depression each week. At the end of the 4 weeks, he breaks the code and compares the two groups.

QUESTIONS

3. *What are some possible threats to validity?*

4. *How should the clinician analyze the data?*

DISCUSSION

Threats to validity include differences in factors that may influence response to treatment between the two experimental groups. The clinician compares the two experimental groups to determine if they differ in their mean age, gender distribution, years of education, or severity of depression at baseline. They do not. He then goes on to look at the distribution of scores that are derived from the scale used to assess depression. Because the scores appear to be normally distributed, he compares the weekly mean scores from each group using a repeated measures analysis of variance (ANOVA). The ANOVA indicates that there is no significant effect of group on outcome. In other words, the two groups do not differ significantly in their mean weekly depression scores.

QUESTIONS

5. *What kind of error could have occurred in the interpretation of the results?*

6. *How does the clinician determine if he has studied enough patients?*

7. *What is another possible explanation for the lack of efficacy of the tea?*

DISCUSSION

Because the clinician did not find a difference, there is a risk of a Type II error [incorrect acceptance of the null hypothesis (no group difference) when the alternative hypothesis is true]. He decides to conduct a power analysis using his estimate of the magnitude of the true effect of the tea, a significance criteria (alpha) of .05 and the sample size of 18. The clinician discovers that his sample had only 25% power to detect an effect. He repeats the study using a sample size with 90% power and still finds no effect of the tea.

An important consideration in psychiatric studies is the problem of etiologic heterogeneity. Patients may exhibit depressive symptoms due to a number of different causes. If there are significant differences in the causes of the depressive symptoms between the two experimental groups, it may be difficult to detect treatment effects.

Case 6: Family Issues in the Life Cycle

The five members of the Smith family are all patients in your primary care practice. Mr. Smith is 45 and an unemployed construction worker. Mrs. Smith is 41 and works as a secretary. They have three sons: John, aged 5; Marcus, aged 9; and Chris, aged 14.

QUESTION

1. *Based on your understanding of the emotional progression through the life cycle, what are the key issues likely to be facing each member of the family at this time?*

DISCUSSION

The youngest son, who is 5 years of age, is probably leaving the security of home for formal schooling for the first time. His social network will be expanding from family alone to family and school friends, and he will have new role models in the form of his teachers. From a psychoanalytical point of view, he is likely to be in the Oedipal phase of psychosexual development. This means that he is likely to feel very attached to his mother and to see his father as somewhat of a competitor.

Marcus, age 9, is well established in his peer group and derives considerable support and recognition from his activities at school and play (sports, musical activities, cub scouts). His life is predictable and relatively serene.

Chris, at age 14, is in the early stages of adolescence and is likely to be testing the limits of his newly acquired independence and his parents' patience. His previously serene and predictable behavior is often otherwise, leading to a series of conflicts with his parents, whom he sees as overprotective. Interest in girls is beginning to develop.

Mrs. Smith is disappointed in her husband but very likely feels guilty for these feelings. Marital tension and arguments are likely to abound as Mrs. Smith sees herself more as the breadwinner and Mr. Smith as a househusband.

Mr. Smith is also in a mid-life transition now and is likely to experience a mid-life crisis with depression and anxiety as he worries about his role in the family, his future employment possibilities, and the family's finances. He might search regressively for comfort via an affair or alcohol.

QUESTION

2. *Mr. Smith has just been diagnosed with cancer and is expected to survive only several months. Considering the different phases of the life cycle and the issues that each member of the family is facing, how is each member likely to respond to this news?*

DISCUSSION

John's cognitive functioning will still be in what is called the preoperational stage. A child at this stage is beginning to develop some symbolic activity but still views the world in an egocentric way and has difficulty distinguishing physical and psychological causality. Particularly, if John has angry feelings about his father spending more time with Mom (the Oedipal conflict), he is likely to believe that he caused the cancer with his thoughts. This may lead to feelings of guilt and depression. He may have difficulty accepting the nonreversibility of death.

Marcus will be able to appreciate his father's illness to a considerable degree psychologically and cognitively. At his father's death, true mourning will not be experienced due to his developmental state; he is still very psychologically dependent on the family.

Chris will begin to experience his father's illness as a permanent loss and will fully mourn his father's death. His school work will suffer. There is the possibility of a behavioral change leading to antisocial acts as he attempts to deal with his depression and resentment.

Mrs. Smith will be anxious and depressed as she struggles with her future as a single parent caring for three children.

Case 7: Difficulty Maintaining an Erection

A 26-year-old man tells his physician during an office visit that he has trouble maintaining an erection. As a result, he has lost interest in having sex.

QUESTIONS

1. What medical illnesses could account for the patient's dysfunction?

2. What medications or drugs could account for the patient's dysfunction?

3. What additional information will you want to gather?

DISCUSSION

Medical illnesses that could account for the patient's symptoms include endocrine disorders (diabetes), neurologic disorders (parasympathetic nerve damage), and peripheral vascular disease. Medications that could account for the patient's symptoms include antihypertensives, antidepressants, and alcohol and other nonprescription drugs of abuse. The review of systems and medical history will help the physician rule out these causes of erectile dysfunction.

At this point in the evaluation, the physician gathers a sexual development history, a relationship history, and an assessment of psychological symptoms. The physician finds no evidence of a psychiatric or medical disorder or a history of substance abuse that would account for the dysfunction. The patient's sexual development history is unremarkable except for anxiety in sexual relationships. The patient says that he has difficulty achieving and maintaining an erection, even when he is alone.

QUESTIONS

4. What is the value of knowing whether the patient has an erection while asleep?

5. What additional tests might help the physician determine the cause of the patient's sexual dysfunction at this point?

DISCUSSION

Testing for nocturnal penile tumescence evaluates whether normal erectile function is demonstrated during rapid eye movement (REM) sleep. This information helps determine the biologic or psychological nature of the dysfunction. For this patient, the result shows normal erectile function. In gathering the patient's sexual history, the physician learns that the patient has been married for 2 years. His difficulty maintaining an erection has been upsetting to his wife and has strained their relationship.

QUESTION

6. What are the next possible steps in the physician's evaluation and treatment plan?

DISCUSSION

At this point, the physician believes that the patient's difficulty maintaining an erection is most likely due to conflictual feelings about his marriage, his wife, or sexuality. Assuming the physician believes it is mostly due to the latter, he might decide to refer the patient and his wife for sexual therapy; or, the physician might decide to try office-based counseling. This approach will involve meeting with the patient and his wife and educating the couple about normal sexual functioning and reasons for sexual dysfunction. Specific behavioral strategies should be suggested to decrease sexual performance anxiety and improve communication.

QUESTION

7. What referrals should be considered and why?

DISCUSSION

In addition to referral to a sex or marital therapist, the physician should consider referral for individual psychotherapy if the physician believes that the patient is noncompliant with the behavioral strategies prescribed. If anxiety is a significant factor, referral for hypnotherapy could be considered.

Case 8: Out-of-Control Asthma

Brian, a 16-year-old Hispanic boy, comes to the emergency room at 8:00 P.M. He is a tenth-grade student from inner-city Chicago. Brian is wheezing and cyanotic, but responds to an epinephrine injection and an aminophylline drip. He is placed in the intensive care unit for the night. His chart shows 17 previous admissions for status asthmaticus during the last year. Although oral theophylline, prednisone, steroids, and an albuterol inhaler were prescribed, the theophylline level on admission is 2 μ/ml (therapeutic level is 10–20 μ/ml. The next morning, Brian's serum cortisol level is 10 μ/dl, indicating no suppression of the hypothalamic-pituitary-adrenal axis by the exogenous corticosteroid. The next morning, his allergist lectures Brian on the importance of taking medications. He states "You've been through our asthma education class three times. You've got to stop acting like a child and take care of yourself. You know what you need to do." Brian sarcastically retorts, "If you'd give me medicine that worked, I'd take it."

QUESTIONS

1. What is an appropriate response to Brian's sarcasm?

2. According to general systems theory, specifically, a biopsychosocial approach to choosing an overall treatment plan, what additional data are relevant?

DISCUSSION

Brian's sarcastic remark is an example of a hostile and controlling statement. This reply can be viewed as a complementary response to the hostile and controlling statement of the allergist. This type of interaction is conventionally labeled a power struggle. An antithetical statement (i.e., one that is opposite in degrees of hostility, control, and focus) often diffuses tension and reinstates a therapeutic conversation. For example, the physician might state, "I'm concerned because your asthma has been out of control lately, and I'm interested in why you think your medications haven't been working right."

A biopsychosocial approach considers a variety of levels of data that may pertain to Brian's problems. For example, on the physiologic level, the patient may have abnormal theophylline or steroid pharmacokinetics that would account for the ineffectiveness of his medications as well as for the laboratory evidence that suggests noncompliance. On the intrapsychic level, the patient may have a learning disability that limits his understanding of information presented in asthma education sessions; or, side effects of the medication (e.g., tremor, altered physical appearance) might be difficult for an image-conscious adolescent to accept. On the interpersonal level, the patient's relationship with his allergist may interfere with optimal compliance and physician–patient communication. On the family level, Brian may have a good reason not to take his medications (e.g., financial difficulties). On the social level, the need to take medications may create the perception of weakness and increase the likelihood of aggressive behavior by peers in the patient's inner-city neighborhood.

After these issues are discussed with Brian's allergist, more information is collected from Brian. During the discussion, Brian complains repeatedly of headaches and back pain. He seems visibly upset when he is asked about his family. Brian lives with his mother, stepfather, and two younger half siblings. When he is asked about his home life, Brian blurts out that his stepfather lost his job 6 months ago and cannot find work. With coaxing, he states that his stepfather began drinking to handle his frustration over being unemployed, and that there is a lot of tension at home. The allergist states that extensive workups of Brian's headaches and back pain have not yielded an organic etiology, and that he is frustrated in his attempts to increase the level of involvement of Brian's parents.

QUESTIONS

3. Is a psychiatric consultation appropriate?

4. Given Brian's noncompliance, what might his parents be like?

DISCUSSION

A psychiatric consultation should be sought for several reasons. First, Brian is endangering his life by noncompliance. His actions reflect a passive suicidal intent. The situation is potentially dangerous, and there is no clear diagnosis or treatment plan. Second, key elements of his social support system, including his allergist and his family, are not working effectively.

Because noncompliance is often associated with a high level of expressed emotion in family members, the patient's parents might be critical and frustrated with him, yet overinvolved with him. In addition, the parents are under considerable additional stress because the stepfather is unemployed. The family may be experiencing additional problems, including domestic violence. If violence is occurring, the stress level may exacerbate asthma in Brian, and the parents may not supervise his self-care thoroughly.

A child psychiatrist is consulted. He obtains the following family history. Two years ago, Brian's mother was hospitalized for 6 weeks for "headaches, fluttery heart, and leg pains" after a period of severe marital conflict. Brian thinks that she had a diagnosis of anxiety disorder. He states that his biological father was diagnosed as having a psychotic depression when Brian's mother divorced him. Brian sees his father every month for an evening, however, and thinks that his father is "just fine."

The psychiatrist convinces Brian's mother and stepfather to attend a meeting so that they can devise a plan to decrease the frequency of Brian's hospitalizations. At the meeting, it is clear that Brian is close to his mother and protective of her. They sit together and whisper to each other. Brian's stepfather is angry and critical, and sits alone. He is upset that Brian's frequent hospitalizations add to the family's financial stress. When he states that Brian is childish and incompetent for not managing his illness better, both Brian and his mother glare at him. Brian's mother puts her arm around Brian and tells

him not to worry about what his stepfather says. She responds to the stepfather by telling the psychiatrist that she is responsible for handling Brian's medications, and that she is sure that he takes them. She cannot understand why he is hospitalized so often, but feels sorry for him because he is so sick and fragile.

QUESTIONS

5. *What cultural factors may explain both Brian's and his mother's somatic symptoms without known cause?*

6. *What risk factors for domestic violence are present in this family?*

7. *What problematic family interactions occur at this meeting?*

DISCUSSION

Brian and his mother, both of whom are Hispanic, deny having emotional symptoms but admit to having physical symptoms. This situation is an example of the effect of cultural factors on medical diagnosis. In many Latin cultures, it is acceptable to admit to physical problems, but not to emotional problems.

Both of Brian's biological parents have psychiatric disorders and they have experienced a divorce. However, these factors do not increase the risk of violence. A more significant risk factor is the stepfather's high level of stress and alcohol abuse. In addition, previous marital conflict may have included violence. A history of violent behavior is a significant risk factor for future violence.

Several signs of problematic family interactions are present. Brian and his mother seem aligned, with the stepfather on the outside. This alignment may indicate a rigid triangle with an inverted power hierarchy. The mother's indirect method of communicating with her husband (she directs a message to the psychiatrist with her husband as the co-receiver) suggests a pattern of unclear communication. Finally, the hostility of the stepfather toward Brian and the overinvolvement of the mother suggest a high level of expressed emotion. Although a high level of expressed emotion does not indicate dysfunction, it is associated with noncompliance in many chronic medical illnesses, including asthma.

QUESTION

8. *What recommendations would be made by each school of family therapy?*

DISCUSSION

The structural–strategic approach would focus on the poor intergenerational boundaries in this family. The therapist would make suggestions that would pull the mother and stepfather together and give that dyad more power over the child. For example, he might suggest that the mother and stepfather set goals for Brian's management of his asthma. The therapist also might suggest that both parents monitor Brian's self-care and jointly enforce consequences for noncompliance.

The behavioral–psychoeducational approach would focus on social learning. The therapist would inform the family that adolescents often do not like to take asthma medications, and suggest that the more involved the parents become in the struggle, the worse the struggle becomes. The therapist might encourage Brian to explain to both the allergist and his parents why he believes his medications are not working and what he dislikes about them. Sharing this information may help Brian to gain empathy from his parents and perform constructive problem solving with his allergist. The therapist would then focus on teaching the family more direct ways to communicate and solve problems.

The intergenerational–experiential approach would focus on how chronic illness was handled in the parent's families of origin. This information helps to identify Brian's expectations. The therapist might encourage the family to develop hobbies or interests together to facilitate bonding. He would also encourage the family to allow Brian to take charge of his asthma care. This step is developmentally appropriate for Brian. The therapist would also ask Brian whether he fears that his family will have trouble if he grows up and leaves home.

Case 9: The Patient Who Requests Physician-assisted Suicide

A 57-year-old married man, father of three, has been undergoing hemodialysis for the past 2 years. He requests that his physician prescribe sufficient hypnotic medication so that he can "go to sleep forever." The patient has contacted an advocacy group that supports physician-assisted suicide. The patient hands the physician materials that he received from the group and asks for the physician's help.

QUESTIONS

1. What is the role of the physician in requests for physician-assisted suicide?

2. What are some of the issues involved in managing this problem?

DISCUSSION

Physician-assisted suicide is illegal in the United States. The role of the physician is to modify pain and suffering, both physical and emotional. Thus, the physician should determine why the patient is requesting assistance for suicide. Does the patient have a major depressive disorder that is causing a cognitive distortion and making him believe that he is causing a family great pain and suffering? Is there conflict within the family that is making this request a cry for attention and help? Is the patient experiencing physical pain that can be better managed? It is essential for the physician to consult with a psychiatric physician and other subspecialists to elucidate the patient's psychological and physical difficulties. Further, discussions with family members can provide a better understanding of the family issues. It is the role of the physician to modify suffering and pain, not to end life.

Case 10: Who Is the Patient's Agent?

A 35-year-old mother of two sees her primary care physician because of increasing weight gain over the past 6 months. The physician examines the patient and finds that she has a coarse, sallow complexion. Examination of the thyroid gland shows no enlargement. The physician's records show that thyroid function tests were performed 6 years ago with normal results. When the physician orders a new set of thyroid screening measures, the patient's insurance company questions why these tests are necessary.

QUESTIONS

1. What is the responsibility of the physician?

2. How should the physician react to the health plan's case manager?

DISCUSSION

The physician is clinically responsible for the care of his patient, regardless of insurance coverage or obstacles that are placed between proper management and questions that arise from the third-party coverage. The fiduciary responsibility of the physician is to carry out the most appropriate investigations to determine the cause of the patient's weight gain. The physician should not become angry or irritated with the case manager, but instead should explain why such a test was ordered. If coverage is still denied, the physician should discuss the matter with a supervisor. Basic clinical guidelines for management of such clinical problems can be found in textbooks of medicine, and they should be discussed with the medical reviewer. Refusal by an insurance company to pay for tests does not relieve the physician of the responsibility to pursue clinical and laboratory investigations in the best interest of the patient.

Case 11: Chronic Physical Complaints Without an Organic Explanation

A 53-year-old woman reports abdominal pain, chronic headaches, difficulty sleeping, and lack of energy. She fears that she has a hidden malignancy. The patient has experienced difficulty sleeping and lack of energy for the past 15 years. She has seen a variety of specialists and has had many evaluations. All findings have been negative, but the negative findings have only reassured her temporarily. Her family states that her main preoccupation is her health. Her current request is for sleep medication.

QUESTIONS

1. What are appropriate management strategies for the hypochondriacal patient?

2. How does the physician address the patient's request for sleeping medication?

DISCUSSION

The hypochondriacal patient uses somatic concerns as a metaphor for emotional distress. Hypochondriacal patients tend to amplify normal visceral sensations. Their conditions have a chronic course, and tend to exacerbate during times of emotional distress. Important comorbid conditions include mood and anxiety disorders. The physician should recognize such depressive states or anxiety disorders and treat them. Regularly scheduled appointments often can modify the hypochondriacal patient's tendency to doctor shop and seek needless laboratory and technological investigations. The patient's insomnia must be viewed as a symptom of another disorder. Sleep difficulties often are a prominent symptom of a depressive disorder. The physician should avoid chronic use of benzodiazepine hypnotics because they may become habituating and foster difficult states that may be confused with an anxiety disorder. The use of antidepressant medication is generally the safest approach in such situations.

Case 12: Should Life Support Be Terminated?

A 78-year-old woman with chronic pulmonary disease is admitted to the hospital with an upper respiratory infection. She chooses not to sign the living will that is routinely offered to her. During the initial part of her hospitalization, she appears alert and understands the nature of her illness. Unfortunately, respiratory failure develops. The patient is intubated and cannot be weaned from a ventilator, despite successful treatment of her infection. After 22 days in the intensive care unit, the patient's daughter requests that life support be terminated. The patient appears confused and cannot respond to questions directed to her.

QUESTIONS

1. Can the patient's daughter, who has power of attorney, demand that life support be terminated?

2. Can the physician decide to withdraw assisted ventilation?

DISCUSSION

The living will directs health professionals not to undertake heroic efforts at life support in a terminal situation. In this case, the patient chose not to sign a living will. Without such a directive, her family cannot order a physician to actively withdraw life support. The physician cannot take this action on his own. It is essential for the primary care physician who knows the patient best to discuss in advance the issue of a living will with the patient with a serious chronic disease who could be hospitalized. The use of the interpretive model of patient–physician interaction can clarify what the patient expects in such a serious medical situation and what she would like done in a dire situation. The fact that the daughter has power of attorney is irrelevant in this situation.

Case 13: The Patient Interview

The patient, a 45-year-old executive, arrives for his first office visit. He is experiencing general malaise.

QUESTIONS

1. How might the interview begin?

2. What are the important elements of the interview?

3. What are the components of the medical history?

DISCUSSION

Early in the interview, it is important to establish rapport and a working relationship with the patient. One approach is the use of open-ended questions. The important elements of the interview are building rapport, gathering information, patient education, and treatment planning. The components of the medical history are patient identification, chief complaint, history of current illness, medical history, family history, social history, and review of systems.

During the social history portion of the interview, the physician inquires about the patient's use of alcohol. The patient becomes defensive and hesitantly admits to drinking more than he should. However, he insists that he does not have a problem with alcohol and can quit drinking any time he wants.

QUESTIONS

4. What interviewing approach is likely to elicit the most useful information?

5. How should the patient be informed about the next steps in the evaluation?

DISCUSSION

Responding to the patient's guardedness is an important first step. The physician might learn more about the patient's drinking behavior and his guardedness by asking how much he drinks and when. The physician might also ask the patient whether he has ever had any drinking-related problems, such as a driving while intoxicated conviction; or whether anyone is concerned about his drinking behavior (e.g., his wife, friends). Acknowledging the patient's concern that the physician might be critical of his drinking may help to establish rapport.

Working with the patient to create an agenda for the visit and generating a variety of options to address each problem is an important step. The patient's potential alcohol abuse should be addressed when the evaluation is completed and the physician has more information and has established rapport with the patient.

Physical examination shows hypertension and hepatomegaly. Laboratory findings show significantly elevated liver function test results. The genogram shows a strong family history of alcohol abuse, impulse-control disorders, and related medical problems. The patient returns for a follow-up visit.

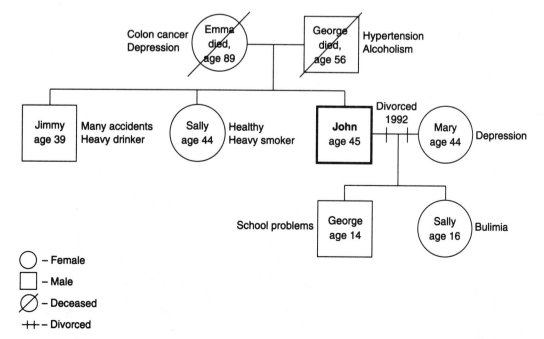

QUESTIONS

6. *What approach is likely to be the most effective in engaging the patient in treatment?*

7. *What techniques might increase treatment adherence and motivation?*

DISCUSSION

Treatment efficacy is increased when the physician takes a collaborative approach and involves the patient as an active participant in treatment planning. In this case, the physician can determine the patient's level of understanding and acceptance of the medical and social complications of his alcohol use. The patient and physician can then generate a list of potential treatment options ranging from self-control and participation in Alcoholics Anonymous (AA) to a hospital-based detoxification program and treatment. The physician can help the patient to make the most appropriate choice by inquiring about his reasons for noncompliance (e.g., social pressure to drink), reasons for previous unsuccessful attempts to control his drinking, and withdrawal symptoms. Patient motivation for treatment adherence and success can be increased by using the stage of treatment progression model (see Chapter 12 IV B 1) and adopting a nonjudgmental, empathic approach that reflects a commitment to the patient and to the importance of an effective approach.

Case 14: Severe Short-term Memory Impairment

A young man is brought to the emergency room by the police after he is found wandering in the middle of a busy street. The police think that he may be intoxicated but did not detect the odor of alcohol on his breath or clothing. In the emergency room, the patient cannot give any coherent answers to questions about his medical history or use of substances. He does not remember that the police brought him to the hospital. The patient performs poorly on the mental status exam. Findings include severe short-term memory impairment, orientation only to self, concrete responses to similarity and proverb testing, inability to reverse three digits, and poor serial seven subtraction.

QUESTIONS

1. *Which of the mental status examination findings would be key in making a diagnosis?*

2. *What is the most likely preliminary diagnosis?*

DISCUSSION

The patient's inability to reverse three digits suggests impaired concentration; the other findings are likely consequences of this observation. Poor concentration or attention, even in the absence of change in the consciousness, suggests delirium. At this point, the cause of the delirium is not known. Further evaluation or change in the patient's course may help to identify the cause of his symptoms.

The physician orders various laboratory tests. Before the results are known, the emergency room nurse reports that the patient is increasingly fearful, restless, and agitated. His temperature rises from normal to 101° F, and his blood pressure and pulse rate are also elevated.

QUESTION

3. *What laboratory studies should be requested?*

DISCUSSION

When delirium is suspected, the differential diagnosis includes an array of medical conditions, substance abuse, withdrawal from medication or substance, and many other causes. A toxicology screen is essential, as are routine urinalysis, a complete blood count, sequential multiple analysis (SMA-6), and blood sugar measurement. In addition, if any clues to the cause are found on physical or neurologic examination, further tests are needed.

The laboratory results are normal. No evidence of trauma or infection is found on examination. The toxicology screen result is negative for alcohol and other substances (i.e., street drugs, medications). Staff carefully search the patient's clothing and find a paper containing several addresses for Alcoholics Anonymous (AA) meetings.

QUESTION

4. *How does this information help to clarify the nature of the patient's delirium?*

DISCUSSION

The patient is not experiencing the dramatic hallucinatory symptoms seen in delirium tremens, but the course suggests an escalating and deteriorating withdrawal syndrome. The laboratory results show no infection, electrolyte disturbance, hypoglycemia, or uremia. The negative toxicology finding and the AA addresses suggest that the patient has stopped his alcohol consumption for several days.

Case 15: Delirium and Hallucinations in a Student

A 20-year-old university student is admitted to the inpatient psychiatry service with a 3-day history of delirium, hallucinations, and increasing agitation and fearfulness. She denies any symptoms of physical illness. The family reports no previous mental problems and insists, as do the patient's friends, that the patient has always deplored all substance abuse and has never even tasted a beer. Mental status examination on admission shows an alert young woman who is frightened by what is happening to her. She has difficulty reversing four digits. Her hair is unkempt, and she wears torn jeans and a food stained T-shirt. Her behavior varies from cooperative to irritable and evasive. She reports hearing a voice but refuses to elaborate on its content. Haltingly, she says that she thinks that people are trying to fool her and explains that she has had trouble for a few days finding her dormitory room. Results of short-term memory testing suggest some impairment. She refuses to give any proverb interpretation, saying that she does not want to play games. She shows some insight and says that some of her perceptions may be mistaken.

QUESTION

1. *Which of the following diagnoses is the least likely: paranoid schizophrenia, delirium, schizophreniform disorder, or drug or toxic reaction?*

DISCUSSION

Paranoid schizophrenia is the least likely diagnosis. It is diagnosed only after a 6-month period in which some symptoms persist despite treatment. Delirium, schizophreniform disorder, and a drug or toxic reaction are all acute syndromes.

The physical and neurologic examination findings are normal, except for a slightly elevated temperature (100° F). Results of laboratory evaluations, including toxicology screen, sequential multiple analysis (SMA-6 and SMA-12), and urinalysis, are normal. Slight lymphocytosis and some unusual lymphocytes are observed. The patient is given a low dose of neuroleptic medication.

QUESTION

2. *Which of the following laboratory examinations could be helpful: computed axial tomography (CAT) scan, glucose tolerance test, heterophil agglutination, thyroid function studies, serologic studies?*

DISCUSSION

The most useful test would be the heterophil agglutination test. The presence of lymphocytosis and some abnormal lymphocytes suggests infectious mononucleosis. This condition occasionally causes psychotic symptoms alone or associated with delirium.

Case 16: Toxic Reaction in the Workplace

A woman is referred to a physician by her attorney for a medical evaluation in preparation for a lawsuit against her employer. The patient claims that her workplace, specifically the materials used in the construction of the building, are causing her to have a toxic reaction. She reports symptoms of headache, eye pain, difficulty breathing, feeling cold and numb in her hands and feet, forgetfulness, difficulty concentrating, and occasional confusion. The physician orders extensive medical tests. All of the results are borderline or negative.

QUESTION

1. *What psychiatric diagnoses would be included in the differential diagnosis?*

DISCUSSION

The primary nonphysiologic diagnosis that must be considered in any situation that includes secondary gain, such as a lawsuit, is malingering. Other possibilities are depression, which often causes multiple nonspecific physical symptoms, and anxiety, which may be accompanied by a variety of physical symptoms that are linked to autonomic hyperarousal. Whenever a patient reports confusion or changes in concentration, or memory, an organic mental disorder must be considered.

QUESTION

2. *What additional procedures could provide more information for the differential diagnosis?*

DISCUSSION

It would be appropriate to refer this patient for a psychological assessment because the diagnosis is not clear, her symptoms are difficult to substantiate through medical evaluation, she may have subtle neurobehavioral changes that are not detected by standard medical tests, and litigation is involved. Obtaining information about her psychiatric and behavioral history is essential. This information could be obtained through a psychiatric examination or as part of a psychological assessment. In addition, psychometric evaluation of her mood state and personality would help to establish the diagnosis and would yield information about the possibility of malingering, based on Minnesota Multiphasic Personality Inventory (MMPI) validity scales. This information would be difficult to obtain otherwise. If the patient is experiencing a toxic reaction that is affecting her brain function, neuropsychological evaluation probably would detect any related cognitive and behavioral changes. Psychological and neuropsychological test data provide the type of detailed documentation about a patient's condition that is often required in legal situations. Further, these baseline data can be used to monitor future change.

QUESTION

3. *What characteristics of the psychosocial assessment would increase the reliability of the results?*

DISCUSSION

Because this case involves litigation, the examination must be complete and the test results must be clear and uncontroversial. The examination should include a careful history and a thorough clinical interview. The patient's medical, psychiatric, and academic records, and work performance evaluations can provide information about prior functioning. The most sound conclusions are based on psychometric tests that have high reliability and validity and well-standardized normative data that are based on a representative population and are administered and stored according to procedures.

The patient's history revealed chronic stomach problems, which she thought to be due to food allergies, and which had been diagnosed by her physician as irritable bowel syndrome. She also complained of skin irritation to many fabrics, detergents, and soaps, and had restricted her exposure to these products significantly. At work she had performed well until 2 years ago, when she was assigned to a new supervisor with whom she has been unable to get along. The patient was aware that two other employees in her building had become ill and that environmental factors had been implicated. There was no history of psychiatric treatment.

The test results included above-average intelligence as measured by the Wechsler Adult Intelligence Scale–Revised, with the only notable subtest scatter to be slightly lower levels of performance on the digit span and arithmetic subtests. Extensive neuropsychological testing of other cognitive functions showed only mild variability in the areas of concentration and new learning. On the MMPI, her scores on all validity scales were within the normal range. Moderate elevations were noted on four clinical scales: hypochondriasis, depression, hysteria, and psychasthenia. The Rorschach test indicated that this was a woman who is experiencing a great deal of situational stress and painful affect. She expends much of her psychological energy in containing her affect, but the results suggest her efforts to do so at this time are unsuccessful.

QUESTION

4. *How would the examiner interpret these findings?*

This is a patient with a history of somatic concerns of the type often thought to have a psychological overlay, and that are sometimes associated with stress and autonomic arousal. She is presumably unhappy in her work setting, and aware that others at her workplace may be experiencing similar problems. The test results show cognitive functions to be intact, but with mild variability in attention, concentration, and new learning. Such variability can result in forgetfulness and is more often associated with emotional interference than organic dysfunction. With normal scores on the MMPI validity scales, no unusual patterns of performance on cognitive tests, nor any obvious inconsistencies between her complaints and the actual test findings, there is little to suggest that she is consciously malingering. Personality testing suggests the presence of anxiety, worry, and depression in a person who is somatically preoccupied. Dynamically, she is expending a great deal of her psychological resources to contain her negative affect, perhaps more than she has available. Her attempts are ineffective, and she appears to cope with painful affect by unconsciously expressing it through somatic channels. Although the phenomenon of environmental illness cannot be ruled out, there is substantial evidence to suggest that psychological distress and dynamics may contribute importantly to her symptom picture. Her unsatisfactory work situation should be explored further as a source of situational stress, and treatment of depression and accompanying anxiety should be recommended.

Case 17: Acute Mental Status Changes in an Elderly Man

A 74-year-old man is brought to a hospital emergency room by his wife. She reports that for several days he has been restless and irritable, and he seems to be hallucinating. He slept little the previous night, but has been taking frequent naps during the day, sometimes drifting off during a meal. One week earlier, he felt well enough to make the travel arrangements for an upcoming vacation. She wonders whether these symptoms indicate that his Parkinson's disease is getting worse.

QUESTIONS

1. *What are the prominent symptoms described by the patient's wife?*

2. *What is the differential diagnosis?*

DISCUSSION

The major symptoms are agitation, probable psychosis (if the patient is hallucinating), and sleep–wake disturbance of acute onset. This behavior is clearly a change from the patient's baseline functioning. These symptoms have many possible explanations. Of greatest concern is the possibility of a cognitive disorder caused by a general medical condition or substance use (i.e., delirium). This diagnosis suggests a serious underlying problem that must be detected and treated. The cause of delirium could be systemic (e.g., sepsis, electrolyte disturbance), a central nervous system (CNS) problem (e.g., subdural hematoma, brain metastases, encephalitis), or a drug-related problem (e.g., withdrawal from alcohol, excessive dosage of medication). Dementia is a possibility, but the acute onset of symptoms suggests another explanation. The patient may have a psychotic disorder. The onset of schizophrenia at his age is highly unlikely, but he may have a long history of this disorder. Manic episodes also cause irritability, insomnia, and hallucinations. However, bipolar illness probably would have been seen earlier. Irritability is seen with some personality disorders, but in such cases it is chronic behavior, not a sudden change. This patient is too ill to have a primary sleep disorder as the sole problem, although sleep disorders may at times precipitate other psychiatric symptoms.

QUESTION

3. What history would help to narrow the differential diagnosis?

DISCUSSION

More information is needed about the patient's psychiatric, medical, and medication histories (particularly recent changes); drug and alcohol consumption; and recent behavior, including trauma or neurologic symptoms. The patient's wife provides the following information.

The patient is a retired engineer. He has been in excellent health, both mentally and physically, except for the onset of Parkinson's disease approximately 5 years ago. He also had prostate enlargement that was complicated by a urinary tract infection several weeks ago. His neurologist has been treating the Parkinson's disease with L-dopa (Sinemet), with moderate success. Because the patient and his wife are planning a trip, the neurologist considered more aggressive use of the medication in an attempt to minimize the patient's stiffness and tremor. The patient's wife brought in the medicine bottle. The patient takes no other medication. He drinks approximately two glasses of wine each week, and his wife reports no illicit drug use. She is unaware of any recent head trauma, seizures, or other neurologic problems.

The patient was sleeping and functioning well until 3 days ago, when he appeared confused and irritable at times. For example, he misplaced things and then blamed his wife. These symptoms have progressively worsened; yet, his condition has fluctuated. He seems clear at times, then he appears confused or suddenly becomes somnolent. He has been restless and has slept poorly at night, which is when he becomes most agitated. Last night, he thought that his wife was someone else, and ordered her out of the house. He also complained about noise in the closet.

QUESTIONS

4. What diagnosis is most likely?

5. What mental status testing would help to confirm the diagnosis?

DISCUSSION

In view of the symptoms, their acute onset, and the lack of psychiatric history, this condition is almost certainly a delirium. Even if the patient had a psychiatric history, mental status findings of a reduced level of consciousness and impaired cognition would confirm the diagnosis of delirium. Delirium can occur in patients with a history of dementia, psychosis, or any other mental disorder. The patient is admitted to the hospital and undergoes a mental status examination.

The patient is disheveled and difficult to interview. He frequently forgets the question and looks around the room or falls asleep. When attention is tested with the digit span test, the patient can repeat only three digits forward. He is irritable. His thought form is noted to show frequent derailment. He denies that he is hallucinating or fearful, but tells the nurse not to poison him. He knows the year and the month but not the date, and he thinks that he is at a hotel. He cannot provide any details about his travel plans, and can only recall one of four words after 5 minutes. He appears to have impaired judgment and insight.

QUESTION

6. *The patient clearly exhibits delirium. What is the next step?*

DISCUSSION

The patient undergoes a complete physical examination, including a thorough neurologic examination.

Other than mild cogwheel rigidity of his arms (a sign of Parkinson's disease), there are no abnormalities other than the mental status findings. Blood samples are drawn for blood count, electrolyte levels, liver and renal function tests, and toxicology screen. In view of his recent urinary tract infection, a urinalysis is done. As the physician is ordering more tests, she notices that the bottle of Sinemet is almost empty, although the prescription was filled only 2 weeks ago. The physician asks the patient's wife about his observation, and she says that her husband was doubling his dose because he wanted to feel his best for their vacation. All of the other test results are normal.

QUESTIONS

7. *What is the cause of the delirium?*

8. *How should it be treated?*

DISCUSSION

The delirium is caused by an overdose of L-dopa. This dopamine agonist alleviates parkinsonian symptoms; however, large doses can cause psychotic symptoms and delirium. The patient's medication is discontinued and then administered at the prescribed dosage as his mental symptoms remit. He and his wife are given more information about his medication and the symptoms of L-dopa toxicity before discharge.

Case 18: Chest Pain

A 30-year-old woman comes to a family practice office. She states that she was referred by the emergency room. She went to the emergency room three times in the past 2 months because of chest pain. The emergency room physicians found no evidence of cardiac disease, so they suggested that she consult a family practice physician. She reports three episodes of what she believes are severe angina or heart attacks. Each time, she had severe chest pain, shortness of breath, and dizziness. She worries daily about having another episode of chest pain. She has brought her records, which indicate that she has undergone thorough and appropriate evaluation of cardiac and other medical explanations. The findings were normal.

QUESTIONS

1. *Because the patient has no medical condition to explain her symptoms, which categories of mental disorder might be considered?*

2. *How would a clinician distinguish between these disorders?*

DISCUSSION

This woman had physical symptoms and anxiety symptoms. The patient may have a so-matoform disorder (e.g., somatization disorder if she frequently presents with different symptoms, or hypochondriasis if she believes that she has a disorder but there is no medical evidence). Alternatively, she may have an anxiety disorder (e.g., panic disorder if her episodes were unexpected, lasted approximately 10 minutes, and included such symptoms as shaking, fear of dying, sweating, or nausea; social phobia if her symptoms always occurred in a social or performance situation, such as when she had to make a presentation; or substance-induced anxiety disorder, such as if the attacks occurred after using cocaine).

Although a physical examination is appropriate for each new patient, such examination or laboratory tests may not help with this differential diagnosis. However, they might provide clues about substance abuse. The key is thorough history. The details of each episode are important, including accompanying symptoms, duration of symptoms, and setting. Medical and psychiatric histories are important. A review of systems may identify a somatization disorder.

The physician gathers the following information about the patient. She is married and has a 3-year-old son. She works as a paralegal. She says that her marriage is stable and reports no legal problems, deaths in the family, or other current stressors. She drinks two to three beers while watching weekend football games, and reports no other drug or alcohol use.

The first episode of chest pain occurred 2 months ago. She was in the grocery store with her son, and she suddenly began to feel nauseated and sweaty. She had sharp, mid-sternal chest pain, tremulousness, shortness of breath, and numbness. She thought that she was dying. An ambulance was called. Her symptoms passed by the time the ambulance arrived, but she was taken to a hospital emergency room and admitted for observation. She had several heart tests and blood studies. She was told that she had not had a heart attack, and was released. The next episode occurred while she was at home reading. The latest episode occurred just after she arrived at work. Each episode was similar and lasted for approximately 10 minutes. She now engages in her usual activities, but feels very distressed about the possibility of having another attack of chest pain. She has had her tonsils and appendix removed. She takes no medication. Her mother and two siblings are alive and well. Her father had a heart attack 3 years ago, at age 54, and has recovered. The patient saw a therapist for depression in college, after the breakup of a romantic relationship. She reports no other psychiatric symptoms or treatment. She has experienced occasional lower back pain since her pregnancy.

QUESTIONS

3. What conclusions can be drawn from this history?

4. What treatment is recommended?

DISCUSSION

The history indicates the patient has panic disorder without agoraphobia. Her episodes have the features of panic attacks: discrete episodes of fear and physical symptoms that last approximately 10 minutes. Panic attacks can occur with several disorders, including panic disorder, agoraphobia, and social phobia, and during drug intoxication. Her episodes have not limited her ability to leave home, so she does not have agoraphobia. Rather than occurring in a stressful social setting, as with social phobia, her episodes occur unexpectedly, which is a hallmark of panic disorder. She reports no drug use, and her hospital records show that drug screen results were negative. Somatoform disorders were considered, but this patient does not have the multiple symptoms typical of somatization disorder. Because there is a medical explanation for her symptoms (i.e., panic disorder), she does not have hypochondriasis. Explaining panic disorder to this patient will probably be reassuring because she has a family history of heart attacks and will appreciate another explanation for her symptoms. Such reassurance is enough for some patients, who can then live with panic attacks if they are brief and infrequent. If treatment is needed, a tricyclic antidepressant will probably stop or significantly decrease the frequency of her panic attacks. Relaxation training may also help. The benzodiazepine alprazolam is another option because it decreases the intensity of the panic attacks and also reduces anticipatory anxiety.

Case 19: Issues Near the End of Life

Ms. Wood was in tears at her husband's bedside when Dr. Clark came into the room. The nursing staff had started cardiopulmonary resuscitation (CPR) on the bluish Mr. Wood and Dr. Clark knew that the only way to save him was with a respirator. However, Mr. Wood was more than 80 years old and his health was rapidly deteriorating. He had congestive heart failure and was dying slowly and painfully of pancreatic cancer. Using a respirator could only prolong his life for a short time, perhaps days or weeks. Dr. Clark was unsure how to proceed.

QUESTIONS

1. Should a respirator be used on this patient?

2. Who should decide?

DISCUSSION

Dr. Clark faces a moral decision. She knows the procedures for initiating the use of the respirator, but is not sure whether it is the right thing to do and who should make the decision. These two fundamental questions of ethical decision making cannot be answered by technical expertise alone.

Consistent with the autonomy model, both Dr. Clark and Mr. Wood have a role in decision making. Dr. Clark brings medical knowledge, and Mr. Wood brings knowledge of his values. Any medical decision, including those at the end of life, may involve conflicting values. Mr. Wood may value longevity, but he may also value life without pain and discomfort. In deciding whether to use a respirator, Mr. Wood would need to determine which value is more important to him. He needs medical information (e.g., whether the respirator is likely to be removed later) to make that decision.

Unfortunately, Dr. Clark and Mr. Wood did not discuss this situation in advance. If they had, Mr. Wood could have signed a living will or designated a durable power of attorney to help guide his physician.

Without advance planning, the next step is normally to identify a surrogate decision maker. Ms. Wood is the likely choice, and she would attempt to assess Mr. Wood's wishes. However, the situation is more complicated. Dr. Clark is facing an emergency, the nursing staff has already started CPR, and there is no time to meaningfully consult with Ms. Wood. After a brief discussion, Dr. Clark and Ms. Wood decide that it is best to go ahead with the respirator.

Mr. Wood survives the CPR, and with the use of a respirator, his vital signs stabilize. He is sad and tearful about the respirator, but he understands why he needed it. He is too weak to talk, but he writes a note to Dr. Clark asking, "How long do I have to use this thing?" Dr. Clark pulls Ms. Wood off to the side and shows her the note. When Dr.

Clark tells Ms. Wood that it is unlikely that her husband will be able to survive without the respirator, Ms. Wood asks her not to tell Mr. Wood the truth because she is afraid that it will upset him too much.

QUESTION

3. Should Dr. Clark tell Mr. Wood the truth?

DISCUSSION

Truth telling is a prima facie duty. Dr. Clark should tell Mr. Wood the truth unless she believes that it would seriously harm him. At this point, Dr. Clark only knows that Ms. Wood believes that the news will upset her husband. Ms. Wood is an important person in the process, but she is not the surrogate decision maker now that Mr. Wood is competent again. Dr. Clark needs more information.

After discussing the situation further with Ms. Wood, Dr. Clark learns that Mr. Wood confided in his wife that he hates respirators, and that if he cannot live without one, he would rather die. When Dr. Clark visits Mr. Wood, he is clearly upset about the respirator. Dr. Clark has some concern that he might try to remove it himself. Dr. Clark decides to tell Mr. Wood that she does not know when they will be able to remove the respirator, but that she hopes that they will be able to do so soon. She discusses with Mr. Wood the sadness that he is feeling and her concern that he may be depressed. Mr Wood does not believe that his sadness about the respirator or his desire to remove it is related to depression, but says that he does not mind talking to a psychiatrist. Dr. Clark obtains informed consent for a psychiatric consultation.

QUESTIONS

4. What ethical principles were in conflict in the truth-telling decision?

5. What ethical model of the physician–patient relationship did Dr. Clark use in that decision?

6. What ethical model did Dr. Clark use in the decision to consult a psychiatrist?

DISCUSSION

Truth telling is grounded in the principle of autonomy (i.e., the physician should respect the patient's self-regarding decisions). In this situation, the principles conflicting with autonomy were nonmaleficence (i.e., a physician should not harm others) and beneficence (i.e., a physician should promote the welfare of others).

By valuing nonmaleficence and beneficence over autonomy and not telling Mr. Wood the full truth, Dr. Clark used the paternalistic model. In deciding to consult a psychiatrist, however, Dr. Clark used the autonomy model. In most medical situations, the autonomy model is most appropriate.

Dr. Clark asks the psychiatrist to assess Mr. Wood for depression. The psychiatrist finds no significant signs of depression. On mental status examination, Mr. Wood, who now has a tracheotomy and can talk, is alert and oriented, has a full range of affect, and becomes animated when discussing his grandchildren. He realistically understands his medical condition, his treatment, and his prognosis. He tells the psychiatrist that he did not believe Dr. Clark when she implied that the respirator could eventually be removed. His sleep and appetite are good. He has no active suicidal thoughts or plans, but he has decided that he wants the respirator removed. Mr. Wood explains, "If I live, great, but if not, that's fine, too. I've had a good life." The psychiatrist asks for permission to hold a conference with his wife and his physician. Mr. Wood agrees, and he repeats his decision to Ms. Wood and Dr. Clark.

QUESTIONS

7. *Is Mr. Wood competent to request removal of the respirator?*

8. *What ethical principles are in conflict for Dr. Clark?*

DISCUSSION

Mr. Wood is competent to make the request. He understands his condition, his treatment, and the possible consequences of refusing treatment. Dr. Clark has a conflict between the principles of autonomy and maleficence.

Dr. Clark is not sure what to do. If the respirator were not in place, it is clear to her that Mr. Wood would have the authority to refuse it. However, because the respirator is in place, the case is more difficult. Because Mr. Wood does not believe that he will survive without the respirator, and because he is not suicidal, he seems to be requesting euthanasia. The question is whether the euthanasia is passive (letting him die) or active (killing him). Dr. Clark knows that this distinction is crucial because the American Medical Association (AMA) holds that active euthanasia, even for humane reasons, is always morally wrong. Dr. Clark refers the case to the hospital ethics committee.

After careful consideration and investigation, the ethics committee decides that removing the respirator is not active euthanasia. The committee explains the general consensus in bioethics that there is no morally relevant difference between stopping treatment and not starting it. If death is expected to result, and does, both stopping treatment and not starting treatment are considered. Both are legal, and neither is active euthanasia; therefore, Dr. Clark can remove the respirator.

QUESTION

9. *Before removing the respirator, what should Dr. Clark do to avoid a similar situation in the future?*

DISCUSSION

Dr. Clark and Mr. Wood should plan what to do if Mr. Wood becomes incapacitated and is unable to make medical decisions.

Comprehensive
Exam

▋QUESTIONS

DIRECTIONS: Each of the numbered items or incomplete statements in this section is followed by answers or by completions of the statement. Select the ONE lettered answer or completion that is BEST in each case.

1. The most common explanation for mental retardation is

(A) chromosomal abnormality
(B) inherited metabolic abnormality
(C) maternal drug or alcohol ingestion
(D) perinatal anoxia
(E) undetermined etiology

2. A patient with fluent aphasia experiences which of the following changes in thought form or content?

(A) Derailment
(B) Word salad
(C) Hallucinations
(D) Flight of ideas
(E) Delusions

3. One concern about genetic research is that it could alter the genetic composition of a population. According to this argument, which ethical principle would be violated in such a situation?

(A) Virtue
(B) Nonmaleficence
(C) Utilitarianism
(D) Egalitarianism
(E) Autonomy

4. Enzymatic degradation is the most important means to stop the signal of which of the following neurotransmitters?

(A) Serotonin
(B) Glutamate
(C) Dopamine
(D) Norepinephrine
(E) Acetylcholine (ACh)

5. A child who views death as abandonment yet fails to appreciate its irreversibility is likely to be at what age?

(A) 3–4 years
(B) 6–7 years
(C) 10–11 years
(D) 14–15 years

6. Which one of the following statements describes health care expenditures relative to the gross national product (GNP) between 1950 and 1988?

(A) They increased at a slightly greater rate than other goods and services
(B) They increased at a slightly lower rate than other goods and services
(C) They increased at approximately the same rate as other goods and services
(D) They approximately doubled
(E) They approximately quadrupled

7. Which method would be most useful for teaching tricks to a seal?

(A) Operant conditioning
(B) Classical conditioning
(C) Autoshaping
(D) Imprinting
(E) Self-stimulation

8. The most common reason for cessation of intercourse in the elderly is

(A) discomfort caused by lack of vaginal lubrication
(B) male sexual dysfunction
(C) loss of interest
(D) depression
(E) substance abuse

Questions 9–10

A patient comes to the emergency room with a sprained ankle. His behavior is demanding, entitled, and arrogant. When seen by a medical student, the patient insists on seeing the head of orthopedic surgery. When told that he will be able to see the orthopedic resident, but only after she completes the casting of a broken leg, the patient bellows, "But can't you see that I'm in pain?"

9. Which pair of diagnoses are most likely to be considered as part of a differential diagnosis?

(A) Manic episode and schizoid personality
(B) Amphetamine intoxication and obsessive-compulsive personality
(C) Posttraumatic stress disorder and borderline personality disorder
(D) Manic episode and narcissistic personality disorder
(E) Panic disorder and borderline personality disorder

10. All of the following will help to differentiate these two disorders EXCEPT

(A) a determination of whether grandiose and irritable behavior is typical for this patient
(B) mental status examination, evaluating distractibility
(C) mental status examination, evaluating thought form
(D) mental status examination, evaluating thought content
(E) mental status examination, evaluating immediate and long-term memory

11. A 25-year-old woman who is pregnant for the first time visits her internist with concerns about her unborn infant. The woman has been treated for skin cancer and reports that several other members of her family have also had skin cancer, including her mother's brother, a maternal cousin, and her maternal grandfather. The woman is afraid of passing cancer on to her child. Which of the following can be most safely concluded regarding the pattern of skin cancer in this family? It is

(A) Familial
(B) Congenital
(C) Heritable
(D) Autosomal dominant
(E) X-linked

12. Explaining the holistic functioning of interdependent parts is the essential goal of

(A) a reductionistic, dualistic model
(B) the biopsychosocial model
(C) the biomedical model
(D) the family life cycle model

Questions 13–14

A 47-year-old married mother of two underwent a mastectomy with positive nodes 3 years prior to evaluation. She presently has been found to have a skeletal metastasis, indicating recurrence of the malignancy. She tearfully tells her physician there is no hope and she might as well go home to die. Her children report that they are alarmed that their mother will hurt herself. The patient has no prior psychiatric history.

13. How does one psychosocially stage this patient with cancer?

(A) Initial diagnosis and treatment
(B) Remission and surveillance
(C) Recurrence
(D) Terminal phase

14. What is the proper management strategy?

(A) Discuss funeral arrangements with the patient
(B) Assuage fears of recurrence by minimizing significance of skeletal metastasis
(C) Explore the patient's suicidal ideation
(D) Ignore the patient's suicidal ideation

15. What ethical principle provides the basis for informed consent?

(A) Virtue
(B) Rights
(C) Autonomy
(D) Egalitarianism
(E) Libertarianism

16. Korsakoff's syndrome may be caused by lesions of the

(A) cerebellum
(B) caudate and putamen
(C) left hippocampus and amygdala
(D) mamillary bodies and adjacent thalamus
(E) nigrostriatal tract

Questions 17–19

A 60-year-old woman is accompanied to her physician's office by her son. The patient denies any significant problems and states that her children do not understand the difficulties associated with aging. The son reports that the patient has insomnia, increased irritability and crying, forgetfulness, and poor attention to hygiene. Recognizing that these symptoms are consistent with a diagnosis of either depression or dementia, the physician refers the patient for psychological evaluation.

17. Which referral statement would help the physician with the differential diagnosis?

(A) Please evaluate the patient's suicide risk.
(B) Please assess the presence and degee of organic impairment.
(C) Please suggest an appropriate therapeutic intervention.
(D) Please document the presence and degree of memory impairment.
(E) Please evaluate the patient's capacity for independent living.

18. Which type of test would be most informative in helping the physician with the differential diagnosis?

(A) Intelligence
(B) Achievement
(C) Mood and personality
(D) Neuropsychological

19. Assuming that this patient will be followed by the psychologist to document any further change, such as might occur after antidepressant therapy is instituted, which test characteristic is most important?

(A) Degree of face validity
(B) Degree of interscorer reliability
(C) Degree of test–retest reliability
(D) Degree of standardization

20. In clinical situations, medical ethics relies heavily on ethical principles for guidance in specific cases. What are the principles?

(A) Responsibility, caring, and duty
(B) Utilitarianism, deontology, and virtue
(C) Autonomy, beneficence, nonmaleficence, and justice
(D) Consequences, rights, duty, and confidentiality
(E) Prudence, benevolence, and truthfulness

21. Which of the following diseases is inherited as an autosomal dominant condition?

(A) Wilson's disease
(B) Phenylketonuria
(C) Tuberous sclerosis
(D) Duchenne's muscular dystrophy
(E) Lesch-Nyhan syndrome

22. Attainment of urinary continence can be described as

(A) a maturational process
(B) the result of growth
(C) reflecting ontogenetic factors
(D) a developmental process

Questions 23–24

A 32-year-old single man calls his physician's office and demands an appointment for a routine physical examination outside regular office hours. The patient states that he has a very important job and cannot readily interrupt his schedule for a medical evaluation. He emphasizes to the physician that any physician would be lucky to have him as a patient because in the future he will become famous and will enhance the physician's reputation as a practitioner. When the physician inquires what type of work the patient does, he states that he is presently working as a clerk in a large warehouse, but that he has written a series of songs and will someday be a celebrity. The patient becomes increasingly irritated as the discussion ensues.

23. Which diagnostic consideration is most applicable to this patient?

(A) Major mood disorder
(B) Schizophrenia
(C) Schizoid personality disorder
(D) Narcissistic personality disorder
(E) Paranoid personality disorder

24. What is the best management strategy?

(A) Terminate the phone conversation
(B) Empathize with the patient
(C) Inform the patient that your time is as valuable as his
(D) Try to rid the patient of his beliefs regarding fame

25. Which statement best describes deontological theories?

(A) They hold that an act is right in accordance with an overriding principle of obligation
(B) They hold that an act is right if it is carried out with good and honest intentions
(C) They hold that an act is right if it is beneficial
(D) None of the above

26. Learned behavioral patterns are advantageous to the survival of a species because they

(A) require a longer period of dependency on the part of the offspring
(B) allow for greater flexibility in response to changes in the environment
(C) guarantee that a behavior will appear in all members of a species
(D) replace innate behavior patterns that have no functional purpose

27. A 45-year-old homeless man comes to the emergency room with severe tremor, confusion, and increased blood pressure. The nursing staff recognize the patient as "an old alcoholic." After other potential medical and psychiatric problems are excluded, the best initial step in the management of the patient is to

(A) give the patient a warm alcoholic drink
(B) give the patient an intramuscular injection of thiamine
(C) let the patient withdraw with no medication
(D) give the patient captopril
(E) give the patient a dose of haloperidol for sedation

28. Which of the following statements is true regarding narcolepsy?

(A) It is a parasomnia
(B) It features sleep attacks and cataplexy
(C) It is another term for sleepwalking disorder
(D) It is a feature of narcotic abuse
(E) It involves delayed onset of rapid eye movement (REM) activity after falling asleep

29. The 95% confidence interval is defined as the sample mean $\pm$ 1.96 $\times$ the standard error. The standard error is defined as

(A) the standard deviation (SD) divided by the square root of the sample size
(B) the square root of the SD
(C) the variance divided by the sample size
(D) the Z score divided by the SD
(E) the frequency of false measurements

30. Which of the following examples best illustrates a complementary interpersonal posture?

(A) Two medical students studying together for a hematology examination
(B) A doctor insisting on giving a blood transfusion to a child whose parents refuse the transfusion for religious reasons
(C) A doctor diligently attending to a moribund patient in the intensive care unit
(D) Two medical colleagues arguing a point during rounds

31. Which of the following tests might be used as an early screening device for dementia during an annual checkup in a patient older than 65 years of age?

(A) Design copying
(B) Serial seven subtraction
(C) Digit repetition
(D) Proverb interpretation
(E) Calculations

32. What is a living will?

(A) A directive signed by a competent patient that authorizes a physician to withhold or discontinue artificial life support if the patient is terminally ill and incompetent
(B) A will completed for a patient who is in an irreversible coma
(C) A directive signed for an incompetent patient that activates a previous will
(D) A durable power of attorney
(E) A requirement of the Patient Self-determination Act

33. Which brain region is most important for learning the motor skills necessary to ride a bicycle?

(A) Hippocampus
(B) Hypothalamus
(C) Cerebellum
(D) Prefrontal cortex
(E) Basal ganglia

34. The most common type of inheritance of mental retardation is

(A) autosomal dominant
(B) autosomal recessive
(C) sex-linked recessive
(D) polygenic
(E) secondary to chromosomal abnormalities

35. A terminally ill patient goes into a coma. Life support is initiated. When is the patient considered dead?

(A) When respiration and heartbeat stop
(B) When the patient is "brain dead"
(C) When respiration stops
(D) When the heartbeat stops
(E) When the patient is in a coma constantly for more than 8 weeks

36. The "family romance" is a common fantasy that is characterized by its

(A) reflection of adolescent infatuation
(B) oedipal nature
(C) occurrence in late adulthood
(D) occurrence in school-age children

Questions 37–38

A 55-year-old man with severe bilateral osteoarthritis is hospitalized after a fall at home. Although his medical condition is quickly stabilized, discharge planning becomes problematic. The patient's sister, who has cared for him since their mother passed away, states that she cannot continue his care. She requests that he be placed in an extended care facility. The medical team social worker learns that the patient's sister considers the patient mentally retarded. This factor affects the type of funding and the type of placement available to the patient. The patient's sister has no documentation of the patient's mental retardation. The medical resident requests a psychological assessment to document the patient's mental retardation and to further discharge planning.

37. Which referral statement is most appropriate?

(A) Please assess reality testing.
(B) Please establish the patient's level of intellectual functioning.
(C) Please assess the presence and degree of organic impairment.
(D) Please evaluate the quality of the patient's relationship with his sister.
(E) Please assess suicide risk.

38. What additional information is necessary to complete the psychological assessment?

(A) Only the psychometric tests are relevant; no additional information is necessary
(B) The patient's hospital course
(C) The patient's social and educational histories
(D) The patient's mood
(E) The patient's genetic history

39. Conditions that have been genetically linked to depression include

(A) alcoholism and antisocial personality disorder
(B) cigarette smoking and epilepsy
(C) somatization disorder and substance abuse
(D) Tourette syndrome
(E) schizophrenia

40. Which one of the following characteristics describes the psychosocial stage of ego integrity versus despair?

(A) The developmental crisis of midlife
(B) A time of generally rapid and consistent decline in tolerance to stress, in physical abilities, and in intellectual capacity
(C) A clash between honesty, values, and ethics, and angry hopelessness
(D) Reaffirmation of parenthood and transmitting values to children
(E) None of the above

41. An investigator tests a new antidepressant drug by giving one group an active drug and another group a placebo. Despite random assignment, the placebo group includes several subjects with a history of spontaneous remission, and the active drug group includes no such subjects. After 6 weeks, the investigator finds no difference in the degree of depression between the two groups. She concludes that the drug is ineffective. This is an example of

(A) type II error
(B) type III error
(C) type I error
(D) low concurrent validity
(E) poor reliability

42. The role of families in major psychiatric illness (e.g., schizophrenia, major depression) is best viewed as

(A) the cause of the illness
(B) a significant factor in treatment outcome
(C) an irrelevant factor
(D) none of the above

43. What type of validity is used when performance on the United States Medical Licensing Examination is compared with the same student's performance in medical school up to the time of the examination?

(A) Concurrent validity
(B) Predictive validity
(C) Content validity
(D) Construct validity

44. An X-linked pattern of inheritance is associated with which of the following disorders?

(A) Schizophrenia
(B) Bipolar disorder
(C) Major depressive disorder
(D) Alcohol abuse
(E) Alzheimer's disease

45. The United States Patient Self-determination Act of 1991 refers to

(A) the patient's right to choose a physician
(B) the patient's right to request a second opinion
(C) the obligation of a health care facility to inform patients of their rights to refuse or discontinue treatment and to complete advance directives
(D) the physician's obligation to respect the principle of patient autonomy

46. A 43-year-old man admits that he has been molesting young children and has recently been caught and charged with child molestation. Which of the following factors is associated with a more favorable prognosis?

(A) Early onset of pedophilic behavior
(B) Frequent pedophilic acts
(C) Guilt associated with pedophilic acts
(D) Easing of legal consequences of molestation
(E) Association with other paraphilias

DIRECTIONS: Each of the numbered items or incomplete statements in this section is negatively phrased, as indicated by a capitalized word such as NOT, LEAST, or EXCEPT. Select the ONE lettered answer or completion that is BEST in each case.

---

47. All of the following statements regarding the treatment of Parkinson's disease are true EXCEPT

(A) L-dopa therapy is used in Parkinson's disease to increase dopamine levels in the striatum
(B) dopamine cannot be used because it cannot cross the blood–brain barrier
(C) because of the dopamine–acetylcholine (ACh) balance in the brain, drugs that increase ACh level, such as acetylcholinesterase inhibitors, are useful in the treatment of Parkinson's disease
(D) the monoamine oxidase-B (MAO-B) inhibitor Deprenyl is a useful adjunct in the treatment of Parkinson's disease
(E) a typical side effect of L-dopa therapy is hypoprolactinemia

48. Innate reflex patterns form a basic concept of cognitive developmental theory. All of the following descriptions of innate reflex patterns are accurate EXCEPT

(A) they exist at or shortly after birth
(B) they require stimulation for activation and stabilization
(C) they represent the foundation for the sensorimotor stage of development
(D) they include sucking, grasping, and eye following
(E) they operate as relatively fixed stimulus–response pathways

49. All of the following statements concerning the association between the use of alcohol and sexual functioning are true EXCEPT

(A) alcohol interferes with sexual functioning by exerting a depressant effect on the central nervous system (CNS)
(B) alcohol may enhance sexual desire by decreasing inhibitions
(C) common types of sexual dysfunction in alcoholic women include inhibited desire, dyspareunia, and orgasmic dysfunction
(D) common types of sexual dysfunction in alcoholic men include inhibited desire, erectile dysfunction, and ejaculatory incompetence
(E) alcohol-related sexual dysfunction reverses with abstinence from alcohol

50. A 63-year-old married man with insulin-dependent diabetes has a stroke. The stroke leaves him incompetent to make decisions about his acute medical care, and his wife is chosen to be the surrogate decision maker. What factor should she NOT consider in making decisions?

(A) A living will
(B) A medical advance directive
(C) Previous conversations with her husband
(D) What she would do in her husband's situation
(E) A patient values history

51. All of the following factors affect drinking behavior EXCEPT

(A) dry mouth
(B) palatability of the fluid
(C) social habits
(D) ingestion of food
(E) calcium intake

52. All of the following are maturationally based ego functions EXCEPT

(A) motor activity
(B) sensory activity
(C) cognition and memory
(D) defenses
(E) language development

53. Which of the following disorders is LEAST likely to be associated with a history of sexual mistreatment or aggression?

(A) Vaginismus
(B) Sexual aversion disorder
(C) Female sexual arousal disorder
(D) Premature ejaculation
(E) Dyspareunia

54. All of the following are designed to decrease health care costs EXCEPT

(A) certificate of need programs
(B) the introduction of new technologies
(C) health care rationing
(D) price controls
(E) managed care programs

55. Which statement does NOT describe paternalism?

(A) It involves interference with the freedom of a competent person
(B) It has been largely replaced by the autonomy model
(C) It is the Hippocratic view of the physician–patient relationship
(D) It is supported by the ethical principle of beneficence
(E) It is currently useful in dealing with competent patients who refuse medical treatment

56. All of the following consequences of behavior increase the probability that the behavioral response will be repeated EXCEPT

(A) positive reinforcement
(B) punishment
(C) negative reinforcement
(D) secondary reinforcers

57. Stimulus generalization can be described as all of the following EXCEPT

(A) a response learned in one situation that can occur in a different but similar situation
(B) determined by resemblances in size, color, or shape
(C) most commonly established by language
(D) a frequent basis for the development of phobias, especially in young children
(E) an effective way of learning classification

58. Innate neonatal reflexes include all of the following EXCEPT the

(A) Moro reflex
(B) anaclitic response
(C) palmar grasp
(D) rooting reflex
(E) Babinski reflex

59. All of the following are examples of the clinical process of the interview, as opposed to the clinical content of the interview, EXCEPT

(A) elucidating the patient's emotional reactions to the subjects being discussed
(B) referring to the specific subjects being discussed
(C) interrupting the conversational flow
(D) using body language
(E) displaying of emotion by the interviewer

60. Developmentally based ego functions include all of the following EXCEPT

(A) object relationships
(B) reality testing
(C) signal anxiety
(D) speech and language
(E) defenses

61. Treatment of alcohol dependence often includes all of the following EXCEPT

(A) evaluation of possible medical complications, including malnutrition and liver dysfunction
(B) evaluation for psychiatric comorbidity (i.e., the presence of problems such as depression, anxiety, or personality disorders)
(C) the use of phenothiazines or other antipsychotic drugs to diminish the symptoms and medical complications of withdrawal
(D) participation in the Alcoholics Anonymous (AA) program
(E) the use of disulfiram

62. All of the following statements about benzodiazepines are true EXCEPT

(A) these drugs work by potentiating the action of γ-aminobutyric acid (GABA)
(B) these drugs are used as anxiolytics
(C) these drugs potentiate the influx of calcium
(D) these drugs have anticonvulsant properties
(E) these drugs are useful in inducing sleep

63. Informed consent may be bypassed in all of the following cases EXCEPT

(A) when the patient insists that she does not want to know the details of treatment
(B) in an extreme emergency
(C) when the patient's family requests it
(D) when there is implied agreement (e.g., in common procedures)
(E) when informing the patient will cause serious and identifiable harm

64. Serotonin transmission is believed to be associated with all of the following EXCEPT

(A) sleep
(B) depression
(C) thermoregulation
(D) obsessive-compulsive disorder
(E) memory loss

65. A 32-year-old woman drops to the ground at a shopping mall and begins shaking her limbs and moaning. The episode lasts 5 minutes. An ambulance takes her to an emergency room, where an electroencephalogram (EEG) performed during a second episode of shaking is normal (i.e., it gives no indication of seizure activity). All of the following statements are true EXCEPT

(A) If it is discovered that she has a history of deliberately feigning illness in order to receive hospital treatment and tests, then the diagnosis is likely to be factitious disorder
(B) If it appears that the symptoms are not being intentionally produced (i.e., she believes she is really having seizures) and that they are caused by emotional conflict related to her husband's infidelity, then the probable diagnosis is conversion disorder
(C) If the woman has amnesia for the 5 minutes of the "pseudoseizure," then the diagnosis is dissociative fugue
(D) If the woman is deliberately faking seizures with the hope that she will begin to receive disability payments, then the diagnosis is malingering
(E) This woman may have a history of seizure disorder

66. Principles of reward and reinforcement propose all of the following EXCEPT

(A) rewarding a behavior on an intermittent, variable basis will establish the strongest and most persistent learning
(B) a continuous and predictable reward is the most satisfactory method to elicit long-term behavior change
(C) disapproval or criticism may either discourage (extinguish) or reinforce a behavior
(D) reward and reinforcement are related to learned needs as well as primary needs
(E) the more closely related in time a response is to a stimulus, the more likely one will be associated as a reward for the other

---

DIRECTIONS: Each set of matching questions in this section consists of a list of four to twenty-six lettered options (some of which may be in figures) followed by several numbered items. For each numbered item, select the ONE lettered option that is most closely associated with it. To avoid spending too much time on matching sets with large numbers of options, it is generally advisable to begin each set by reading the list of options. Then, for each item in the set, try to generate the correct answer and locate it in the option list, rather than evaluating each option individually. Each lettered option may be selected once, more than once, or not at all.

Questions 67–71

Match each description with the psychometric test it most accurately describes.

(A) Rorschach test
(B) Minnesota Multiphasic Personality Inventory (MMPI)
(C) Halstead-Reitan Battery (HRB)
(D) Wechsler Adult Intelligence Scale-revised (WAIS-R)
(E) Thematic Apperception Test (TAT)

67. Test that measures the potential for adaptive functioning and has good standardization, reliability, and validity

68. Objective test that measures the patient's current emotional state and enduring personality characteristics and has good standardization, modest reliability, and acceptable validity

69. Projective test that measures thought process and cognitive style and has good standardization and acceptable reliability and validity

70. Projective test that assesses unconscious conflicts and has marginal reliability and validity

71. Cognitive tests that measure integrity of brain–behavior relations and have good standardization and validity and adequate reliability

Questions 72–75

Match the neuroanatomic region and type of manipulation with the corresponding type of behavior exhibited.

(A) Affective attack
(B) Quiet biting attack
(C) Taming in animals
(D) Aggressive behavior in humans

72. Lesions to the orbital prefrontal cortex

73. Stimulation of the medial hypothalamus

74. Removal of the amygdala

75. Stimulation of the lateral hypothalamus

Questions 76–81

Match each aspect of family life with the corresponding current demographic trend.

(A) Increasing
(B) No significant change
(C) Decreasing

76. The number of children born per couple in the United States

77. The importance of extended family members as sources of social support

78. The number of single-parent families

79. The percentage of the American population that eventually marries

80. The number of children whose father is the sole family wage-earner

81. The reported rate of family violence

Questions 82–83

Match the research examples with the appropriate statistical test.

(A) Chi-squared
(B) Analysis of variance (ANOVA)
(C) Paired *t*-test
(D) Unpaired *t*-test
(E) Fisher exact test

82. The prevalence of posttraumatic stress is determined in a group of 200 men and women. Twenty-seven of one hundred women are given the diagnosis, but only ten of one hundred men are given the diagnosis.

83. Pulse rate is measured in 10 patients before and after the administration of a new antianxiety drug. The mean pulse rate before the drug is given is 84, and after the drug is given it is 72.

Questions 84–87

Match each region of the brain with the neurotransmitter found there.

(A) Norepinephrine
(B) Serotonin
(C) Dopamine
(D) Glycine
(E) Acetylcholine (ACh)

84. Substantia nigra

85. Locus coeruleus

86. Raphe nuclei

87. Nucleus basalis

Questions 88–92

Match each statement or question with the interviewing technique that it exemplifies.

(A) Exploration
(B) Open-ended questions
(C) Direct questions
(D) Interpretation
(E) Empathy

88. Where is your pain located?

89. You say your pain occurs only at work? Tell me more about the nature of your work.

90. The injury must have been very painful.

91. You seem to be angry about your illness. Perhaps you feel that your mother is responsible for it?

92. How did this pain begin?

Questions 93–96

Match each psychiatric disorder with its corresponding behavioral model.

(A) Maternal separation
(B) Grooming behavior disorders
(C) Amphetamine-induced hyperactivity
(D) Geller-Seifter conflict test

93. Anxiety disorder

94. Depression

95. Schizophrenia

96. Obsessive-compulsive disorder

Questions 97–99

Match each situation with the type of physician reimbursement it describes.

(A) Fee for service
(B) Capitation
(C) Salary
(D) Resource-based relative value scale
(E) Preferred provider organization (PPO)

97. An ophthalmologist agrees that, in exchange for five thousand dollars, he will provide all necessary ophthalmologic care for 1 year to the employees of Company A

98. A neurosurgeon in Los Angeles is paid more by Medicare to spend 30 minutes evaluating a man's severe headache than a family practitioner in Arizona is paid to spend 30 minutes evaluating a man's persistent cough

99. A pediatrician charges seventy five dollars for a checkup for a 2-year-old child and one hundred dollars for a hospital visit

Questions 100–103

Match each variable with the correct classification.

(A) Ordinal
(B) Nominal
(C) Interval
(D) Ratio

100. Clinician's ratings of improvement on a 6-point scale

101. Diagnosis

102. Correct responses on a test of memory

103. Weight

Questions 104–108

Match each dimension of personality (from the five-factor model) with the proper description.

(A) High-spirited, outgoing
(B) Organized, with a clear plan
(C) A worrier who feels vulnerable
(D) Always wishes to please, can be a "doormat"
(E) Appreciative of modern abstract art

104. Neuroticism

105. Extroversion

106. Openness

107. Agreeableness

108. Conscientiousness

ANSWERS AND EXPLANATIONS

1. The answer is E [Chapter 15 II A]. For the majority of cases of mental retardation there is no obvious cause. Attributable causes of mental retardation include chromosomal abnormalities (e.g., Down syndrome), inherited metabolic problems (e.g., phenylketonuria), maternal drug or alcohol ingestion, prenatal and perinatal anoxia, trauma, infections, and malnutrition.

2. The answer is B [Chapter 13 IV D 2 a (12)]. Word salad, a form of disorganized speech characterized by an incoherent mixture of words or phrases, is usually caused by fluent aphasia. Word salad may be mistakenly classified as derailment, tangentiality, or flight of ideas. Derailment is a shift in thinking in which the patient's ideas move from one unrelated topic to another. Tangentiality is shifts in topic that are related initially, but move progressively further from the initial topic. Flight of ideas is a speech pattern that includes accelerated speech and rapid shifts in topic. All of these thought form disorders are examples of loosened associations. Hallucinations and delusions are thought content disorders; therefore, they affect what is said, not how it is said.

3. The answer is B [Chapter 16 IV C]. Nonmaleficence is the principle that a physician should not harm others. Genetic research that alters genetic composition could harm others. Autonomy would not be involved directly in the situation and virtue, utilitarianism, and egalitarianism are not ethical principles.

4. The answer is E [Chapter 1 II D 3 f; V B 1; VI B 2]. Acetylcholine (ACh) is hydrolyzed to choline and acetate by the swift action of the enzyme acetylcholinesterase. Choline is subsequently taken up into the nerve terminal. Glutamate and monoaminergic neurotransmitters, such as serotonin, dopamine, and norepinephrine, are removed from the synaptic cleft largely by reuptake. Metabolism of these transmitters is secondary in importance to the rapid and specific uptake process.

5. The answer is A [Chapter 8 VII A 1]. Children younger than 5 years of age tend to see death as abandonment. They may also believe that the deceased person will come back. A child of 6 or 7 years of age is more likely to

appreciate the finality of death, but may continue to have egocentric thoughts and thus feel responsible for the death. By midadolescence, most children have a clear understanding of death.

6. The answer is D [Chapter 17 II D 2]. Between 1950 and 1988, health care expenditures, as a percentage of the gross national product (GNP), grew from 5.3% to 11.6%. This growth, significant as it is in absolute terms, has focused the attention of policymakers, in both the government and the private sector, on health care expenditures, largely because it has outstripped the rate of growth of the consumer price index. The implications of such a growth rate, if unchecked, are seen as threatening to both the government's fiscal balance and private industry's international competitive position.

7. The answer is A [Chapter 5 III B 2 a–b]. Seals and other animals that are trained to perform tricks for an audience are trained according to the principles of operant conditioning. For this reason, animal trainers always have at hand a bucket of fish or a bag of treats.

8. The answer is B [Chapter 9 I D 1–2]. Although loss of interest, depression, substance abuse, and discomfort caused by lack of vaginal lubrication are all possible reasons for the cessation of intercourse in the elderly, the most common reasons for cessation of intercourse in the elderly are male sexual dysfunction and poor health in one of the partners.

9–10. The answers are: 9-D, 10-E [Table 15-7; Chapter 11 IV B 2]. Demanding, entitled behavior is characteristic of both mania and narcissistic personality disorder. Schizoid personality features emotional detachment. Whereas individuals with borderline personality may be demanding, due in part to the intense rage that they feel when abandoned, more characteristic symptoms are impulsivity, mood swings, and the use of a defense called splitting. People with obsessive-compulsive personalities are workaholics who are stubborn and preoccupied with rules and schedules. Patients who are intoxicated with either amphetamines or cocaine often experience hallucinations and euphoria, which can resemble mania, but demonstrate other symptoms such as hypervigilance, tension, confusion, and dilated pupils. Posttraumatic stress disorder and panic disorder are anxiety disorders and do not feature entitled, arrogant behavior.

A mental status examination evaluating immediate and long-term memory will not help to differentiate mania from narcissistic personality disorder. On the other hand, a mental status examination of this patient evaluating thought form and content and distractibility should help differentiate mania and narcissistic personality disorder. Narcissistic personality disorder will not feature flight of ideas, distractibility, or delusions, all of which are typically seen in mania. The history will also be of help, because in mania the grandiosity and irritability represent a change in behavior, whereas personality disorders describe persistent behavior. If the apparent diagnosis is mania, a psychiatric consultation would be appropriate.

11. The answer is A [Chapter 4 I B 3 b]. When a disorder is seen to aggregate in a family, it can be described as familial. It is not safe to assume, however, that it is heritable. While there may be inherited factors involved (e.g., fair skin), it is also possible that environmental factors are entirely responsible. For instance, family members may spend each summer together at the beach and suffer repeated sunburns. The pattern would not be described as congenital, because the cancer is not present at birth. Even if genes are responsible, then neither autosomal dominant nor X-linked transmission is likely. An autosomal dominant pattern would not be expected to skip a generation (neither of the woman's parents have cancer). In X-linked disorders, the women are carriers and half of their sons are affected.

12. The answer is B [Chapter 10 I B 1–2; IV C]. General systems theory is a holistic model that was developed to explain how a wide variety of systems function as complete entities. The biopsychosocial model applies general systems theory to the field of medicine. The biopsychosocial model was developed as an alternative to the reductionistic, dualistic biomedical model that is most prominent in the field of medicine. The family life cycle model is a normative model of family life that identifies specific tasks that families face during different stages of development.

13–14. The answers are: 13-C, 14-C [Chapter 11 V D]. This patient had previously been treated for carcinoma of the breast; therefore, she now has recurrent disease. There is not enough data to indicate that she is in the terminal phase of the disease.

The task in recurrence is to achieve maximal treatment and foster hope. Aggressive treatment of pain, anxiety, and depression is mandatory. Careful evaluation of suicidal ideation and potential is also necessary. The patient should be given accurate data about her condition while maintaining an element of hope (e.g., by discussing available therapies). It is important for the physician to understand the patient's ideas, fears, and outlook for treatment. To this end, it is essential for the physician to understand the patient's prior experience with similar diseases.

15. The answer is C [Chapter 16 IV A 1]. Autonomy is the ethical principle of respecting the self-determining decisions of others. Virtue, rights, egalitarianism, and libertarianism are not ethical principles.

16. The answer is D [Chapter 2 III E 1 a]. Untreated, Wernicke's encephalopathy can advance to damage the mamillary bodies and neighboring areas of the thalamus, producing a disorder known as Korsakoff's amnesia, Korsakoff's psychosis, or Korsakoff's syndrome. The disorder features retrograde and anterograde amnesia. The tendency of some amnestic patients to confabulate, or make up stories when they cannot remember the truth, can make them appear psychotic. Bilateral, but not unilateral, temporal lobe lesions can also cause an amnestic syndrome.

17–19. The answers are: 17-B [Chapter 14 I A 2], **18-D** [Chapter 14 I B 2 a (6), II E], **19-C** [Chapter 14 I B 1 a, b (1), (3)]. The most appropriate referral statement might be: Please provide evidence relevant to a differential diagnosis of dementia versus depression. The differential diagnosis is concerned with whether the symptoms are caused by a functional (e.g., mood, personality, situation-based) disorder or by neurologic dysfunction. Memory may be affected in both depression and dementia, and it may be important to determine whether other abilities (e.g., attention, abstract reasoning) are also impaired. Evaluation of suicide risk, recommendation of therapy, and determination of the patient's capacity for independent living will not provide the physician with the necessary information to make the differential diagnosis. However, a psychological evaluation can provide this information, and it may be offered in the report.

A neuropsychological examination can provide the necessary information to differentiate between underlying depression and dementia (i.e., presence or absence of neurologic disorder). An examination that focuses on the cognitive abilities that are affected by dementia and depression would provide the most information. Many comprehensive neuropsychological examinations include measures of intelligence and mood and personality. These measures alone cannot fully address the differential diagnosis. Achievement tests are of little help in this case, although they may be used in the context of a comprehensive neuropsychological examination if there was doubt about a patient's educational skills.

If the patient will be reevaluated, test–retest reliability is important. A high level of test–retest reliability ensures that changes in the score are caused by psychological or neuropsychological changes in the patient, and not by expected variation of the test. Face validity has little bearing on this issue, unless it is determined that the patient intentionally exaggerates or minimizes symptoms at one evaluation but not the other. Interscorer reliability has little relevance if the same psychologist examines the patient at both evaluations. If different technicians administer and score the test, however, then this characteristic has more importance. Although standardization is important for the interpretation of any psychometric test, it will presumably remain constant during the follow-up period, and thus merits no special consideration in this example.

20. The answer is C [Chapter 16 IV A–D]. Autonomy, beneficence, nonmaleficence, and justice are the most commonly cited ethical principles. Utilitarianism, deontology, and virtue are ethical theories, not principles. Prudence, benevolence, and truthfulness are character traits that are often cited in virtue theory.

21. The answer is C [Chapter 4 I B 7 a (1); I B 7 b]. Tuberous sclerosis is transmitted via an autosomal dominant mode of inheritance. Phenylketonuria and Wilson's disease are transmitted via an autosomal recessive mode. Duchenne muscular dystrophy and Lesch-Nyhan syndrome are X-linked recessive disorders.

22. The answer is D [Chapter 8 I C, D]. Maturation is the biologically and phylogenically based sequential evolution of functions. When these are combined with experience and result in new, learned behaviors, the process is known as development. Thus, myelinization that permits toilet training to proceed is a maturational step. The process of achieving continence is a learned, developmental process.

23–24. The answers are: 23-D, 24-B [Chapter 11 IV B 2 d]. Although more data is needed to definitively diagnose the patient's personality style, many patients with narcissistic personality disorders have an inflated sense of self-importance and often request special privileges. The patient does not appear to be paranoid (for example, he readily told the physician about his job). Although additional evaluation is necessary to confidently rule out a mood disorder or schizophrenia, there was no evidence over the phone that these disorders were present.

This patient would be best managed by empathizing with his scheduling difficulties, while suggesting that he look at his schedule carefully and try to arrange an office visit within the regular hours of operation. Thus, firm limits should be set without arguing with the patient or directly confronting his grandiosity.

25. The answer is A [Chapter 16 III B]. Deontological theories recommend acting in accordance with an overriding duty or principle. Virtue theories hold that an act is right if it is carried out with good and honest intentions. Utilitarian theories maintain that an act is right if it is beneficial.

26. The answer is B [Chapter 5 I B 2]. The greatest advantage of learned behavioral patterns is that they allow greater adaptability on the part of the individual to changes in the environment. Long periods of offspring dependency are not advantageous to the survival of a species.

27. The answer is B [Chapter 3 V D 1 c; X B 3]. Excluding other medical or psychiatric problems and withdrawal from other drugs is an essential first step. Once the diagnosis is established as alcohol withdrawal, the patient should be given an intramuscular dose of thiamine. Alcoholic patients often have malnutrition and malabsorption problems. A 3-day regimen of thiamine will prevent potentially significant damage that might be caused by Wernicke's encephalopathy. Supportive medical treatment should be given. A detoxification program should be established with the use of a long-acting benzodiazepine. Spontaneous withdrawal can be dangerous to the patient. Antihypertensive medications and antipsychotic agents are not usually needed.

28. The answer is B [Chapter 15 XIV A 3]. Narcolepsy is a dyssomnia that features sudden, daytime sleep attacks, cataplexy (i.e., a sudden loss of muscle tone when awake), and the almost immediate onset of rapid eye movement (REM) activity when the patient falls asleep. Thus, a careful history and an electroencephalogram (EEG) usually lead to the correct diagnosis. Parasomnias are disorders that occur during either REM or non-REM sleep phases, and include nightmare disorder, sleep terror disorder, and sleepwalking. Narcolepsy is unrelated to narcotic abuse.

29. The answer is A [Chapter 6 II B 3 d]. The standard error is defined as the standard deviation (SD) divided by the square root of the sample size. As the sample size increases, the standard error decreases.

30. The answer is C [Chapter 10 II C 3 a]. Dyadic behavior is composed of a sequence of successive dyadic postures. These postures typically are defined in terms of the focus and degrees of interdependence and affiliation of the behavior observed. Complementary and symmetric postures are two patterns of recurrent behavioral pairings that have special clinical import. Complementary postures are those in which the observed behaviors show similar degrees of affiliation and interdependence, but differing focus (e.g., a relationship in which one person is dominant and the other is submissive). Symmetric postures are pairings of behaviors that show similar degrees of affiliation and interdependence as well as similar focus (e.g., a relationship in which both participants regard each other as equals, regardless of whether they are cooperating or fighting).

31. The answer is A [Chapter 13 IV E 2 a]. Design copying might be used an as early screening device for dementia. Skillful design copying requires intactness of the visual cortex, parietal association areas, frontal lobe motor and extrapyramidal systems, and connecting nerve pathways. The diffuse cortical

damage that characterizes Alzheimer's dementia makes integrity of all these neural structures unlikely.

32. The answer is A [Chapter 16 V A 3 c]. A living will is a directive that describes an individual's wishes in the event that the individual becomes terminally ill and incompetent to make medical decisions. Once a patient is in an irreversible coma it is too late for a living will. A durable power of attorney is when an individual names a person to act on her behalf should the individual be incompetent to make medical decisions. The Patient Self-determination Act requires health care facilities that receive federal funding to provide patients with written information about relevant state laws regarding their rights to refuse or discontinue treatment.

33. The answer is E [Chapter 2 III E 2]. Learning motor skills, such as bicycle riding, is known as procedural memory. It requires intact functioning of the basal ganglia. The hippocampus is important in declarative learning. The mamillary bodies of the hypothalamus also have a role in declarative memory. Damage in this area is seen in Korsakoff's amnesia. The prefrontal cortex is important for immediate memory and planning. The cerebellum would be important for maintaining balance and coordination on a bicycle, but not for learning how to ride.

34. The answer is D [Chapter 4 III D]. Specific forms of mental retardation may result from chromosomal abnormalities (e.g., Down syndrome) as well as autosomal dominant conditions (e.g., tuberous sclerosis), autosomal recessive conditions (e.g., phenylketonuria), and sex-linked recessive disorders (e.g., Hunter's mucopolysaccharidosis). The most commonly observed form of mental retardation is, however, polygenic in transmission (i.e., a number of genes contribute to the abnormality).

35. The answer is B [Chapter 16 V B 1]. The definition of death has changed from a focus on the heart and lungs to a focus on the brain. A comatose patient is considered dead when there is irreversible cessation of all brain function (i.e., he is "brain dead"). A patient may be in a coma without being "brain dead."

36. The answer is D [Chapter 8 III B 1 b (2)]. Latency is a period of psychosocial development that extends from the end of the oedipal stage to the beginning of puberty. Fantasies are common during this period. The "family romance" fantasy arises from a child's disillusionment with his real parents. The child often imagines ideal parents who are rich and powerful.

37–38. The answers are: 37-B [Chapter 14 I A 2, I B 2 (a) (1)], **38-C** [Chapter 14 I, A 3; II A 1 b]. The goal of the referral is to determine the patient's level of intellectual functioning, specifically, whether it is in the mentally retarded range. The Wechsler Adult Intelligence Scale-revised (WAIS-R) is the standard test for the assessment of adult intelligence, and would most likely be used in this case. Another test of intelligence, the Stanford-Binet Scale, is usually used with children and adolescents, but it is also used with the severely impaired and mentally retarded adults.

A psychological assessment should integrate psychometric testing with information about the patient's prior functioning. In this case, it is important to know the patient's previous level of adaptive functioning. For example, was he able to live independently, to care for himself, to cook and clean, to handle money or finances, to make decisions by himself? Mental retardation is a developmental disorder and must be evident before the age of 18 years. If a social and educational history showed that the patient had previously functioned at a much higher level, then mental retardation would not be an appropriate diagnosis and an alternate diagnosis such as dementia should be considered. Although social services may request only the patient's intelligence quotient (IQ), a single IQ can be a misleading indicator of adaptive functioning unless it is considered in the context of the patient's history. The patient's hospital course and mood do not directly relate to the referral question. Genetic history may uncover the cause of observed mental retardation, but a genetic factor is not a necessary nor a sufficient condition for the diagnosis. Therefore, these issues are not *necessary* features of the assessment.

39. The answer is A [Chapter 4 III B 4 C]. Depression, alcoholism, and antisocial personality disorder have been genetically linked in what has been termed depressive spectrum disease. This term may represent a condition that is different from other depressive disorders. In affected families, depression occurs

primarily in women, whereas alcoholism and antisocial personality disorder occur more commonly in men. Somatization disorder and substance abuse have been linked to antisocial personality disorder. Tourette syndrome is a tic disorder that has been linked to obsessive-compulsive disorder. There is no evidence linking smoking, epilepsy, or schizophrenia to depression.

40. The answer is E [Chapter 7 V G, H]. The stage of ego integrity versus despair is associated with older age and maturity, not with midlife (generativity). This is a time of gradual and variable decrements in physiologic and intellectual status. It is a time of satisfaction with one's life and family versus a sense of failure, futility, and lack of pride (despair). Reaffirmation of self and transmitting of values to the next generation are characteristic of the previous stage of generativity.

41. The answer is A [Chapter 6 II C 1 b]. A type II error is the incorrect acceptance of the null hypothesis (no group differences exist) when the alternative hypothesis is correct. The example shows a problem with internal validity. The presence of an extraneous variable (history of spontaneous remission) leads to effects that are confounded with the effect of the independent variable (drug versus placebo).

42. The answer is B [Chapter 10 I B 2 c; III B 1 a–d]. Social support systems have a significant effect on the course of medical illness. Families are typically central in an individual's network of social support, and they usually influence a number of variables that are related to the outcome of major psychiatric disorders (e.g., medication compliance, modulation of emotional environment). Theories that emphasize the causal role of families in major psychopathology (e.g., schizophrenogenic mother hypothesis) have little empirical validation.

43. The answer is A [Chapter 6 III A 2 a; Chapter 14 I B 1 c]. Concurrent validity is a type of criterion-based, or empirical, validity. It is used to validate a test against an existing criterion. In this example, the existing criterion is the student's performance in medical school before the examination. Another type of empirical validity, predictive validity, is the degree of association between performance on a test and an outcome criterion that is measured at some point in the future. Content validity is the judgment by experts that the test content accurately reflects the specific area that it is intended to measure. Construct validity examines the meaning of the test results by determining their relation to similar and dissimilar theoretical constructs.

44. The answer is B [Chapter 4 III B 1 b (2)]. There may be X-linked transmission in some forms of bipolar (manic–depressive) disorder. No pattern suggestive of X-linked transmission has been reported for schizophrenia, major depression, Alzheimer's disease, or alcohol abuse.

45. The answer is C [Chapter 16 V A 3 c (1)]. The United States Patient Self-determination Act requires health care facilities that receive federal funding to provide patients with written information about their rights to refuse or discontinue treatment. The act is not related to choosing a physician or obtaining a second opinion. The act follows principle of autonomy.

46. The answer is C [Chapter 9 VI A 3]. Poor prognosis in the treatment of paraphilias is associated with deficient guilt, early onset, and high frequency of behavior. Legal consequences usually improve the prognosis. The association of pedophilia with other paraphilias does not necessarily affect prognosis.

47. The answer is C [Chapter 1 III B 3 a, c, 4 a (1)–(3)]. Acetylcholine (ACh) and dopamine occur in a type of functional balance in the neostriatum. Therefore, a lack of dopamine produces hyperactivity in the striatal cholinergic cells. Anticholinergic drugs are successfully used to treat Parkinson's disease. In Parkinson's disease, the dopamine neurons in the substantia nigra degenerate. Therefore, they do not supply adequate amounts of dopamine to the neostriatum. Orally administered L-dopa, the immediate precursor of dopamine, is converted to dopamine in the surviving dopamine neurons and increases the dopamine level in the brain. Dopamine cannot be administered because it cannot cross the blood–brain barrier, whereas L-dopa can. Carbidopa, a peripheral decarboxylase inhibitor, is often administered with L-dopa to prevent decarboxylation of L-dopa in peripheral tissues, thereby ensuring that a greater amount of L-dopa reaches the brain. Deprenyl (selegiline), a specific inhibitor of monoamine oxidase B (MAO-B), may prevent the metabolism of dopamine. It also re-

duces the severity of symptoms of Parkinson's disease. Because dopamine is a prolactin-inhibiting factor (PIF) in the tuberinfundibular tract, administration of exogenous L-dopa suppresses the secretion of prolactin from the hypothalamus by raising local levels of dopamine.

48. The answer is E [Chapter 7 IV A 1 b]. There are two types of reflexes identified in cognitive developmental theory: classic reflexes and innate reflex patterns. Classic reflexes are fixed stimulus–response pathways that involve neurologic maturation, and they are relatively unable to be modified by experience or learning. Examples include the Babinski reflex, the knee jerk, the triceps reflex, and cranial nerve reflexes. Innate reflex patterns, on the other hand, form the basis for initial interactions with the environment and are significantly modified by experience and learning.

49. The answer is E [Chapter 9 VII F 1]. Chronic abuse of alcohol can cause irreversible sexual dysfunction. Small amounts of alcohol can enhance sexual desire by decreasing inhibitions, but larger amounts depress the central nervous system (CNS) and interfere with sexual excitement and performance in both men and women.

50. The answer is D [Chapter 16 V A 3 b (2)]. The role of the surrogate decision maker is to decide, as much as possible, what the patient would want. A living will, medical advance directive, or patient values history would all be useful in determining the patient's wishes. The wife could also consider previous conversations with her husband when making decisions on his behalf. The wife's wishes in the same situation do not necessarily reflect what the patient wants.

51. The answer is E [Chapter 5 II B 2–3]. Calcium is an important nutrient that may be involved in regulating certain homeostatic functions (e.g., eating, temperature), but calcium is not thought to regulate drinking behavior. Dry mouth influences the frequency of drinking, but not the total amount of fluid consumed. The palatability of the fluid cause alterations in drinking behavior. Social habits affect when and what humans drink. Both humans and animals drink when they eat to counteract the dehydration that the ingestion of food produces.

52. The answer is D [Chapter 7 II A 6 b]. Maturationally based ego functions are those that depend on and emerge out of neurologic maturation and, as such, develop along a more or less predetermined sequential timetable. Defenses, on the other hand, are individualized and dependent on the interaction with the environment and the influence of specific experience.

53. The answer is D [Chapter 9 V A 2, B 2, C 3, D 1 –2]. Premature ejaculation is usually caused by the interference of anxiety, but is not usually the result of sexual mistreatment. Vaginismus, sexual aversion disorder, female sexual arousal disorder, and dyspareunia may have multiple causes that result in fear, disinterest, or anxiety. One such cause is a history of sexual mistreatment or aggression.

54. The answer is B [Chapter 17 II D 5]. New technologies are not usually designed to have an impact on medical costs, and the net effect can be either increased or decreased costs. For instance, increases come from technologies that create a new demand [e.g., magnetic resonance imaging (MRI) scans to evaluate headaches]. On the other hand, a new surgical technique that shortens recovery time would decrease costs. In light of rapidly rising health care costs, a number of programs have been designed to try to reverse the trend. Certificate of need programs prevent unnecessary expansion of expensive medical services in locales that already have such services available. Rationing is the decision to spend limited resources on certain health care services (often preventive programs, such as well-baby care) at the expense of other services that are less likely to save lives (e.g., expensive surgery for terminally ill patients). Price controls limit what hospitals and doctors can charge, thus limiting costs to the government and insurers. Managed care provides overseers who decide what the insurance company thinks is "medically necessary," and then exclude payments for any other services. Such decisions often conflict with the judgment of the clinician, but tend to shorten hospital stays and to lower the use of expensive services.

55. The answer is E [Chapter 16 V A 1 a (1)–(2)]. Competent patients may refuse medical treatment based on the autonomy model. Paternalism does not help in this situation. Paternalism does interfere with the freedom of competent persons, has been largely replaced

in medical ethics by the autonomy model, and is supported by the Hippocratic view and by the principle of beneficence.

56. The answer is B [Chapter 5 III B 2 a (2)]. Positive and negative reinforcement increase the probability that the behavioral response occurring before the reinforcement will be repeated. It is important not to confuse negative reinforcement with punishment. When a response is negatively reinforced, it prevents or avoids an unpleasant consequence, such as changing the television channel when an obnoxious commercial appears. In the same situation, punishment would be watching the commercial. Secondary reinforcers also increase the probability of a response by their association with a primary reinforcer.

57. The answer is E [Chapter 7 III A 6]. Stimulus generalization is a concept used to explain a universe of both desirable and undesirable behaviors. It is not an effective way of learning classification, because it may combine objects into classes on the basis of irrelevant characteristics. Stimulus generalization is based either on concrete similarities (color, size, and shape)—especially in young children (fear of one dog is fear of all dogs)—or on language (e.g., the word "dog" may mean all four-footed animals and later only a certain kind of four-footed animal).

58. The answer is B [Chapter 8 II A 2 b, B 3 b]. The anaclitic response is not an innate neonatal reflex. Rather, it is the apathy and emotional withdrawal demonstrated by infants who are separated from their mother between 6 and 12 months of age. Innate neonatal reflexes include the Moro reflex, the palmar grasp reflex, rooting and sucking reflexes, and the Babinski reflex. The Moro reflex, also known as the startle reflex, involves flexion of the arms and legs in response to abrupt movement or a loud noise. The palmar reflex causes an infant's fingers to grasp an adult finger which is placed in the palm. Rooting and sucking reflexes facilitate feeding. The Babinski reflex is hyperextension of the toes in response to stroking the sole of the foot.

59. The answer is B [Chapter 12 II D 1–3]. The content of the clinical interview is the actual verbal exchange. The process of the interview is the means by which the message is conveyed. It involves attention to underlying messages that are often revealed through an abrupt stop in the activity in which the patient was engaged, body language, symbolic reference to past events, avoidance of certain topics, and the interviewer's emotional reaction.

60. The answer is D [Chapter 7 II A 6 b]. Developmentally based ego functions are individually shaped (learned) out of the combination of maturation and experience. Maturational function, such as sensory development, proceeds in a relatively similar fashion for each individual, but reality testing combines sensory experience, memory, perception, and personal experience, especially with the parents. Speech and language are maturationally based and are dependent primarily on neurologic integrity.

61. The answer is C [Chapter 15 V G; Chapter 3 X B]. Benzodiazepines, rather than phenothiazines, are commonly used to ease withdrawal from alcohol and to decrease the likelihood of serious complications such as seizures and delirium tremens. Benzodiazepines, like alcohol, have GABAergic effects but can be withdrawn slowly and systematically. Evaluation of the medical and psychiatric condition of alcohol-dependent patients is very important, because concomitant illness is so common. Participation in 12-step recovery programs, such as Alcoholics Anonymous (AA), is recommended for patients with many types of substance abuse. Disulfiram helps many alcoholics maintain sobriety because it alters the metabolism of alcohol in such a way as to induce an uncomfortable (and potentially dangerous) reaction if the patient drinks.

62. The answer is C [Chapter 1 VI A 1 c (1)]. Benzodiazepines and barbiturates bind to a recognition site on the γ-aminobutyric acid-A (GABA-A) receptor and potentiate the inhibitory action of GABA. These agents have anxiolytic, anticonvulsant, hypnotic (sleep-inducing), and muscle relaxant properties. The GABA-A receptor is a ligand-gated ion channel that allows the influx of chloride ions (Cl^-).

63. The answer is C [Chapter 16 V A 2 b (1)–(4)]. If the patient is competent and there is no other reason to bypass informed consent, then a request from the family would not be sufficient reason to bypass informed consent. Informed consent may be bypassed when the patient insists that he does not want to know the details of treatment, in emergency situa-

tions, when there is implied agreement, or when informing the patient will cause serious and identifiable harm.

64. The answer is E [Chapter 1 IV E 1–3]. Memory loss is not consistently associated with aberrations of the serotonergic system. Serotonergic neurotransmission is believed to be important in sleep, thermoregulation, and mood, and may be involved in the pathogenesis of obsessive-compulsive disorder.

65. The answer is C [Chapter 15 IX B; X; XI B]. Dissociative fugue describes the behavior of a patient who travels from home and cannot recall his or her past. The determination that motor activity that resembles a seizure is not of neurologic etiology (a so-called pseudoseizure) still leaves a number of possible explanations. Factitious disorder, conversion disorder, and malingering can be difficult to differentiate, because correct diagnosis requires the clinician to know whether the patient is deliberately producing the symptoms (malingering, factitious disorder) or unconsciously producing the symptoms (conversion disorder). It is also necessary to know whether deliberately faked symptoms are done for external gain (e.g., drug prescriptions, insurance benefits), as is seen in malingering, or because the patient has a psychological need to be treated for illness, as is seen in factitious disorder. Pseudoseizures may certainly occur in patients with prior histories of seizures.

66. The answer is B [Chapter 7 III A 5 b (3)]. Empiric studies document that unpredictably intermittent rewards are the most effective reinforcement for behavior and that continuous reward is an effective short-term, not long-term, reinforcement. Disapproval or criticism may be experienced as attention and be reinforcing of behavior. A reward, as defined by the subject, is reinforcement for behavior and is related to the gratification of both primary and learned needs.

67–71. The answers are: 67-D [Chapter 14 I B 2 a (1), II A], **68-B** [Chapter 14 II C 1, a], **69-A** [Chapter 14 II C 2, a–b], **70-E** [Chapter 14 II C 3, II C 3 a], **71-C** [Chapter 14 II E, 1, a]. The Wechsler Adult Intelligence Scale-Revised (WAIS-R) is a test of potential ability for adaptive functioning. The test does not necessarily indicate a patient's normal level of functioning. The WAIS-R is the standard test for the measurement of intelligence in adults, and excellent validity may therefore be presumed. Standardization is excellent, and reliability is good.

The Minnesota Multiphasic Personality Inventory (MMPI) is an objective self-report test that has been extensively validated. It has highly standardized administration, scoring, and interpretive procedures. Although the reliability is modest and variable because of the variability in some of the characteristics that are measured (e.g., depression, worry), the test has been extensively validated. The focus of the test is the identification of problem areas rather than the explanation of positive and healthy aspects of personality.

The Rorschach test is a projective test designed to measure various elements of thought process (e.g., reality testing, thought form and content) and cognitive style as well as personality dynamics and organization. The Exner comprehensive system, used by most psychologists, is well standardized and has acceptable reliability and validity.

The Thematic Apperception Test (TAT) is a widely used projective test that assesses unconscious needs, conflicts, drives, and interpersonal issues. Consistently adequate reliability and validity have not been demonstrated. Nonetheless, the test may generate useful hypotheses and provide information that contributes to the overall understanding of the patient.

The Halstead-Reitan Battery (HRB) is a well-known standardized test battery that is used in the evaluation of brain injury and dysfunction. It has good validity and reasonable reliability.

72–75. The answers are: 72-D, 73-A, 74-C, 75-B [Chapter 5 II D 1–3]. Lesions caused to the orbital prefrontal cortex may result in aggressive behavior and disregard for societal rules in humans. In cats, stimulation of the medial hypothalamus elicits an affective attack, and stimulation of the lateral hypothalamus elicits a quiet biting attack. Removal of the amygdala in monkeys and rats results in a reduction of aggressive behavior.

76–81. The answers are: 76-C, 77-B, 78-A, 79-B, 80-C, 81-A [Chapter 10 IV B 1–2]. Demographic trends suggest that the American family is in a state of flux. Whether these changes represent crisis or progress is a widely debated issue. The many changes in American society are likely to be important in the future practice of medicine. Marriage remains as popular as ever, with 95% of individuals marrying at least once. Married couples are having fewer children, and more couples are

remaining childless. Both the number of working mothers and the number of single-parent families (most of which are headed by women) are increasing. Only 20% of children younger than 18 years have a father who acts as the sole family wage-earner. Although the average geographic distance between extended family members continues to increase, extended families continue to be major sources of social support. The rate of family violence continues to increase, but this increase may be the result of improved detection and reporting rather than an increase in intrafamily violence.

82–83. The answers are: 82-A [Chapter 6 II C 3 a], **83-C** [Chapter 6 II C 2 a (2)]. Because both of the variables (sex and diagnosis) are nominal, a nonparametric test such as chi-squared should be used. Chi-squared tests the statistical significance of the difference between the observed and expected frequencies. It is the most commonly used nonparametric test. The paired t-test compares sample means from paired observations of the same individuals. Difference scores for each pair are computed, and the mean of these scores is divided by the square root of the variance of the difference scores over the number of pairs.

84–87. The answers are: 84-C, 85-A, 86-B, 87-E [Chapter 1 III B 3 a, C 3 a; IV D; V D]. Dopamine is the neurotransmitter of the cells in the cell-dense zona compacta of the substantia nigra.

Norepinephrine is used by cells in and around the nucleus locus coeruleus.

Serotonin is synthesized by neurons located along the midline raphe area of the brain stem.

Acetylcholine (ACh) is contained in a population of cells known as the basal nucleus (of Meynert).

88–92. The answers are: 88-C, 89-A, 90-E, 91-D, 92-B [Chapter 12 II A 1–2, C 1–2; III B 1]. A number of techniques can be used to ensure that the communication in a physician–patient interview is productive. Direct questions ask for specific information and usually elicit brief, concise answers.

Open-ended questions allow the patient to describe his symptoms and speak generally about his illness.

Exploration invites the patient to explain a remark or conclusion.

Empathy implies understanding and can be

an effective technique; it is best used after the patient expresses how he feels.

Interpretation should be used with caution and only after the interviewer and the patient establish a good relationship.

93–96. The answers are: 93-D, 94-A, 95-C, 96-B [Chapter 5 V B 2, C, E 1, F 1–2]. The Geller-Seifter conflict test is used to test antianxiety drugs. In this paradigm, animals are trained to press a lever to obtain food. Sometimes, they are shocked when they press the lever. This situation represents an approach–avoidance conflict that is analogous to anxiety-provoking situations for humans.

Maternal separation in nonhuman primates resembles depressive behavior. The animals initially protest, but eventually despair and depression occur. Animals then appear socially withdrawn and hypoactive.

Amphetamine- and phencyclidine (PCP)-induced hyperactivity is used as a model of schizophrenia. In nonpsychotic humans, amphetamine and PCP intake cause behavior and symptoms similar to those observed in schizophrenic patients.

Grooming behavior disorders in animals resemble obsessive-compulsive disorder in humans and share similar physiologic and ethological bases.

97–99. The answers are: 97-B, 98-D, 99-A [Chapter 17 I B 2 c]. Capitation (from the Latin *caput,* head) means that a clinician receives a fixed amount of money (a "price per head") to provide services to a group of patients for a set period of time. The payment is the same regardless of how many patients see the clinician.

Medicare's resource-based relative value scale sets maximum clinician fees based upon a number of factors, including practice expenses, the difficulty of the work, and the years of training. Thus, a specialist in an expensive city can charge more than a generalist in a rural area for what might appear to be a similar service.

Fee for service, traditionally the standard means of physician reimbursement, means that the clinician sets a fee for each service and the fee is paid by the patient or the insurance company.

Preferred provider organizations (PPOs) use a variety of physician reimbursement schemes.

Under a salary-based system [commonly employed by health maintenance organizations (HMOs)], a clinician is paid a salary to see patients. This removes the financial motive to provide extra services.

100–103. The answers are: 100-A, 101-B, 102-C, 103-D [Chapter 6 II A 1–2]. Ordinal variables are sets of ordered categories.

Nominal variables represent named categories.

Interval variables are sets of ordered measurements in which the difference between any two measurements is known and is equal.

For ratio variables, the existence of a true zero point allows the ratio of numbers to have meaning.

104–108. The answers are: 104-C, 105-A, 106-E, 107-D, 108-B [Chapter 11 IV C]. Neurotic individuals tend to worry and feel vulnerable. They experience depression and anxiety.

An extrovert is an outgoing, high-spirited individual who likes being with other people.

Open people like new and different experiences; they are often politically liberal and aesthetically avant-garde. Open people often have a rich fantasy life.

Agreeable people try to please others and avoid interpersonal hostility.

Conscientious people are goal-directed, timely, and organized.

Index

Note: Page numbers in italics denote illustrations, those followed by (t) denote tables, those followed by Q denote questions, and those followed by E denote explanations.

A

Absorption, of drugs, 47, 48
Abstract thinking, in mental status examination, 232–233, *233*
Abuse of drugs, 62–65
  alcohol, 62
  caffeine, 65
  cannabis, 64
  cross-dependence on hypnotics, 63
  hallucinogenics, 64
  opioids, 63
  sedative hypnotic agents, 63
  stimulants, 63–64
  tobacco, 65
Abuser, characteristics of, 179
Acetylcholine, 13–15
  muscarinic receptors, 14
  as neurotransmitter, 47
  nicotinic receptors, 13, 22Q, 23E
  synthesis of, *14*
ACTH. *See* Corticotropin
Action potential, 3
Active listening, in communication
  with patient, 204, 213Q, 214Q,
  215E
Addiction, to stimulants, 64
Addison's disease, pituitary hormone, 18
Adenosine triphosphate (ATP), 4
Adenylate cyclase, 4
ADH. *See* Antidiuretic hormone
ADHD. *See* Attention deficit hyperactivity disorder
Adjustment disorder, 274
Adolescence
  anxiety disorder in, 61
  biologic factors, 140–141
  depression, 60
  drugs, 60, 69Q, 71E
  ego identity, development of, 141
  mania, 60
  mood disorders, 60
  obsessive-compulsive disorder, 61
  panic disorder, 61
  psychiatric symptoms in, 60–61
  psychological factors, 141
  psychosis in, 60
  puberty, 140
  sexuality, 151, 152(t), 166Q, 169E
  sociocultural factors, 141
  turmoil during, 141
Adoption study, in genetics, 77–78
Adrenergic receptor, 4
Adulthood
  early, 141–142
  late, 143–144
  middle, 142–143
  midlife transition, 142–143
  sexuality, 151–152

Affect, isolation of, in psychoanalytic
  theory, 123
Age, and sleep cycles, 30
Agency issues, case study, 328–329
Aggression
  animal models, 92–93
  in child, 61
Aging
  mental status changes, case study,
  336–338
  sexuality and, 152
Agoraphobia, 269
Agreeableness, as dimension of personality, 194
Alcohol, abuse of, 62
  genetics and, 81
Allergic reactions to drugs, 50
α-adrenergic receptor, 4
α-methyltyrosine, 6
Alzheimer's disease
  basal forebrain and, 26
  genetics of, 80, 84Q, 86E
  and positron-emitting technique (PET),
  41–42
Amino acids, 5, 15–16
  synthesis, *16*
Amino-4-phosphonobutyric acid
  (AMPA), 4
Amnesia, 262
  dissociative, 271
AMPA. *See* Amino-4-phosphonobutyric
  acid
Amphetamines, and norepinephrine,
  11
Analgesics, behavioral effects of, 66
Analysis of variance (ANOVA), 111
Anatomy of brain, 25
Animal models
  aggression, 92–93
  behavior patterns, learned, 87
  brain self-stimulation, 93
  conflict situations, 97–99
    behaviors, 98
    classification, 98
    inhibitory avoidance, 98–99
    schedule-induced behavior, 98
  consummatory behavior, 88–94
  dementia, 100
  depression, 100
  drinking behavior, 89–90
  eating behavior, 88–89
  evolution, 87
  human behavior and, 87–105
  imprinting, 94
  inherited behavior patterns, 87
  learned helplessness, 100
  learning, 94–97
    associative, 95–97
    conditioning, 95–97

autoshaping, 97
  biofeedback, 97
  classical, 95
  instrumental, 95–97
motivation, 88–94
  neuroses, conditioned, 99
  obsessive-compulsive disorder, 99
  of psychiatric disorders, 99–100
  reproductive behavior, 90–92
  response–suppression paradigm, 99
  schizophrenia, 100
  sexual behavior, 90–92
  substance abuse, 93–94
Anorexia nervosa, 59–60, 272
  and magnetic resonance imaging, 37
ANOVA. *See* Analysis of variance
Antianxiety agent
  absorption of, 57
  clinical uses of, 57–58
  dosage, 57–58
  excretion of, 57
  metabolism of, 57
  pharmacokinetics of, 57
  pharmacology of, 57
  side effects, 58
  tolerance for, 58
Antiarrhythmic agents, behavioral
  effects of, 65
Antibacterial agents, behavioral effects
  of, 66
Anticholinergic drugs, behavioral
  effects of, 65
Anticipatory mourning, 144
Antidepressants, 51–53
  absorption, 52
  for anxiety disorder, 57
  for attention deficit disorder, 53
  bipolar illness, 52
  for bulimia, 53
  for chronic pain, 53
  classes of, 51–52
  clinical use of, 52–53
  and cognitive disturbance, 51
  dosage, 53
  elimination, 52
  for enuresis, 52
  heterocyclic antidepressants, 51
  mechanism of action, 52
  monoamine oxidase inhibitors, 52
  for narcolepsy, 52
  and neurovegetative signs, 51
  and obsessive-compulsive disorder, 52
  and panic disorder, 52
  poisoning, 53
  and psychotherapy, 51
  serotonin reuptake inhibitors, 52
  serotonin–norepinephrine reuptake
  inhibitors, 52
  side effects, 53, 54(t)

toxicity, 53
triazolopyridines, 51
tricyclic antidepressants, 51
Antidiuretic hormone (ADH), 19
Antiemetic drugs, behavioral effects of, 66
Antihistamines
 for anxiety disorder, 57
 and sleep patterns, 32
Antihypertensive drugs, behavioral effects of, 65
Anti-inflammatory drugs, behavioral effects of, 66
Antimanic agents, 56
 antipsychotic drugs, 55
 carbamazepine, 55, 56
 classes of, 55
 clinical use, 55–56
 lithium, 55, 56
 for organic brain syndrome, 55
 pharmacokinetics of, 55
 pharmacology of, 55
 for schizophrenia, 55
 side effects of, 56
 toxicity of, 56
 valproate, 55, 56
Antimicrobial drugs, behavioral effects of, 66
Antipsychotic agents, 10, 47–51, 55, 68Q, 70E
 and bipolar disorder, 48
 and delirium, 48
 and depression, 48
 neuroleptics, 48
 psychosis and, 47
 and schizophrenia, 48
 and sleep patterns, 32
Antitubercular drugs, behavioral effects of, 66
Anxiety disorder, 56–57, 57, 268–270, 269(t)
 in adolescent, 61
 agents for, 56–57
 antidepressants for, 57
 antihistamines for, 57
 azaspirones for, 56
 barbiturates for, 57
 benzodiazepines, 56, 69Q, 70E
 β blockers for, 57
 buspirone for, 57
 in child, 61
 drugs for, 61
 in elderly, 62
 meprobamate for, 57
 panic disorder, 61
 school phobia, 61
 and sleep patterns, 31
 stranger, 137
Arteriovenous vascular malformation, and magnetic resonance imaging, 36
Aspartate, as neurotransmitter, 47
Asthma, out-of-control, case study, 325–327
ATP. See Adenosine triphosphate
Attachment style, in social behavior, 175–176
Attention, in mental status examination, 223, 223
Attention deficit hyperactivity disorder, 60–61, 260
 antidepressants for, 53
 dietary manipulation for, 61
 genetics and, 82
 stimulants for, 61
Autism, 260

Autonomic nervous system, and pain, 33
Autonomy
 development of, 138
 and ethical theory, 283
Autoreceptor, 5
Autoshaping, 97
Aversive conditioning, in behaviorism, 126
Avoidance, inhibitory, animal models, 98–99
Azaspirones, for anxiety disorder, 56

B

Babinski reflex, 136
Barbiturates, for anxiety disorder, 57
Basal ganglia, 25
Beck Depression Inventory, for psychological assessment, 247
Behavior
 aggression, 92–93
 brain self-stimulation, 93
 drinking, 89–90
 eating, 88–89
 familial, 171–188
 inherited, 87. See also Genetics
 interpersonal, 172–176, 174
 learned, 87
 in mental status examination, 224, 225–226
 reproductive, 90–92
 sexual, 90–92
 social, 171–188
 substance abuse, 93–94
Behavioral disorders, genetics and, 73–86
Behaviorism. See Learning
 aversive conditioning, 126
 desensitization, 126
 modeling, 126
 positive reinforcement, 126
Bender Visual-Motor Gestalt Test, for psychological assessment, 249
Beneficence, and ethical theory, 283
Benzodiazepines
 for anxiety disorder, 56
 as hypnotic agents, 58
 and sleep patterns, 32
β blockers, for anxiety disorder, 57
β-adrenergic receptor, 4, 22Q, 23E
Biofeedback, 97
Biomedical theory, 130–131
Biopsychosocial model, of medical science, 172
Bipolar disorder, 267–268
 antidepressants for, 52
 and antipsychotic agents, 48
Body dysmorphic disorder, 271
Borderline personality disorder, and electroencephalogram (EEG), 37, 38, 39(t), 40
Brain, anatomy of, 25
Bulimia, 59–60, 272
 antidepressants for, 53
 and magnetic resonance imaging, 37
Buspirone, for anxiety disorder, 57, 58
Butyrophenone compounds, 48, 49(t)

C

Caffeine, abuse of, 65
Calcium channel
 inhibitors, behavioral effects of, 65
 voltage-dependent, 4

Calculations, in mental status examination, 231, 231–232
California Verbal Learning Test, for psychological assessment, 249
CAMP. See Cyclic adenosine 3′,5′-monophosphate
Cancer, patient with, physician–patient relationship, 196–197
Cannabis, 64
Carbamazepine, 55, 56
Cardiovascular disease, and sexuality, 163
Cardiovascular drugs, behavioral effects of, 65
Catecholamine theory of mood disorders, 11
Catecholamines, 6–11, 7, 8
 antipsychotic drug therapy, 10
 catechol-O-methyltransferase (COMT), 8
 dopamine, 8–9
  β-hydroxylase, 6
 mesocortical tract, 8
 mesolimbic tract, 8
 metabolism of, 8
 3-methoxy-4-hydroxyphenylglycol (MHPG), 10
 neuroleptics, 10
 nigrostriatal pathway, 8
 norepinephrine, 6, 10–11
 parkinsonism, 9
 schizophrenia, 9
 synthesis of, 7–8, 8
 tardive dyskinesia, 9
 tuberoinfundibular tract, 9
 tyrosine hydroxylase, 6
Catechol-O-methyltransferase (COMT), 8
Caudate nucleus, neuroanatomy, 25
CCK. See Cholecystokinin (CCK)
Cerebral blood flow, regional, 40–41
CGMP. See Cyclic guanosine 3′,5′-monophosphate (cGMP)
Chest pain, case study, 338–340
Child. See also Childhood
 aggressiveness in, 61
 anxiety disorder, 61
 attention deficit hyperactivity disorder, 60–61
 depression, 60
 enuresis, treatment of, 61
 impulsiveness in, 61
 mood disorders, 60
 obsessive-compulsive disorder, 61
 panic disorder, 61
 psychosis in, 60
 tantrums in, case study, 320–321
Child Behavior Checklist, for psychological assessment, 247
Child rearing tasks, in family life cycle, 180–181
Childhood
 cognitive maturation, 139
 development of sexuality, 151
 latency period, 140
 motor development, 138
 physical growth, 138
 play, 140
 psychological development, 139–140
 psychosexual development, 139–140
 social development, 139–140
Cholecystokinin (CCK), 17–18
Chromosomes
 and behavioral disorders, 73–74, 84Q, 85E
 dominance, 75

expressivity, 74–75, 84Q, 86E
genocopy, 74
genome, 76
genotype, 74
heritability, 74
homozygosity, 75
intermediate inheritance, 75
penetrance, 74
phenocopy, 74
phenotype, 74
recessivity, 75
terminology, 74–75
Chronic illness, and sexuality, 163
Chronic pain, antidepressants for, 53
Cimetidine, behavioral effects of, 66
Classical conditioning, 95, 125–126
Clinical study design, 321–322
Clinical syndromes, 259–277
Clozapine, 48, 49(t)
Cognition, and serotonin, 14–15
Cognitive disturbance
  and antidepressant agents, 51
  patient with, physician–patient relationship, 195, 196(t)
Cognitive theory, 126–128
Communication with patient, 190, 203–217
  active listening, 204, 213Q, 214Q, 215E
  building rapport, 203–205
  emotion of patient, responding to, 203–204
  information gathering, 205–206
  medical history, 205–210, 208(t), 209(t)
  patient education, 206–207
  positive regard, 204
  treatment planning, 206–207
Computed tomography (CT), 35–36, 44Q, 45E
COMT. *See* Catechol-O-methyltransferase
Conditioning
  animal models, 95–97
  autoshaping, 97
  biofeedback, 97
  classical, 95
  instrumental, 95–97
Conflict
  animal models, 97–99
  behaviors, animal models, 98
  classification, animal models, 98
  ethics and, 280–281
  inhibitory avoidance, animal models, 98–99
  schedule-induced behavior, animal models, 98
Conscientiousness, as dimension of personality, 195
Consciousness, in mental status examination, 222–223
Construct validity, research design, 113
Constructional ability, in mental status examination, *231*, 231–232
Consumers in health care system, 305–306
Consummatory behavior, animal models of, 88–94
Contraceptives, oral, behavioral effects of, 66
Conversion disorder, 271
Corpus striatum, 25
Correlation, in statistics, 111, 118Q, 120E
Correlational research study, example of, 116–117

Cortex, 25, *26*
  telencephalon, 25
Corticosteroids, behavioral effects of, 66
Corticotropin (ACTH), 18
Corticotropin-releasing factor (CRF), 18
Cortisol, for hypothyroidism, 34
Countertransference
  in physician–patient relationship, 192, 199Q, 201E
  in psychoanalysis, 124
CRF. *See* Corticotropin-releasing factor
Crisis, and family life cycle, 181
Cross-dependence
  hypnotic agents, 63
  with opioids, 63
CT. *See* Computed tomography
Cultural gap, in physician–patient relationship, 190
Cultural influences on sexuality, 155
Cushing's syndrome, pituitary hormone, 18
Cyclic adenosine 3′,5′-monophosphate (cAMP), 4
Cyclic guanosine 3′,5′-monophosphate (cGMP), 4
Cyclic nucleotide, 4

D

Death/dying
  adult's perspective, 145
  case study, 340
  child's death, parental response to, 144–145
  child's perspective, 144–145
  ethical issues and, 286–287
  physician response to, 145
Defenses, in psychoanalytic theory, 122–123
Delirium, 234Q, 236E, 260–261, 261(t)
  and antipsychotic agents, 48
  case study, 333–334
  physician–patient relationship, 195, 196(t)
Delusional disorder, 266
  and pain, 33
Dementia, 261, 262(t)
  animal models, 100
  and computed tomography, 35
  drug treatments for, 61–62
  and magnetic resonance imaging, 37
  physician–patient relationship, 195, 196(t)
  and regional cerebral blood flow, 40–41
  and single-photon-emitting radionuclides (SPECT), 41
  and sleep patterns, 31–32
Denial, process of, 122, 132Q, 134E
Deontology, 281–282
Dependence
  on drugs, 62
  on hypnotic agents, 59
Depersonalization disorder, 272
Depolarization, 3
Depression, 266–267, 268(t)
  adolescent, 60
  animal models, 100
  antidepressants, 51, 52
  and antipsychotic agents, 48
  child, 60
  in elderly, 62
  and pain, 32–33
  and pituitary hormone, 18

and single-photon-emitting radionuclides (SPECT), 41
Desensitization, in behaviorism, 126
Despair, *vs.* ego identity, in later adulthood, 143–144
Detoxification, 263
Development, 135
Diagnosis, genetic, prenatal, 82–83
Diagnostic and Statistical Manual of Mental Disorders, 259
Diencephalon, 26–27
  hypothalamus, 27
  limbic structure, 27
  thalamus, 26–27
Dietary manipulation, for attention deficit hyperactivity disorder (ADHD), 61
Digitalis, behavioral effects of, 65
Diphenhydramine, behavioral effects of, 66
Dissociative disorders, 271–272
Distribution, of drugs, 47
Disulfiram
  in abuse of alcohol, 62
  behavioral effects of, 66
Doctor. *See* Physician
Dominance, genetic, 75
Dopamine, 4, 8–9, 21Q, 23E
Dopamine D$_2$ receptor, 4, 22Q, 23E
Dopamine β-hydroxylase, 6
Dopamine receptor, 4
Dopaminergic drugs, behavioral effects of, 66
Dosage of drugs, 50
Down syndrome, 73–74
Drawing, projective, for psychological assessment, 247
Drinking behavior, 89–90
Drives, in psychoanalytic theory, 121
Drugs
  absorption of, 47, 48
  abuse of, 62–65
  adolescent, 60–61, 69Q, 71E
  affecting sexual functioning, 164
  for aggressiveness, in child, 61
  allergic reactions to, 50
  analgesics, 66
  antianxiety agents, 56–58
  antibacterial agents, 66
  anticholinergic drugs, 65
  antidepressant agents, 51–53
  antiemetic drugs, 66
  antihypertensive drugs, 65
  anti-inflammatory drugs, 66
  antimanic agents, 53–56
  antimicrobial drugs, 66
  antipsychotic agents, 47–51
  antitubercular drugs, 66
  anxiety disorder, 61
  attention deficit hyperactivity disorder (ADHD), 60–61
  and behavior, 47–71
  butyrophenone compounds, 48, 49(t)
  cardiovascular drugs, 65
  child, 60–61 , 69Q, 70E
  classes of, 48, 49(t)
  clinical use of, 50
  corticosteroids, 66
  dependence on, 62
  distribution of, 47
  dopaminergic drugs, 66
  dosage of, 50
  effect on sleep patterns, 32, 68Q, 70E
  elderly, 61–62, 69Q, 70E
  and electroconvulsive therapy (ECT), 51

elimination of, 47
for enuresis, 61
excretion of, 50
extrapyramidal side effects of, 50, 68Q, 70E
hormones, 66
hypnotic agents, 58–59
hypothalamic temperature regulation and, 50
for impulsiveness, in child, 61
individualization of treatment, 67, 68Q, 70E
informing patient, 66
interactions of, 66
mechanism of action, 48
metabolism of, 50
mood disorders, 60–61
neurochemical response to, overview, 3
and neuroleptic malignant syndrome, 51
and neurotransmitters, of central nervous system, 47, 48(t)
nonpsychiatric, 65–66
obsessive-compulsive disorder, 61
oral contraceptives, 66
overdose of, 51
panic disorder, 61
patient noncompliance, 67
pharmacodynamic interactions, 67
pharmacokinetic principles, 47, 47(t)
pharmacokinetics of, 48–50
pharmacologic properties, 48
pharmacology, 48–50
phenothiazines, 48, 49(t)
and pigmentary retinopathy, 50
placebo effect, 67
prescribing, 66–67
psychopharmacology, 60–61
psychotropic, effect on neurotransmitters, 48(t), 68Q, 70E
and receptors, of central nervous system, 47, 48(t)
reevaluation of prescription, 67
response to, overview, 3
school phobia, 61
and seizure threshold, 50
sexual dysfunction, pharmacologic agents implicated in, 158(t)
side effects of, 50–51
tardive dyskinesia and, 51
therapeutic index, 47
thioxanthene compounds, 48, 49(t)
thyroid hormones, 66
toxicity of, 50–51
DSM. *See Diagnostic and Statistical Manual of Mental Disorders*
Dysfunction, sexual, 156–160, 158(t)
Dysrhythmia, and electroencephalogram (EEG), 37
Dyssomnias, 272–273

E

Eating behavior, 88–89
Eating disorders, 59–60, 272
Economics of health care system, 307–309
ECT. *See* Electroconvulsive therapy
Education of patient, 206–207
EEG. *See* Electroencephalogram
Ego, in psychoanalytic theory, 123
Ego identity
development of, 141
in later adulthood, 143–144
Eicosanoids, 16

Elderly
anxiety in, 62
dementia, 61–62
depression, 62
drug treatments for, 61–62
dementia, 61–62
pharmacokinetics, 61
toxicity, 61
Electroconvulsive therapy (ECT), 51
Electroencephalogram (EEG), 37, *38*, 39(t), *40*, 44Q, 45E
Elimination, of drugs, 47
Emotion of patient, responding to, 203–204
Empathy, in physician–patient relationship, 190
Enuresis
antidepressants for, 52
treatment of, 61
Environment, influence on behavior, 172
Epilepsy, and sleep patterns, 32
Erectile dysfunction, 157(t), 156–157
case study, 324–325
Ethics, 279–293
autonomy, 283
beneficence, 283
conflict and, 280–281
controversies in, 284–288
death, 286–287
deontology, 281–282
and health care allocation, 288
Hippocratic oath, 279, 289Q, 292E
justice and, 283–284
medical technology and, 287–288
nonmaleficence, 283
physician–patient relationship, 284–286
value theory, 281
virtue theory, 283
Evoked potentials, electroencephalogram (EEG), 37
Evolution, 87
Excretion of drugs, 50
Experimental research study, example of, 116
Explosive disorder, 273
Expressivity
chromosomes, 74–75, 84Q, 86E
genetic, defined, 74–75
Extinction, in behaviorism, 125, 133Q, 134E
Extrapyramidal motor system, 25
Extrapyramidal side effects of drugs, 50
Extroversion, as dimension of personality, 194

F

Factitious disorder, 271
Family, definitions of, 178
Family behavior, 178–182
abuser, characteristics of, 179
crisis in, 181
demographic analysis, 178–180
in family life cycle, 180–181
family therapy, 181–182, 182(t), 186Q, 187E
life cycle of, 180–181
violence, 179
Family history of patient, 209, 209(t)
Family life cycle, crisis in, 181
Family study, in genetics, 76–77
Family therapy, 181–182, 182(t)
Female, sexual response cycle, 153(t), 153–154

Financing of health care system, 301–304
Follicle-stimulating hormone (FSH), 18
FSH. *See* Follicle-stimulating hormone
Fugue, dissociative, 271

G

Gambling, pathological, 273
Gender
awareness, development of, 151
identity, disorder, 161
Genes
and behavioral disorders, 73–74
dominance, 75
expressivity, 74–75
genocopy, 74
genome, 76
heritability, 74
homozygosity, 75
intermediate inheritance, 75
penetrance, 74
phenocopy, 74
phenotype, 74, 85Q, 86E
recessivity, 75
terminology, 74–75
Genetic counseling, 82
Genetics
adoption study, 77–78
and alcohol abuse, 81
Alzheimer's disease, 80, 84Q, 86E
attention deficit disorder, 82
basic principles of, 73–76
and behavioral disorders, 73–86
clinical family study, 76–77
Down syndrome, 73–74
genetic counseling, 82
genome, 76
Klinefelter syndrome, 74
LOD score, 76
mental retardation, 80–81
methods of study, 76–78
molecular, 75–76
molecular family study, 77
mood disorders, 79–80
obsessive-compulsive disorder, 82, 85Q, 86E
personality disorder, 81
prenatal diagnosis, 82–83
and psychiatric disorders, 78–82
restriction fragment length polymorphisms (RFLP), 75–76
risk patterns for mental illness, 78(t)
schizophrenia, 78–79
Tourette syndrome, 82, 85Q, 86E
twin study, 77
Globus pallidus, neuroanatomy, 25
Glucose, hypoglycemia and, 34
Glutamate, 22Q, 23E
as neurotransmitter, 47
Glycine, amino acid, 15, 22Q, 23E
G-protein-coupled receptors, 4–5
Growth, 135
Guanylate cyclase, 4
Gut peptide, 17–18

H

Hallucinations, case study, 333–334
Hallucinogenics, abuse of, 64
Haloperidol, 50
Halstead-Reitan neuropsychological test battery, for psychological assessment, 247–249, 248(t)
Health care allocation, and ethics, 288

Health care system, 295–315, 313Q,
  314E
  consumers of, 305–306
  economics of, 307–309
  financing of, 301–304
  history of, 295–301
  management, 304–305
  political issues, 306–307
  reform of, 309–310
  structure of, 295–301
Heritability factors, 74
Heterocyclic antidepressants, 51
Hippocratic oath, 190, 279, 289Q, 292E
Homosexuality, 155–156, 167Q, 169E
Homozygosity, 75
Hormones
  behavioral effects of, 66
  influence on sexuality, 154
5-HT$_1$, and serotonin, 12
5-HT$_2$, and serotonin, 12
Huntington's disease
  and magnetic resonance imaging, 36
  and memory, 34, 84Q, 86E
5-hydroxytryptamine$_3$, 4, 22Q, 23E
Hypercortisolism, and hypothyroidism,
  34
Hyperdopaminergic state, 21Q, 23E
Hyperglycemia, and insulin, 34
Hyperthyroidism, 33
Hypnotic agents
  absorption of, 59
  abuse of, 63
  benzodiazepines, 58
  classes of drugs, 58
  clinical uses of, 59
  cross-dependence, 63
  dependence on, 59
  excretion of, 59
  for insomnia, 58
  oversedation with, 59
  pharmacokinetics of, 58–59
  pharmacology of, 58
  rebound insomnia with, 59
  side effects of, 59
  withdrawal, 63
  zolpidem, 58
Hypochondriacal patient, 271
  physician–patient relationship, 195
Hypocortisolism, and hypothyroidism, 34
Hypoglycemia
  and glucose, 34
  and insulin, 34
Hypothalamic hormone, 20
Hypothalamic temperature regulation
  and drugs, 50
Hypothalamus, 27
  diencephalon, 27
Hypothesis testing, 110
Hypothyroidism, 33, 34(t)
  hypercortisolism, 34

I

Id, in psychoanalytic theory, 123
Identity disorder, dissociative, 271–272
Imprinting, 94
Impulse control disorders, 273
Impulsiveness, in child, 61
Infancy, development of sexuality, 151
Infancy to toddlerhood
  autonomy, 138
  development in, 135–138
  object relations, 137
  play, 137–138
  self-awareness, 138
  smile, development of, 137

  sociocultural factors in, 138
  stranger anxiety, 137
Information, neuronal transmission of,
  3–6
Inheritance, intermediate, 75
Insomnia, hypnotic agents for, 58
Instincts, in psychoanalytic theory, 121
Instrumental conditioning, 95–97
Insulin
  and hyperglycemia, 34
  hypoglycemia and, 34
Intellectualization, in psychoanalytic
  theory, 123
Intelligence tests, 240–243
Interactions of drugs, 66
Interpersonal behavior, 172–176, *174*
Interviewing skills, 204–205
  case study, 330–332
Intoxication, 263, 276Q, 277E
  from stimulants, 64
Ion, 21Q, 23E
Isolation of affect, in psychoanalytic
  theory, 123

J

Justice, and ethical theory, 283–284

K

Kainate, amino acids, 16
Kindling, amino acids, 16
Kleptomania, 273
Klinefelter syndrome, 74

L

Lactation, sexuality during, 162–163
Language, in mental status examination, 225–228, *227–228*
Learned helplessness, animal models,
  100
Learning
  animal models, 94–97
  associative, 95–97
  conditioning, 95–97
    autoshaping, 97
    biofeedback, 97
    classical, 95
    instrumental, 95–97
  imprinting, 94
Learning theory, 124–126
Life cycle, 135–148
  adolescence, 140–141
  adulthood, 141–143
  childhood, 138–140
  death/dying, 144–145
  development, 135
  family issues in, case study, 322–323
  growth, 135
  infancy to toddlerhood, 135–138
  later adulthood, 143–144
  maturation, 135
  old age, 143–144
Life support, termination of, case study,
  330
Ligand-gated ion channel, 4
Limbic structure, diencephalon, 27
Limbic system, 27, *28,* 28(t)
Lithium, 55, 56, 69Q, 71E
Loxapine, 48, 49(t)
Luria-Nebraska neuropsychological
  battery, for psychological assessment, 249
Luteinizing hormone (LH), 18

M

Magnetic resonance imaging (MRI), 36
Magnetic resonance spectroscopy
  (MRS), 39–40, 40(t)
Magnetoencephalography (MEG), 37,
  39
Male, sexual response cycle, 153(t),
  153–154
Managed competition, and health care
  system reform, 310
Management of health care system,
  304–305
Mania
  adolescent, 60
  antimanic agents for, 53
  and electroencephalogram (EEG), 37
  overview, 53
Manic-depressive disorder, and magnetic resonance imaging, 37
MAO. *See* Monoamine oxidase
Maturation, 135
Measurement, and statistics, 107–112
  analysis of variance, 111
  correlation, 111
  descriptive statistics, 108–110, *109*
  hypothesis testing, 110
  inferential statistics, 110–112
  meta-analysis, 112
  multivariate technique, 112
  nonparametric test, 111
  paired test, 111
  parametric test, 110–111
  regression, 111, *112*
  unpaired test, 111
  variables, types of, 107–108
Mechanism of action, of drug, 48
Medical condition, mental disorder due
  to, 262
Medical history, 205–206, 207–210,
  208(t), 209(t)
  technique variations, 210–211
Medical science model, biopsychosocial, 172
Medical technology and ethics,
  287–288
Medication. *See* Drugs
MEG. *See* Magnetoencephalography
Melanocyte-stimulating hormone
  (MSH), 20
Melatonin, 20
  and seasonal mood disorder, 20
  and serotonin, 11
Memory, 34
  declarative, 34
  Huntington's chorea and, 34, 84Q,
    86E
  impairment, short-term, case study,
    332–333
  in mental status examination,
    227–228, 230–231
  procedural, 34
  and serotonin, 14–15
Mental process, unconscious, 121,
  132Q, 134E
Mental retardation, 259–260
  genetics of, 80–81
Mental status examination, 219–236
  abstract thinking, 232–233, *233*
  attention, 223, *223*
  behavior, 224, *225–226*
  calculations, *231,* 231–232
  components of, 222–233
  consciousness, 222–223
  constructional ability, *231,* 231–232
  language, 225–228

memory, 230–231
score sheet, *220–221*
structure of, 222, *222*
thought, 228–230
vigilance, 223, *223*
Meprobamate, for anxiety disorder, 57
Mesencephalon, 27–28
Mesocortical tract, 8
Mesolimbic tract, 8
Meta-analysis, in statistics, 112
Metabolism, of drugs, 50
Metencephalon, 29
3-methoxy-4-hydroxyphenylglycol
    (MHPG), 10
MHPG. *See* 3-methoxy-4-
    hydroxyphenylglycol (MHPG)
Midlife transition, during adulthood,
    142–143
Millon Clinical Multiaxial Inventory II,
    for psychological assessment, 247
Minnesota Multiphasic Personality In-
    ventory, 243–245, 245(t)
Modeling, in behaviorism, 126
Molecular genetics, 75–76
Molindone, 48, 49(t)
Monoamine oxidase (MAO), 52
Monoamines, 5
    as neurotransmitter, 47
Mood disorder, 266–268, 267(t)
    adolescent, 60
    child, 60
    genetics of, 79–80
    and serotonin, 13
Motivation, animal models of, 88–94
Mourning, anticipatory, 144
MRI. *See* Magnetic resonance imaging
MRS. *See* Magnetic resonance spec-
    troscopy
MSH. *See* Melanocyte-stimulating hor-
    mone
Multiple personality disorder. *See* Iden-
    tity disorder, dissociative
Multiple sclerosis, and magnetic reso-
    nance imaging, 36
Multivariate technique, in statistics,
    112
Muscarinic acetylcholine, 4
Muscarinic receptor, 4
    acetylcholine, 14
Myelencephalon, 29
Myers-Briggs Type Indicator, for psy-
    chological assessment, 247

N

Narcolepsy, antidepressants for, 52
Neuroanatomy, 25–29
    basal forebrain, 26
    basal ganglia, 25
    corpus striatum, 25
    cortex, 25, *26*
    diencephalon, 26–27
    hypothalamus, 27
    limbic system, 27, *28,* 28(t)
    memory, 34
    mesencephalon, 27–28
    metencephalon, 29
    myelencephalon, 29
    neuroendocrinology and, 33–34
    and pain, 32–33
    raphe nuclei, 27–28, 44Q, 45E
    rapid eye movement (REM), 29(t),
        29–32
    reticular formation, 28
    sleep, 29(t), 29–32
    substantia nigra, 27

telencephalon, 25–26
ventral segmental area, 27
Neurochemistry
    acetylcholine, 13–15
    action potential, 3
    adenosine, 16
    adenosine triphosphate (ATP), 4
    adenylate cyclase, 4
    adrenergic receptor, 4
    α-adrenergic receptor, 4
    amino acids, 15–16
    antipsychotic drug therapy, 10
    autoreceptor, 5
    β-adrenergic receptor, 4
    calcium, 5
    catecholamines, 6–11
    catechol-O-methyltransferase
        (COMT), 8
    cyclic adenosine 3,′5′-
        monophosphate (cAMP), 4
    cyclic guanosine 3,′5′-
        monophosphate (cGMP), 4
    cyclic nucleotide, 4
    depolarization, 3
    dopamine, 8–9
    receptor, 4
    dopamine D_2 receptor, 4
    dopamine β-hydroxylase, 6
    drugs, response to, 3
    5-hydroxytryptamine$_3$, 4
    ligand-gated ion channel, 4
    mesolimbic tract, 8
    metabolism of, 8
    3-methoxy-4-hydroxyphenylglycol
        (MHPG), 10
    monoamine oxidase (MAO), 6
    monoamines, 5
    muscarinic acetylcholine, 4
    muscarinic receptor, 4
    neuron, 3–6
    neuronal transmission of information,
        3–6
    neuropeptides, 17–20
    neurotransmitter, 5–6
    disturbance, 3
    nigrostriatal pathway, 8
    nonpeptide neurotransmitter candi-
        dates, 16
    norepinephrine, 6
    opiate receptor, 4
    pertussis toxin, 6
    phosphatidylinositol, 5
    phosphodiesterase inhibitor, 6
    prostaglandins, 16
    purines, 16
    receptor, 4–5
    second messenger, 4
    serotonin, 11–13
    synapse, chemical, 4
    thromboxanes, 16
    transmission of information, neuronal,
        α-methyltyrosine, 6
    types of, 5
    voltage-dependent calcium ion chan-
        nel, 4
Neuroendocrinology, 33–34
    thyroid, 33
Neuroimaging techniques
    and behavioral functioning, 42
    computed tomography (CT), 35–36,
        44Q, 45E
    electroencephalogram (EEG), 37,
        44Q, 45E
    functional, 37–42
    magnetic resonance imaging (MRI),
        36

magnetic resonance spectroscopy
    (MRS), 39–40, 40(t), 44Q, 45E
magnetoencephalography (MEG), 37,
    39
positron-emitting technique (PET),
    41–42, 44Q, 45E
regional cerebral blood flow, 40–41
single-photon-emitting radionuclides
    (SPECT), 41, 44Q, 45E
structural, 35–37
Neuroleptic, 10, 21Q, 23E
    malignant syndrome, and drugs, 51
Neuron, 3
Neuronal transmission of information,
    3–6
Neuropeptide, 17–20
    antidiuretic hormone (ADH), 19
    cholecystokinin (CCK), 17–18
    corticotropin, 18, 43Q, 45E
    corticotropin-releasing factor (CRF),
        18
    endogenous opioid peptide, 17
    follicle-stimulating hormone (FSH), 18
    gut peptide, 17–18
    hypothalamic hormone, 20
    luteinizing hormone (LH), 18
    melanocyte-stimulating hormone
        (MSH), 20
    melatonin, 20
    neurotensin, 18
    oxytocin, 19–20
    pineal hormone, 20
    pituitary hormone, 18–20
    prolactin, 18, 19
    somatostatin, 18
    substance P, 17
    thyroid-stimulating hormone (TSH),
        18
    vasoactive intestinal polypeptide
        (VIP), 18
    vasopressin, 19–20
Neuropsychological assessment,
    247–250
Neuroses, conditioned, animal models,
    99
Neurotensin, 18
Neuroticism, as dimension of personal-
    ity, 194
Neurotransmitter, 5–6
    of central nervous system, drugs and,
        47, 48(t)
    disturbance, 3
    release, 4
Neurovegetative signs, and antidepres-
    sant agents, 51
Nicotinic receptors, 13, 22Q, 23E
    acetylcholine, 13
Nigrostriatal pathway, 8, 21Q, 23E
Nonmaleficence, and ethical theory,
    283
Nonparametric test, in statistics, 111
Nonpeptide neurotransmitter candi-
    dates, 16
Nonpsychiatric drugs
    antiarrhythmic agents, 65
    antihypertensives, 65
    behavioral effects of, 65–66
    cardiovascular drugs, 65
    digitalis, 65
Norepinephrine, 6, 10–11
    β receptors, 10–11
    α receptors, 10
    amphetamines, 11
    brain tracts, 11
    catecholamine theory of mood disor-
        ders, 11

effect on behavior, 11
propranolol, 11
reserpine, 11
tricyclic antidepressants, 11

O

Object relations, 137
Obsessive-compulsive disorder, 270
  animal models, 99
  antidepressants for, 52
  in child, 61
  and computed tomography, 35
  genetics, 82, 85Q, 86E
  and positron-emitting technique (PET),
    41–42
  and serotonin, 13
Openness, as dimension of personality,
  194
Operant conditioning, 126
Opiate receptor, 4
Opiates, role of, and pain, 32
Opioid peptide, endogenous, 17
Opioids
  abuse of, 63
  cross-dependence, 63
  overdose, 63
  withdrawal from, 63, 68Q, 70E
Oral contraceptives, behavioral effects
  of, 66
Organic brain syndrome, antimanic
  agents for, 55
Overdose
  of drugs, 51
  opioids, 63
Oversedation, with hypnotic agents, 59
Oxytocin, 19–20

P

Pain, 32–33
  chronic, patient with, physician–
    patient relationship, 196
  with mental disorder, 32–33
  types of, 32
  without organic cause, case study,
    329–330
Pain disorder
  with psychological factors, 271
  sexual, 159
Panic attacks, and sleep patterns, 31
Panic disorder, 61, 268–269
  antidepressants for, 52
Parametric test, 110–111
Paraphilia, 161
Parasomnias, 273
Parkinsonism, 9, 22Q, 23E
  and memory, 34
Patient, relationship with physician.
  See Physician–patient relationship
Patient history. *See* Medical history
Patient noncompliance, to drug pre-
  scription, 67
Pavlovian conditioning. *See* Classical
  conditioning
p-chlorophenylalanine, 6
PCPA. *See* p-Chlorophenylalanine
Penetrance, genetic, 74
Peptide
  as neurotransmitters, 47
  subunit, 4
Personality, dimensions of, *194*,
  194–195
Personality disorder, 274
  categories of, 193(t)

genetics and, 81
  patient with, physician–patient rela-
    tionship, 195
Personality types, physician–patient
  relationship, 192–194, 193(t)
Pertussis toxin, 6
PET. *See* Positron-emitting technique
Pharmacodynamic interactions, 67
Pharmacokinetics
  of drugs, 48–50
  principles of, 47, 47(t)
Pharmacologic properties, of drugs, 48
Pharmacology of drugs, 48–50
Phencyclidine, amino acids, 16
Phenothiazines, 48, 49(t)
Phenylephrine, behavioral effects of,
  66
Phobia, 269–270
Phosphatidylinositol, 5
Phosphodiesterase, 4
Phosphodiesterase inhibitor, 6
Physician-assisted suicide, 197
Physician–patient relationship,
  189–201
  cancer, patient with, 196–197
  chronic pain, patient with, 196
  communication, 190
  components of, 190
  countertransference, 192
  defined, 189
  delirium, 195, 196(t)
  dementia, 195, 196(t)
  ethics and, 284–286
  Hippocratic oath, 190, 279, 289Q,
    292E
  hypochondriacal patient, 195
  models of, 191(t), 191–192
  noncompliant patient, 196
  patient with cognitive impairment,
    195, 196(t)
  personality, dimensions of, *194*,
    194–195
  personality disorder
    categories of, 193(t)
    patient with, 195
  personality types, 192–194, 193(t)
  physician-assisted suicide, 197
  "sick role" of patient, 189–190
  under stress, 195–197, 196(t)
  transference, 192
Physostigmine, 6
Pigmentary retinopathy, and drugs, 50
Pineal hormone, 20
Pituitary hormone, 18–20
  Addison's disease, 18
  Cushing's syndrome, 18
  depression and, 18
Placebo effect, 67
Play, development through, 137–138
Political issues, health care system,
  306–307
Polysomnography, 30
Positive regard, in communication with
  patient, 204
Positive reinforcement, in behaviorism,
  126
Positron-emitting technique (PET),
  41–42, 44Q, 45E
Postpartum period, sexuality during,
  162–163
Posttraumatic stress disorder, 270
Potassium, 21Q, 23E
Pregnancy, sexuality during, 162–163
Prescribing drugs, 66–67
  informing patient, 66
  patient noncompliance, 67

placebo effect, 67
Projection, in psychoanalytic theory,
  122, 132Q, 134E
Projective drawing, for psychological
  assessment, 247
Prolactin, 18, 19
Propranolol, and norepinephrine, 11
Prostaglandins, 16
Psychiatric disorders
  animal models of, 99–100
  genetics and, 78–82
Psychic determinism, 121
Psychoanalysis, 124
Psychoanalytic theory, 121–124
  basic concepts of, 121–123
  defenses, 122–123
  denial, 122
  drives, 121
  ego, 123
  id, 123
  instincts, 121
  intellectualization, 123
  isolation of affect, 123
  perspectives of, 123–124
  projection, 122
  psychic determinism, 121
  psychoanalysis, 124
  psychosexual stages, 122
  rationalization, 123
  reaction formation, 123
  regression, 123
  repression, 122
  splitting, 122
  structural model, 123
  superego, 123
  unconscious mental process, 121
  undoing, 123
Psychodynamic theory. *See* Psychoanalytic theory
Psychological assessment, 237(t),
  237–238, 240–250, 241(t), 242(t),
  243(t), 244(t), 246(t), 248(t)
  achievement, 243
  analysis of test data, 250
  Beck Depression Inventory, 247
  Bender Visual-Motor Gestalt Test, 249
  California Verbal Learning Test, 249
  Child Behavior Checklist, 247
  classification of measurements,
    239–240
  Halstead-Reitan neuropsychological
    test battery, 247–249, 248(t)
  intelligence, 240–243
  Luria-Nebraska neuropsychological
    battery, 249
  Millon Clinical Multiaxial Inventory II,
    247
  Minnesota Multiphasic Personality
    Inventory, 243–245, 245(t)
  of mood state, 243–247
  Myers-Briggs Type Indicator, 247
  neuropsychological assessment,
    247–250
  of personality functioning, 243–247
  projective drawing, 247
  reporting of test data, 250
  Rey-Osterrieth Complex Figure Test,
    249
  Rorschach inkblot test, 245, 245(t),
    253Q, 256E
  sentence completion test, 246
  Sixteen Personality Factor Inventory,
    247
  Stanford-Binet Scale, 243
  Thematic Apperception Test, 245–246
  vocational testing, 247

WAIS-R intelligence scale, 241–243, 242(t)
Wechsler Memory Scale-Revised, 249–250
Wisconsin Card Sorting Test, 250
Psychological influences on sexuality, 155
Psychometric evaluation, 238(t), 238–240
Psychopathology, defining, 259
Psychopharmacology
  adolescent, psychiatric symptoms in, 60–61
  child, psychiatric symptoms in, 60–61
Psychosexual stages, in psychoanalytic theory, 122
Psychosis
  in adolescent, 60
  and antipsychotic agents, 47
  in child, 60
  and pain, 33
Psychosocial theory, 128–130
Psychotherapy, and antidepressant agents, 51
Psychotic depression, case study, 317–318
Psychotic disorder
  brief, 266
  shared, 266
Puberty, development during, 140
Purines, 16
Putamen, neuroanatomy, 25
Pyromania, 273

R

Radioactive tracer, and regional cerebral blood flow, 40–41
Raphe nuclei, 27–28, 44Q, 45E
Rapid eye movement (REM), 29(t), 29–32
Rationalization, in psychoanalytic theory, 123
Reaction formation, in psychoanalytic theory, 123
Rebound insomnia, with hypnotic agents, 59
Receptor, 4–5
  of central nervous system, drugs and, 47, 48(t)
Recessivity, genetic, 75
Reform, of health care system, 309–310
Regional cerebral blood flow, 40–41
Regression
  in psychoanalytic theory, 123
  in statistics, 111, *112*
Reinforcement
  in behaviorism, 125
  positive, in behaviorism, 126
Reliability, of research design, 112–114, 252Q, 255E
REM. *See* Rapid eye movement
Repression, in psychoanalytic theory, 122
Reproductive behavior, 90–92
Research design, 112–117
  examples of, 116–117
    correlational study, 116
    experimental study, 116
  measures of, 113–114
  reliability of, 112–114, 252Q, 255E
  types of studies, 114–115
  validity of, 112–114
Reserpine, 11

Response-suppression paradigm, animal models, 99
Restriction fragment length polymorphisms (RFLP), 75–76
Reticular activating syndrome, 43Q, 45E
Reticular formation, 28
Retirement, and later adulthood, 143
Rey-Osterrieth Complex Figure Test, for psychological assessment, 249
RFLP. *See* Restriction fragment length polymorphisms
Risperidone, 48, 49(t)
Rorschach inkblot test, 245, 245(t), 253Q, 256E

S

Schizoaffective disorder, 266
Schizophrenia, 9, 265(t), 265–266
  animal models, 100
  antimanic agents for, 55
  and antipsychotic agents, 48
  case study, 318–319
  and computed tomography, 35
  and electroencephalogram (EEG), 37
  genetics and, 78–79
  and magnetic resonance imaging, 36
  serotonin and, 13
  and single-photon-emitting radionuclides (SPECT), 41
  and sleep patterns, 31
  transmethylation hypothesis of, 13
Schizophreniform disorder, 266
School phobia, 61
Seasonal mood disorder, melatonin and, 20
Second messenger, 4
Sedative hypnotic agents, abuse of, 63
Seizure
  amino acids, 16
  threshold, effect of drugs, 50
Self-awareness, development of, 138
Self-stimulation, of brain, 93
Sentence completion test, for psychological assessment, 246
Serotonin, 11–13
  5-HT$_1$, 12
  5-HT$_2$, 12
  memory and, 14–15
  and mood disorder, 13
  and obsessive-compulsive disorder, 13
  and schizophrenia, 13
  synthesis of, *12*
Serotonin reuptake inhibitors, 52
Serotonin-norepinephrine reuptake inhibitors, 52
Sexual behavior, animal models, 90–92
Sexual dysfunction, 156–160
  pharmacologic agents implicated in, 158(t)
Sexual response cycle, 153(t), 153–154
Sexuality, 151–170
  adolescence, 151, 152(t)
  adulthood, 151–152
  and aging, 152
  cardiovascular disease and, 163
  childhood, 151
  chronic illness and, 163
  cultural influences on, 155
  development of, 151–153
  drugs affecting sexual functioning, 164
  dysfunction, 156–160, 158(t)

  erectile dysfunction, 157(t), 156–157
  gender awareness, development of, 151
  gender identity disorder, 161
  homosexuality, 155–156
  hormonal influence on, 154
  infancy, 151
  in medical practice, 161–164
    during pregnancy, 162–163
    sexual counseling, 162
    sexual history, 161–162
  pain disorders, 159
  paraphilia, 161
  sexual dysfunction, 156–160
    pharmacologic agents implicated in, 158(t)
  sexual response cycle, 153(t), 153–154
  "Sick role" of patient, 189–190
Side effects of drugs, 50–51
Single-photon-emitting radionuclides (SPECT), 41, 44Q, 45E
Sixteen Personality Factor Inventory, for psychological assessment, 247
Sleep, 29(t), 29–32
  disorders of, 31–32, 272–273
  history, 31
  stage sequence, 30, *30, 31*
Smile, development of, 137
Social behavior
  attachment style, 175–176
  emotion, expressed, 173–174
  interaction in group, 176–178
  interpersonal behavior, 172–176, *174*
  structural analysis model, 173, *174*
  support system, 177–178
Social phobia, 269–270
Sodium, 21Q, 23E
Somatization disorder, 270
Somatoform disorder, 270–272
  and pain, 33
Somatostatin, 18
Somatotropin, 19
Splitting, in psychoanalytic theory, 122
Stanford-Binet Intelligence Scale, 243
Statistics, 107–112
  analysis of variance, 111
  correlation, 111
  descriptive statistics, 108–110, *109*
  hypothesis testing, 110
  inferential statistics, 110–112
  measurement and, 107–112
  meta-analysis, 112
  multivariate technique, 112
  nonparametric test, 111
  paired test, 111
  parametric test, 110–111
  regression, 111, *112*
  unpaired test, 111
  variables, types of, 107–108, 118Q, 119E, 119Q, 120E
Stimulants
  abuse of, 63–64
  for attention deficit hyperactivity disorder (ADHD), 61
  central nervous system activity, 63–64
  medical complications with, 64
  tolerance for, 64
Stranger anxiety, 137
Stress
  and pain, 33
  and physician–patient relationship, 195–197, 196(t)
Structural analysis model, of social behavior, 173, *174*
Substance abuse, 263

animal models, 93–94
Substance dependence, 263
Substance P, 17
Substantia nigra, 27
Suicide, physician-assisted, 197
  case study, 328
Superego, in psychoanalytic theory,
  123
Support system, 177–178
Synapse, 4
  chemical, 4
  electrotonic, 4
Systems theory, 171

T

Tantrums in child, case study, 320–321
Tardive dyskinesia, 9
  and drugs, 51
Telencephalon, 25–26
Temperature regulation, hypothalamic,
  and drugs, 50
Thalamus, and diencephalon, 26–27
Thematic Apperception Test, 245–246
Theophylline, behavioral effects of, 66
Therapeutic index, of drugs, 47
Thioxanthene compounds, 48, 49(t)
Thought, in mental status examination,
  228–230
Thromboxanes, 16
Thyroid
  hyperthyroidism, 33
  hypothyroidism, 33, 34(t)
Thyroid hormones, behavioral effects
  of, 66
Thyroid-stimulating hormone (TSH), 18
Thyrotropin (TSH), 19
Thyroxine, 19
Tobacco, abuse of, 65
Tourette syndrome, genetics, 82, 85Q,
  86E
Toxic reaction to workplace, case
  study, 334–336
Toxicity of drugs, 50–51
Transference
  in physician–patient relationship, 192
  in psychoanalysis, 124
Transmethylation hypothesis of schizo-
  phrenia, 13
Transmission of information
  binding of neurotransmitter, 6, 7(t)
  neuronal, 3–6

action potential, 3
adenosine triphosphate (ATP), 4
adenylate cyclase, 4
adrenergic receptor, 4
α-adrenergic receptor, 4
α-methyltyrosine, 6
amino acids, 5
amino-4-phosphonobutyric acid
  (AMPA), 4
autoreceptor, 5
β-adrenergic receptor, 4
calcium, 5
cyclic adenosine 3′,5′-
  monophosphate (cAMP), 4
cyclic guanosine 3′,5′-
  monophosphate (cGMP), 4
cyclic nucleotide, 4
depolarization, 3
dopamine, 4
dopamine D_2 receptor, 4
dopamine receptor, 4
G-protein-coupled receptors, 4–5
guanylate cyclase, 4
5-hydroxytryptamine₃, 4
ligand-gated ion channel, 4
monoamine oxidase (MAO), 6
monoamines, 5
muscarinic acetylcholine, 4
muscarinic receptor, 4
neuron, 3–6
neurotransmitter, 4, 5–6
opiate receptor, 4
p-chlorophenylalanine (PCPA), 6
peptide subunit, 4
pertussis toxin, 6
phosphatidylinositol, 5
phosphodiesterase, 4
phosphodiesterase inhibitor, 6
physostigmine, 6
receptor, 4–5
repolarization, 3
second messenger, 4
synapse, 4
  chemical, 4
  electrotonic, 4
  types of, 5
Treatment planning, 206–207
Triazolopyridines, 51
Trichotillomania, 273
Tricyclic antidepressants, 51
  and norepinephrine, 11
  and sleep patterns, 32

TSH. *See* Thyroid-stimulating hormone;
  Thyrotropin
Tuberoinfundibular tract, 9
Twin study, in genetics, 77
Tyrosine hydroxylase, 6

U

Undoing, in psychoanalytic theory, 123
Unpaired test, in statistics, 111

V

Validity, of research design, 112–114
Valproate, 55, 56
Value theory, 281
Variables, types of, in statistics, 108
Vasoactive intestinal polypeptide (VIP),
  18
Vasopressin, 19–20
Ventral segmental area, 27
Vigilance, in mental status examina-
  tion, 223, *223*
Violence, in family, 179
VIP. *See* Vasoactive intestinal polypep-
  tide
Virtue theory, 283
Vocational testing, 247

W

Wechsler Intelligence Scale, 241–243,
  242(t)
Wechsler Memory Scale-Revised, for
  psychological assessment, 249–250
Wernicke's encephalopathy, 43Q, 45E
Wilson's disease, and magnetic resonance imaging, 36
Wisconsin Card Sorting Test, for psychological assessment, 250
Withdrawal, 263, 264(t)
  from hypnotic agents, 63
  from opioids, 63
Workplace, toxic reaction to, case
  study, 334–336
Worthlessness, feelings of, case study,
  319–320

Z

Zolpidem, hypnotic agents, 58